Second Ed

ASP

Associate Safety Professional

EXAM STUDY WORKBOOK

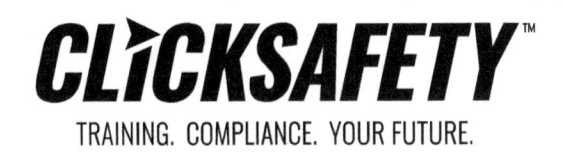

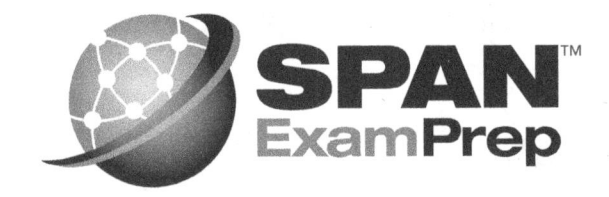

CLICKSAFETY
TRAINING. COMPLIANCE. YOUR FUTURE.

SPAN ExamPrep

CLICKSAFETY™
TRAINING. COMPLIANCE. YOUR FUTURE.

ClickSafety, Inc.
5 Wall Street
Burlington, MA 01803
www.ClickSafety.com

Information about ClickSafety books, workshops, online courses, and other products can be found by contacting ClickSafety directly by phone at 800-971-1080, by email at Sales@ClickSafety.com, or by visiting our website at www.clicksafety.com.

Copyright © 2021 by ClickSafety, Inc.

All rights reserved. No part of the material protected by this copyright may be reproduced or utilized in any form, electronic or mechanical, including photocopying, recording, or by any information storage and retrieval system, without written permission from the copyright owner.

The content, statements, views, and opinions herein are the sole expression of the respective authors and not that of Jones & Bartlett Learning, LLC. Reference herein to any specific commercial product, process, or service by trade name, trademark, manufacturer, or otherwise does not constitute or imply its endorsement or recommendation by Jones & Bartlett Learning, LLC and such reference shall not be used for advertising or product endorsement purposes. All trademarks displayed are the trademarks of the parties noted herein. *Associate Safety Professional Exam Study Workbook, Second Edition* is an independent publication and has not been authorized, sponsored, or otherwise approved by the owners of the trademarks or service marks referenced in this product.

There may be images in this book that feature models; these models do not necessarily endorse, represent, or participate in the activities represented in the images. Any screenshots in this product are for educational and instructive purposes only. Any individuals and scenarios featured in the case studies throughout this product may be real or fictitious, but are used for instructional purposes only.

This publication is not intended to guarantee that the user will pass an exam or become certified. It may not cover every aspect of the certification process. The information contained in this study workbook is intended to be used in preparation for the Associate Safety Professional (ASP®) certification and should not be used as an authority in the professional practice of safety, health, or environmental compliance. The Associate Safety Professional (ASP®) certification is a registered trademark of the Board of Certified Safety Professionals (BCSP). The opinions expressed are those of the authors, and no guarantee, warranty, or other representation is made as to the absolute correctness or sufficiency of the information contained in this study workbook.

ISBN: 978-1-284-22862-5

Production Credits

Product Manager: Teresa Malmberg
Content Development Manager: Haritha Treadway
Manager, Project Management: Kristen Rogers
Director of Marketing: Mindy Michalek
Marketing Manager: Liz Bormida
Content Services Manager: Colleen Lamy
VP, Manufacturing and Inventory Control:
  Therese Connell
Product Fulfillment Manager: Wendy Kilborn

Composition and Project Management:
  S4Carlisle Publishing Services
Cover Design: Kristin E. Parker
Text Design: Kristin E. Parker
Rights & Permissions Manager: John Rusk
Senior Media Development Editor: Troy Liston
Rights Specialist: Maria Leon Maimone
Cover Image (Title Page): © Studio-Pro/Getty Images
Printing and Binding: LSI

6048

Printed in the United States of America
24 23 22   10 9 8 7 6 5 4 3 2

Table of Contents

Introduction ... 1

The Safety Professional ... 2
Professionalism, Ethics, and Codes of Conduct ... 4
About the ASP Exam ... 6
Accredited Certification vs. Certificate Program ... 7
Benefits of Certification ... 7
Overview of the ASP Certification Process ... 8
ASP/GSP/CSP Qualifications ... 8
Taking the Computer-Based Exam ... 10
    Frequently Asked Questions About the Computer Exam ... 10
    General Comments ... 12
Applied Study and Testing Techniques ... 12
The Question-and-Answer Study Method ... 14
    Applied Logic: Socratic Method ... 14
    Question ... 14
Exam Graphic User Interface Examples ... 16
Select Study References for the ASP Exam ... 17

Domain 1: Advanced Sciences and Math ... 19

ASP Math Equations and Formulas ... 19
    Structural and Mechanical Calculations ... 22
Engineering Control Calculations ... 22
    Financial Principles Formulas ... 25
    Statistics Calculations ... 26
Domain 1 Quiz 1 Questions ... 30
Domain 1 Quiz 1 Answers ... 33
    Alternate Solution ... 35
Domain 1 Quiz 2 Questions ... 40
Domain 1 Quiz 2 Answers ... 43
Domain 1 Quiz 3 Questions ... 52
Domain 1 Quiz 3 Answers ... 57
    Recordable Incident Rate ... 64
    Fleet Formulas ... 64
    DART Rate (Days Away/Restricted or Job Transfer Rate) ... 64

Domain 2: Safety Management Systems ... 66

Domain 2 Quiz 1 Questions ... 67
Domain 2 Quiz 1 Answers ... 69
Domain 2 Quiz 2 Questions ... 80
Domain 2 Quiz 2 Answers ... 83
Domain 2 Quiz 3 Questions ... 87
Domain 2 Quiz 3 Answers ... 91

Domain 3: Ergonomics ... 99

Domain 3 Quiz 1 Questions ... 100
Domain 3 Quiz 1 Answers ... 102

Domain 4: Fire Prevention and Protection ... 110

Domain 4 Quiz 1 Questions ... 110
Domain 4 Quiz 1 Answers ... 113
Domain 4 Quiz 2 Questions ... 118
Domain 4 Quiz 2 Answers ... 120

Domain 5: Emergency Response Management (ERM) ... 124

Domain 5 Quiz 1 Questions ... 124
Domain 5 Quiz 1 Answers ... 128

Domain 6: Industrial Hygiene and Occupational Health ... 138

Domain 6 Quiz 1 Questions ... 138
Domain 6 Quiz 1 Answers ... 141
Domain 6 Quiz 2 Questions ... 144
Domain 6 Quiz 2 Answers ... 146
Domain 6 Quiz 3 Questions ... 152
Domain 6 Quiz 3 Answers ... 154

Domain 7: Environmental Management ... 159

Domain 7 Quiz 1 Questions ... 160
Domain 7 Quiz 1 Answers ... 163

Table of Contents (continued)

Domain 8: Training, Education, and Communication 171

Domain 8 Quiz 1 Questions 171
Domain 8 Quiz 1 Answers 174
Domain 8 Quiz 2 Questions 181
Domain 8 Quiz 2 Answers 183

Domain 9: Law and Ethics... 189

Domain 9 Quiz 1 Questions 189
Domain 9 Quiz 1 Answers 193

Introduction 197

Self-Assessment Exam 1 Questions 197
Self-Assessment Exam 1 Answers 212
Self-Assessment Exam 2 Questions 226
Self-Assessment Exam 2 Answers 239
Self-Assessment Exam 3 Questions 251
Self-Assessment Exam 3 Answers 265
Self-Assessment Exam 4 Questions 275
Self-Assessment Exam 4 Answers 288
Self-Assessment Exam 5 Questions 297
Self-Assessment Exam 5 Answers 311
Self-Assessment Exam 6 Questions 324
Self-Assessment Exam 6 Answers 338

Reference List 353
Index 355

About the Author

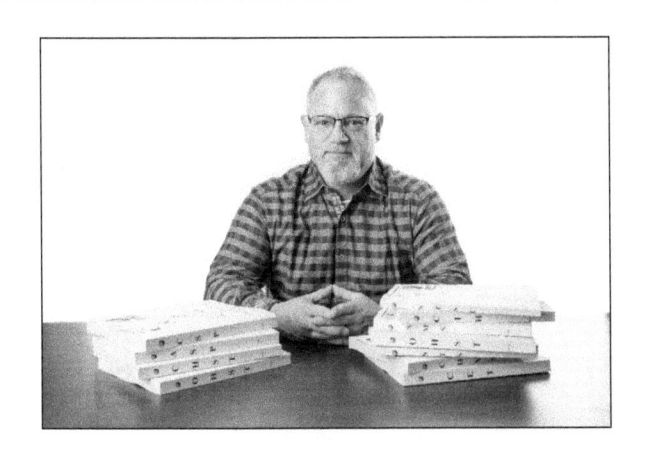

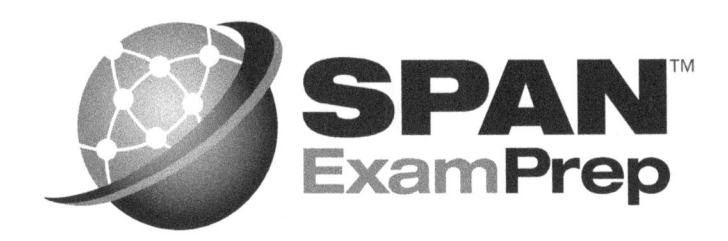

Daniel J. Snyder, EdD, CSP, SMS, OHST, CHST, CIT

With 28 years of global occupational safety and health consulting experience, Dr. Snyder partners with stakeholders to develop strategies for improving safety and health management systems by conducting workplace evaluations, facilitating research to improve safety performance, and designing customized educational curriculum. Daniel served in the Army in military intelligence and as a safety liaison for implementing field expedited safety training as part of the National Incident Management System for disaster response. He holds a doctorate degree in Human Resource Development and Adult Lifelong Learning from the University of Arkansas. As the former owner of SPAN, he is a subject-matter expert on certification exam blueprints, safety and health management systems, and safety training, and is currently a consultant to ClickSafety.com. He is the author of the SPAN Exam study workbooks and serves on several standards and professional development committees, including the Chairperson for the ANSI/ASSP Z490.1 Criteria for Accepted Practices in Safety, Health and Environmental Training Standard. Daniel is a member of the U.S. Technical Advisory Group to the ISO Technical Committee 283 responsible for the ongoing development and enhancement of *ISO 45001, (OHSMS), international standard*. Dr. Snyder's research-based consultancy and curriculum help organizations develop influential safety leaders. Daniel is an accomplished speaker and author whose works include the Ethics chapter in the American Society of Safety Professionals' *Consultants Business Development Guide (2015)* and the National Safety Council's *Pocket Guide to Safety Essentials, 2nd Edition (2014)*. Dr. Snyder is dedicated to advancing health and safety professional development by offering safety expert services. He can be contacted at expert@danielsnyder.com.

Introduction

There are two major objectives of the ASP workbooks and workshops:

1. Provide candidates the knowledge and skills to successfully attain the Associate Safety Professional® (ASP) certification.
2. Enhance skills, knowledge, and abilities as a safety professional.

This workbook is designed to be used as a resource for self-directed study in preparation for the ASP exam. In the fast-track, three-day workshop conducted by SPAN™ Safety Workshops, participants are provided expert guidance and use the same content presented in these workbooks. This curriculum is also used in the online SPAN CertBoK™ Exam Learning Management System (LMS).

Workshops are conducted periodically throughout the year so that professionals can take the examination as soon as they are prepared. Visit the SPAN website for workshop dates and locations: www.spansafety.com.

The exam is designed for candidates with 1 year of professional safety experience where safety is at least 50% preventive, professional level, with breadth and depth of safety duties. Candidates must also hold a bachelor's degree in any field or an associate degree in safety, health, or the environment that includes at least four courses with at least 12 semester hours of study in the safety, health, and environmental domains covered in the BCSP ASP examination blueprint. Depending on the university, candidates may qualify as a Graduate Safety Professional (GSP). Generally, it takes the average safety and health practitioner about 40–100 hours of dedicated self-study, in addition to a workshop, to adequately prepare for the examination. The self-study can generally be accomplished in about 4 to 12 weeks, depending on individual needs.

The workbook is divided into two sections designed for self-study and facilitated professional development workshops. After each section of the workbook, there are fully developed explanations for the answer selected for each question. In many cases information about all the selections offered as possible answers will be included to assist in developing a better understanding of the subject. These sessions are designed to allow the safety professional to measure progress during the extended program of self-study that is normally required to pass the certification exams.

Considerable effort has been made to fully develop and explain the concepts and techniques discussed. However, given the differences in the background and experience of the safety practitioners sitting for the ASP examination, it is impossible to explain all concepts to all candidates. The materials are based on the exam blueprint and subject-matter expertise.

Browse through the rest of the workbook, stopping and actually reading whenever a subject or question is of interest. Study the explanations of all the answers, as these represent much of the exam philosophy and may add significant value in preparation. These are only suggestions.

After reviewing the workbook, establish a study plan. There are voluminous resources available for each domain of the exam blueprint. Simply stated, chance favors the prepared mind and candidates should have a study plan. Budget adequate time to master the material.

This workbook is designed to optimize study time. There is no extraneous or "nice to know" information in this workbook. All of the information is important. Concentrating on the areas emphasized in the text should reduce research and study time considerably.

The BCSP exams have changed dramatically in the past few years and SPAN® conducts ongoing research and development to ensure the accuracy and quality of the curriculum based on the actual exam blueprint. **This workbook does not contain actual ASP test questions** and uses a question-and-answer format with detailed explanations. Difficult concepts or theories may have material presented in a table, diagram, illustration, or a paraphrased format. This method is used to allow broad coverage of the material and optimize study efforts.

The beginning sections of the workbook are devoted to enhancing knowledge and skills in:

- The exam process
- Study and testing techniques
- Applied math and science problems

Content may serve as preliminary exercises to engage the analytical portions of the brain and help prepare candidates for the mathematical components of the exam. The problems are representative of the exam based on the blueprint.

From the introductory section, the workbook progresses to individual segments covering each of the nine ASP exam blueprint domains. These nine blueprint domains utilize the question-and-answer format designed to mimic the types of questions offered on the exam. Explanations are offered to reduce research time, considering that the examination covers a tremendous amount of subject matter.

The questions presented are representative of the questions found on the actual examination(s). For this reason, candidates must understand the area (or areas) to which the question pertains. Refer to the exam references for additional study resources.

Approximately 60.5% of the scored questions must be answered correctly to pass the ASP examination. Master the concepts contained herein. Become familiar with the subject areas contained in the workbook. Repetition will help to identify areas of strength and weakness unique to every individual.

The assumption is made that only fully qualified safety practitioners will attempt to sit for the ASP examination, which means everyone using this workbook has a solid foundation in the safety and health field. Given this assumption, no attempt has been made to provide a basic safety text. Rather, the problems presented in this book are representative of questions that may be expected to appear on the ASP examination and are based on the exam blueprint. The workbook is designed as a guide; depending on an individual's knowledge baseline, additional research may be required.

Achieving certification is a challenging task. Embrace the journey of professional development in preparation for the exam. The modern safety professional must be an adaptive leader and lifelong learner.

This curriculum has been carefully checked for accuracy, but errors may exist. Should an error be discovered, contact the author via info@spansafetyworkshops.com.

The Safety Professional

A **safety professional** is one who applies the expertise gained from a study of safety science, principles, and other subjects and from professional safety experience to create or develop procedures, processes, standards, specifications, and systems to achieve optimal control or reduction of the hazards and exposures that may harm people, property, or the environment.

A **Certified Safety Professional**® (CSP) is a safety professional who has met and continues to meet the criteria established by the Board of Certified Safety Professionals (BCSP) and is authorized by the BCSP to use the Certified Safety Professional® title and the CSP credential.

The primary focus of the safety profession is prevention of harm to people, property, and the environment. It uses appropriate methods and techniques of loss prevention and loss control. "Safety science" is a twenty-first-century term for everything that goes into the prevention of accidents, illnesses, fires, explosions and other events that harm people, property, and the environment (ANSI/ASSP, 2007).

To perform their professional functions, individuals practicing in the safety profession generally have education, training, and experience from a common body of knowledge (**Table 1**). They need to have a fundamental knowledge of physics, chemistry, biology, physiology, statistics, mathematics, computer science, engineering mechanics, industrial processes, business, communication, and psychology. Professional safety studies include industrial hygiene and toxicology, design of engineering hazard controls, fire protection, ergonomics, system and process safety, safety and health program management, accident investigation and analysis, product safety, construction safety, education and training methods, measurement of safety performance, human behavior, environmental safety and health, and safety, health, and environmental laws, regulations, and standards. Many have backgrounds or advanced study in other disciplines, such as management and business administration, engineering, education, physical and social sciences, and other fields. Others have advanced study in safety, and this additional background extends their expertise beyond the basics of the safety profession.

An American national standard sets forth common and reasonable parameters of the professional safety position in the ANSI/ASSP Z590.2-2003 *Criteria for Establishing the Scope and Functions of the Professional Safety Position* publication. Safety professionals must plan for and manage resources related to their functions. By acquiring the knowledge and skills of the profession, developing the mind-set and wisdom to act responsibly in the occupational context, and keeping up with changes that affect the safety profession, the required safety professional functions are able to be performed with confidence, competence, credibility, and respected authority (ANSI/ASSP, 2017).

Safety professionals' precise roles and responsibilities depend on the companies or organizations for which they work. Different industries have different hazards and require unique safety expertise. However, most safety professionals do at least several of the following:

- **Hazard Recognition**: Identifying conditions or actions that may cause injury, illness, or property damage
- **Inspections/Audits**: Assessing safety and health risks associated with equipment, materials, processes, facilities, or abilities
- **Fire Protection**: Reducing fire hazards by inspection, layout of facilities and processes, and design of fire detection and suppression systems
- **Regulatory Compliance**: Ensuring that mandatory safety and health standards are satisfied
- **Health Hazard Control**: Controlling hazards such as noise, chemical exposures, radiation, or biological hazards that can create harm

- **Ergonomics**: Improving the workplace based on an understanding of human physiological and psychological characteristics, abilities, and limitations
- **Hazardous Materials Management**: Ensuring that dangerous chemicals and other products are procured, stored, and disposed of in ways that prevent fires, exposure to, or harm from these substances
- **Environmental Protection**: Controlling hazards that can lead to undesirable releases of harmful materials into the air, water, or soil
- **Training**: Providing employees and managers with the knowledge and skills necessary to recognize hazards and perform their jobs safely and effectively
- **Accident and Incident Investigations**: Determining the facts related to an accident or incident based on witness interviews, site inspections, and collection of other evidence
- **Advising Management**: Helping managers establish safety objectives, plan programs to achieve those objectives, and integrate safety into the culture of an organization
- **Record Keeping**: Maintaining safety and health information to meet government requirements, as well as to provide data for problem solving and decision-making
- **Evaluating**: Judging the effectiveness of existing safety- and health-related programs and activities
- **Emergency Response**: Organizing, training, and coordinating skilled employees with regard to auditory and visual communications pertaining to emergencies such as fires, accidents, or other disasters
- **Managing Safety Programs**: Planning, organizing, budgeting, and tracking completion and effectiveness of activities intended to achieve safety objectives in an organization or to implement administrative or technical controls that will eliminate or reduce hazards
- **Product Safety**: Assessing the probability that exposure to a product during any stage of its life cycle will lead to an unacceptable impact on human health or the environment and determining the appropriate auditory and visual hazard warnings
- **Security**: Identifying and implementing design features and procedures to protect facilities and businesses from threats that introduce hazards

Safety professionals work virtually anywhere people might be exposed to hazards. They provide technical assistance in identifying, evaluating, and controlling hazards globally. Because safety is an element in all human endeavors, the performance of these functions, in a variety of contexts in both public and private sectors, often requires specialized knowledge and skills. Typical settings are manufacturing, insurance, risk management, government, education, consulting, construction, health care, engineering and design, waste management, petroleum, facilities management, retail, transportation, and utilities. Within these contexts, safety professionals must adapt their functions to fit the mission, operations, and climate of their employer. Not only must individuals practicing in the safety profession acquire the knowledge and skills to perform these functions effectively in their employment context, but through continuing education and training they must stay current with new technologies, changes in laws and regulations, and changes in the workforce, workplace, and world business, political, and social climate.

Table 1 10 Basic Principles of Safety (Petersen, 2003)

1.	An unsafe act, an unsafe condition, and an accident are all symptoms of management systems problems.
2.	Circumstances that will produce severe injuries are predictable and can be identified and controlled.
3.	Safety should be managed like any other company function. Management should direct the safety effort by setting achievable goals and by planning, organizing, and controlling to achieve them.
4.	The key to effective line safety performance is management procedures that fix accountability.

5.	The function of safety is to locate and define the operational errors that allow accidents to occur. This function can be carried out in two ways:
	    a. By asking why accidents happen; searching for their root causes
	    b. By asking whether certain known effective controls are being utilized

(Continues)

Table 1 10 Basic Principles of Safety (Petersen, 2003) (Continued)

6. The causes of unsafe behavior can be identified and classified. Some of the classifications are overload (the improper matching of a person's capacity with the load); traps; and the worker's decision to err. Each cause is one that can be controlled.

7. In most cases, unsafe behavior is normal human behavior; it is the result of normal people reacting to their environment. Management's job is to change the environment that leads to unsafe behavior.

8. There are three major subsystems that must be dealt with in building an effective safety system: the physical; the managerial; the behavioral.

9. The safety system should fit the culture of the organization.

10. There is no one right way to achieve safety in an organization; however, for a safety system to be effective, it must meet certain criteria. The system must force supervisory performance; involve middle management; have top management visibly showing their commitment; have employee participation; be flexible; and be perceived as positive.

Reproduced from Petersen, D. (2003). *Techniques of Safety Management: A Systems Approach* (4th ed.). Des Plaines, IL: American Society of Safety Engineers.

Professionalism, Ethics, and Codes of Conduct

Is it safe? How safe is safe enough? Who decides? These are perhaps the most critical and frequently asked questions posed to OSH professionals. A primary role of the safety professional is to advise stakeholders and decision-makers in defining acceptable risk (INSHPO 2017, ASSP) and helping find tolerable solutions.

The art and science of occupational health and safety requires a dynamic mix of technical competencies and interpersonal skills. The epistemology of the safety profession was discussed earlier (**Table 2**). The art of professional practice is grounded in ethics, politics, and esthetics. Together, "the art and science of safety" provide the competencies required to influence those decision-makers impacting occupational health and safety (Snyder, 2018).

Table 2 Philosophy of Safety

Philosophical Branch	Philosophical Focus	Speculative Question	Operative Question
Metaphysics	Study of Existence	What is reality?	What is the perceived reality of the organizational safety and health culture?
Analytics	Study of History	Is there meaning in the historical process?	Will predictive analytics prevent future mishaps?
Epistemology	Study of Knowledge	How do I know?	How do communication, training, and education inform workers about workplace hazards and risk-control measures?
Politics	Study of Force	What can I do?	How is decision-making power influenced?
Logic	Study of Reason	How do I validate reasoning?	What evidence is needed to accept or reject hypotheses?
Ethics	Study of Action	What should I do?	Who is impacted by the outcome of this decision?

- Do we think differently when thinking scientifically than when thinking ethically?
- Can you find scientific answers to the questions "What is reasonable?" or "What is fair?"

A professional is defined as a member of a group of colleagues who have articulated a set of standards and values and can enforce them, at the very least, by exclusion from the group. Aim to show several different ways to think through a problem in professional ethics, rather than merely describe what professionals say are their problems (sociology of ethics). Professionalism can be defined as skill, or competency in work. The ethical element is "Will the work be beneficial to others?" Work itself doesn't have moral status; the execution of work has moral status. Professional ethics helps a professional decide when faced with a problem that raises a moral issue. Complexity arises from there being many people, with many issues involved, the history of the issues, and who decides, not just what is decided (Strahlendorf, 2004).

Often, the terms "ethics" and "morality" are used interchangeably, but they are different.

- Morality: Making choices with reasons
- Ethics: The study of *how* choices are made (ethics is the study of morality)

Ethics is a rational reflection upon good and evil (without weighing in on the question of heaven or hell, angels and demons). The word *ethics* refers to our identification of the "good" in any given situation, as well as the rationale for the identification. Ethics engages each of us at the level of the thought, the reasoning process that goes into every decision we make, whether for our own happiness or that of another. Sound ethical judgment arises when proper habits of thought have given way to confidence in the right conduct and in doing it.

As safety consultants (and mature adults), there is no flight from precisely this kind of deliberation. Professionals must make choices that are responsible, defensible, and appropriate. Decide upon the highest good and order all the others, the lesser goods, in a hierarchy. This could be applied to a risk assessment or matrix (Keys, Rodriquez, & Walaski, 2015).

Reflecting on professional ethics and codes of conduct assists with choices about what one ought to do (**Table 3**).

- Descriptive ethics: What IS
- Prescriptive ethics: What OUGHT to be

Codes of ethics require objectivity, which means that there are principles and values outside of the individual that the members of the community share and that individuals will be measured against.

There are rigorous professional guidelines and regulations regarding ethics for a safety professional. Below is a list of some of them:

- Board of Certified Safety Professionals Code of Ethics and Professional Conduct
- American Society of Safety Professionals' Code of Professional Conduct
- American Industrial Hygiene Association and American Conference of Governmental Industrial Hygienists Joint Ethical Principles
- American Board of Industrial Hygiene Code of Ethics
- International Code of Ethics for Occupational Health Professionals
- Federal Contractor Code of Business Ethics and Conduct (48 CFR 3.10)
- American Society of Civil Engineers Code of Ethics
- National Society of Professional Engineers Code of Ethics
- Institute of Hazardous Materials Management Code of Ethics

As a safety professional, you should be familiar with the codes of conduct pertinent to your work. However, in and of themselves, they are insufficient. You must also develop a robust code of personal ethics. The avoidance of wrong is not the same as doing right. As safety professionals, we must honor a high ethical standard, one that encompasses not just ourselves but our clients, colleagues, and community. You must not only behave ethically; you must strive to encourage ethical behavior in others.

Table 3 BCSP Code of Ethics Standards

HOLD paramount the safety and health of people, the protection of the environment, and protection of property in the performance of professional duties and exercise their obligation to advise employers, clients, employees, the public, and appropriate authorities of danger and unacceptable risks to people, the environment, or property.
BE honest, fair, and impartial; act with responsibility and integrity. Adhere to high standards of ethical conduct with balanced care for the interests of the public, employers, clients, employees, colleagues, and the profession. Avoid all conduct or practice that is likely to discredit the profession or deceive the public.
ISSUE public statements only in an objective and truthful manner and only when founded upon knowledge of the facts and competence in the subject matter.

(Continues)

Table 3 BCSP Code of Ethics Standards (*Continued*)

UNDERTAKE assignments only when qualified by education or experience in the specific technical fields involved. Accept responsibility for their continued professional development by acquiring and maintaining competence through continuing education, experience, professional training, and keeping current on relevant legal issues.
AVOID deceptive acts that falsify or misrepresent their academic or professional qualifications. Do not misrepresent or exaggerate their degree of responsibility in or for the subject matter of prior assignments. Presentations incident to the solicitation of employment shall not misrepresent pertinent facts concerning employers, employees, associates, or past accomplishments with the intent and purpose of enhancing their qualifications and their work.
CONDUCT their professional relations by the highest standards of integrity and avoid compromise of their professional judgment by conflicts of interest. When becoming aware of professional misconduct by a BCSP certificant, take steps to bring that misconduct to the attention of the Board of Certified Safety Professionals.
ACT in a manner free of bias with regard to religion, ethnicity, gender, age, national origin, sexual orientation, or disability.
SEEK opportunities to be of constructive service in civic affairs and work for the advancement of the safety, health, and well-being of their community and their profession by sharing their knowledge and skills.

Reproduced with permission from the Board of Certified Safety Professionals.

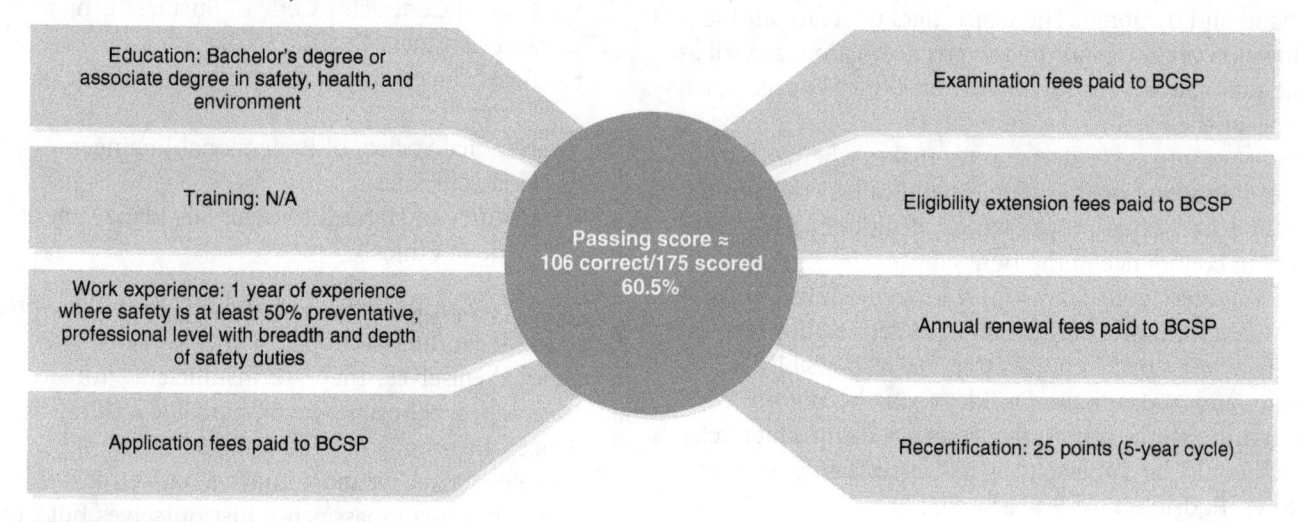

- Education: Bachelor's degree or associate degree in safety, health, and environment
- Training: N/A
- Work experience: 1 year of experience where safety is at least 50% preventative, professional level with breadth and depth of safety duties
- Application fees paid to BCSP

Passing score ≈ 106 correct/175 scored 60.5%

- Examination fees paid to BCSP
- Eligibility extension fees paid to BCSP
- Annual renewal fees paid to BCSP
- Recertification: 25 points (5-year cycle)

ASP Certification Overview

About the ASP Exam

Safety practitioners come from different academic backgrounds and work experience ranging from operations to engineering. They all had one common goal: promoting the safety and health of employees. Until the Certified Safety Professional® certification program began, they also had no standard measure of qualification.

The Associate Safety Professional® (ASP) is currently its own certification by the Board of Certified Safety Professionals (BCSP). With few exceptions, one must attain the ASP before achieving the Certified Safety Professional® (CSP) designation, which is the gold standard in safety certification.

The BSCP was chartered in 1969 to establish a method of measuring qualifications for the safety profession. The Board established qualification standards and began issuing certification shortly after being founded. Although chartered as an independent, separately incorporated board, the BCSP has several sponsoring organizations that provide members to the BCSP Board of Directors. These sponsoring organizations are as follows:

- American Society of Safety Professionals (ASSP)
- American Industrial Hygiene Association (AIHA)
- National Safety Council (NSC)
- Institute of Industrial Engineers (IIE)
- Society of Fire Protection Engineers (SFPE)
- International System Safety Society (ISSS)
- National Fire Protection Association (NFPA)
- National Environmental Training Association (NESHTA)

Accredited Certification vs. Certificate Program

Accredited Certification	Certificate Program
Results from an assessment process	Results from an educational process
Typically requires some amount of professional experience	For novice and experienced professionals
Awarded by a third-party, standard-setting organization	Awarded by training and educational programs or institutions
Indicates mastery/competency as measured against a defensible set of standards, usually by application or exam	Indicates completion of a course or series of courses with a specific focus; is different than a degree-granting program
Standards set through a defensible, industry-wide process (job analysis/role delineation) that results in an outline of required knowledge and skills	Course content set a variety of ways (faculty committee; dean; instructor; occasionally through defensible analysis of topic care)
Typically results in a designation to use after one's name; may result in a document to hang on the wall or keep in a wallet	Usually listed on a résumé detailing education; may result in a document to hang on the wall
Has ongoing requirements to maintain; individual must demonstrate knowledge of content; holder must demonstrate he/she continues to meet requirements	Is the end result; individual may or may not demonstrate knowledge of course content at the end of a set period in time

The BCSP's certifications are accredited by independent, third-party organizations that regularly evaluate certification requirements. Accreditation assures:

1. Governance
   - Nominations/elections
   - Peer participation
   - Public participation
2. Financial disclosure
   - Stability and financial condition
   - Budget details
3. Fairness to candidates
4. Examinations
   - Validity
   - Reliability
   - Passing scores
5. Recertification
6. Independence from preparation
7. Management systems

International Accreditation is provided by the American National Standards Institute (ANSI 17024/ISO)17F[1]. National Accreditation is achieved through both the National Commission for Certifying Agencies (NCCA)18F[2] and the Council of Engineering and Scientific Specialty Boards (CESB)19F[3].

The ASP is the first step in attaining the CSP designation, which is the premier certification in the safety profession. No other single means of measuring safety and health practitioners' qualifications is as widely accepted or respected. At publication of this workbook, there are over 12,000 Associate Safety Professionals® and over 14,000 Certified Safety Professionals®.

Benefits of Certification

The process of certification commands a considerable amount of effort. Many safety practitioners wonder if the advantages of certification justify all the effort. The average person holding the CSP credential today earns nearly $25,000 more than others in the safety field who hold no certification. The latest survey from the BSCP indicated that the average salary of those holding the CSP certification is approximately $98,000.

The primary advantage of certification is that it provides a credential. The ASP/CSP indicates that a safety professional has achieved a standard level of qualification as judged by their professional peers. This level of qualification is important in establishing credibility within the ever-growing field of occupational health and safety management. Employment opportunities are much greater for personnel holding CSP certification, the courts recognize the certification as a step toward authentication as an expert witness, and it is almost always required to do consultant work in the field of safety today. There are several reasons that should cause candidates to think about starting the process of obtaining certification *right now*.

---

[1] ASP, CSP
[2] ASP, CSP, OHST, CHST, STS
[3] CET

- A growing trend by states to license safety professionals, much like physicians, engineers, architects, and other professionals. Some states have that authority under their duty to "protect the health, safety, and welfare of the public."
- Substantial support to modify existing safety and health laws to acknowledge certified "safety specialists." Some projects require a certified professional to be on staff.
- Certified safety and health professionals obtain employment earlier and receive greater compensation than noncertified employees.
- As the requirements increase, the examinations may become even more dynamic, complex, difficult to pass, and expensive both in time and financial investment.

These and other recent developments add up to a future environment where a certification is going to be the desired/required credential. Being an ASP will become much more important, more lucrative, and more difficult to attain. Like the other professional certification/registration examinations, the ASP and CSP exams should be taken as early in one's career as possible.

Overview of the ASP Certification Process

The following information concerning the requirements for certification may have changed after publication. It is strongly suggested that candidates contact the BCSP for current information. For exact requirements, go to the BCSP website at www.bcsp.org and review the ASP complete guide. There are common questions by potential candidates, such as "What do I have to do to get the ASP?"

The ASP is a certification awarded by the BCSP to individuals who meet all of the requirements established by the Board. It is one of several approved credentials that can qualify an individual to sit for the CSP examination. Along with the education and experience requirements, candidates must successfully complete the examinations.

ASP/GSP/CSP Qualifications

Those candidates possessing other acceptable registrations or certifications may waive the ASP exam.

All others must successfully complete the ASP prior to receiving the CSP certification.

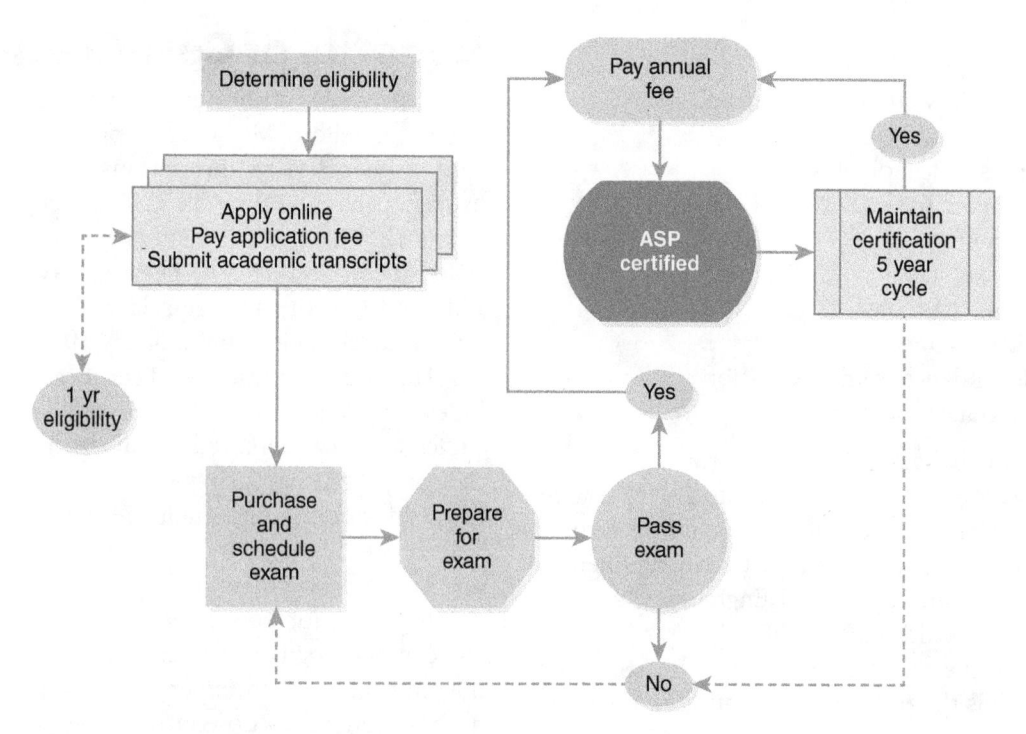

Figure 1 Certification Process

Minimum Academic Requirement:
- Associate's in Safety (SH&E-related and from an accredited school)
- Bachelor's in any field (from an accredited 20F[4] school)
- Bachelor's from a QAP School (BCSP Qualified Academic Program for GSP)
  - The Graduate Safety Practitioner (GSP) designation is a path offered to the CSP certification for qualifying ABET-ASAC21F[5] or AABI22F[6] graduates.
  - GSPs receive a waiver of the ASP examination

Experience Requirement:
- At least 1 year of experience where safety is at least 50% of the duties
- Qualifying criteria for experience
  - Full-time position (or part-time ≥ 900 hrs/yr)
  - Professional safety is primary function (≥ 50% of position)
  - Primary responsibility must be the prevention of harm to people, property, or the environment
  - Must be at professional level (responsible charge)
  - Breadth: Safety tasks, hazard types, etc.
  - OHST/CHST count as one year of experience

Pass the ASP and CSP examinations leading to the CSP certification (with some exceptions that waive the ASP exam, including the GSP designation).

Recertification Requirements:
- 25 points every 5 years
- 10 point categories (some with point limitations)
- Practice
- Membership
- Service
- Publishing, presenting, patents
- Writing exam questions
- Professional development conferences
- Safety-related courses, seminars, quizzes
- Continuing education

- New advanced degree
- Other certifications/re-examination

A candidate for certification may take the ASP exam after meeting the academic/experience requirements. The ASP is truly a safety fundamentals test. It covers the basic academic knowledge expected of a safety professional at the entry level.

Before taking the Comprehensive Practice Exam, the academic/experience requirements must be met, passing scores must be recorded on the ASP (unless waived by other registration or certification), and the candidate must have four years of acceptable professional safety experience. When a candidate has successfully completed the Comprehensive Practice Examination, he or she is designated a Certified Safety Professional® (CSP).

The entire process of certification generally takes from 3 to 6 months, allowing plenty of time to plan an individual study program. Costs associated with the certification process are as follows:

ASP Criteria	
Minimum formal education	Minimum bachelor's degree in any field or an associate's in safety, health, or the environment
Training prerequisite	N/A
Work experience	At least 1 year of experience where safety is at least 50%, preventive, professional level, with breadth and depth of safety duties
Application fees	$160
Examination fees	$350
Eligibility extension fees	$100
Renewal fees	$170
Passing scores	60.5%
Recertification (5-year cycle)	25 points

The above information is accurate as of this printing. For more current information, candidates should contact the Board at:

Board of Certified Safety Professionals
8645 Guion Road
Indianapolis, IN 64268
Phone (317) 593-4800
Fax (317) 593-4400
www.bcsp.org

---
[4]Accredited School is one that is recognized by the US Department of Education or the Council for Higher Education Accreditation (CHEA).
[5]Accreditation Board for Engineering and Technology (ABET)-Applied Science Accreditation Commission (ASAC)
[6]Aviation Accreditation Board International (AABI)

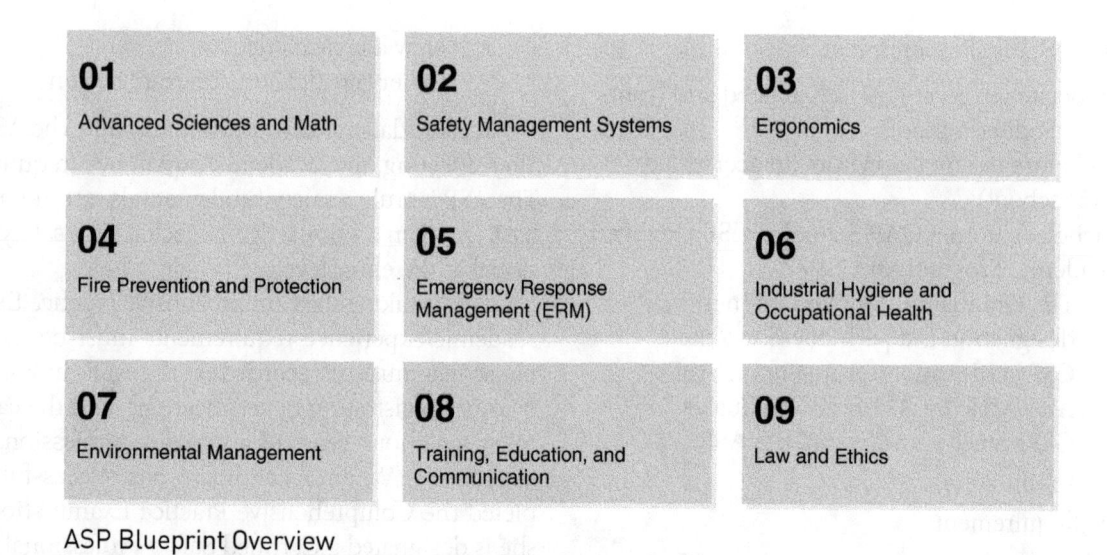

01 Advanced Sciences and Math	02 Safety Management Systems	03 Ergonomics
04 Fire Prevention and Protection	05 Emergency Response Management (ERM)	06 Industrial Hygiene and Occupational Health
07 Environmental Management	08 Training, Education, and Communication	09 Law and Ethics

ASP Blueprint Overview
Modified from from ASP® Exam Blueprint (ASP10), November 10, 2019.

Taking the Computer-Based Exam

One major goal of the BCSP is to offer certification examinations with a high degree of validity and reliability to promote a fair assessment of a candidate's competency as a safety and health practitioner.

Testing on computer is done via Pearson VUE (www.pearsonvue.com).

Examinations can be taken every business day at many locations throughout the world. Many locations also have evening and Saturday hours.

Candidates must complete an application and return it, with supporting information and the application fee ($160), to the Board of Certified Safety Professionals (BCSP). Once a candidate has been approved and has paid the examination fee ($350), the Board will mail an examination authorization letter. Once the application is approved, candidates have 1 year to arrange for an actual examination date. Arrangements are made directly with Pearson VUE online or via the national toll-free number (**888) 269-2219**. Some Pearson VUE testing centers are busier than others, so schedule early if possible.

At the Pearson VUE centers, a candidate signs in, presents identifications, and is seated at a computer workstation. The center provides laminated graph paper and a marker. There is a short orientation and practice program to acquaint candidates with the examination procedure. During actual testing, a small clock in the monitor screen corner keeps track of the remaining time.

ABSOLUTELY NO NOTES OR REFERENCE MATERIALS ARE ALLOWED! Laminated graph paper and writing utensils will be provided. After finishing the computerized examination, a pass/fail grade will be given. A detailed score report will be mailed at a later date from the BCSP.

For worldwide locations, look at the website www.pearsonvue.com.

Frequently Asked Questions About the Computer Exam

Note: Remember, the best and most current source of information on procedures and policies for the computer test is directly from the BCSP at (317) 593-4800 and www.bcsp.org.

Question How do the questions appear on the computer screen? How do I make answer selections? Can I back up or mark questions so that I can come back to them? Do I need to be a computer whiz to take this test?

Answer Examination questions appear one at a time and look very similar to the questions in the workbook. With a mouse or keys, the candidate selects the preferred answer and moves on to the next question. Questions may be marked for further review or skipped and revisited later. After the last question, a list appears and shows item numbers, answers selected, and questions marked or skipped. Since the computer test is very "friendly," candidates do not have to be computer literate to take this exam.

Question Can you bring food or drinks into the exam room?

Answer No. All candidates are given a small locker for personal belongings, including snacks,

Introduction

ASP Exam Domains

Domain 1: Advanced Sciences and Math	Domain 2: Safety Management Systems	Domain 3: Ergonomics	Domain 4: Fire Prevention and Protection	Domain 5: Emergency Response Management (ERM)	Domain 6: Industrial Hygiene and Occupational Health	Domain 7: Environmental Management	Domain 8: Training, Education, and Communication	Domain 9: Law and Ethics
Chemistry concepts, electrical principles, radioactivity principles, calculations of storage capacities, calculations for rigging and load, ventilation and system design, noise hazards, environmental and climate conditions, calculations for fall protection, physics concepts, financial principles, descriptive statistics, lagging indicators, leading indicators	Hazard control hierarchy; risk transfer; change management; methods for hazard and risk analysis; process safety management; principles of fleet safety; hazard communication; hazardous energy control; excavation/trenching/shoring; confined space; physical security; fall protection; machine guarding; powered industrial vehicles; scaffolding; use methods of hazard identification; assess and analyze risk; give financial justification of hazard controls; implement hazard controls; monitor and reevaluate hazard controls; conduct incident investigation; conduct audits and inspections; evaluate cost, schedule, performance, and project risk	Fitness for duty, stressors, risk factors, work design, material handling, work practice controls, use qualitative and quantitative analysis methods	Chemical knowledge, electrical knowledge, hot work, combustible dust, fire science, detection systems, suppression systems, knowledge of segregation and separation, housekeeping	Emergency management response, incident command system (ICS), pre-planning and practice, violence in the workplace, emergency action plans, emergency response plans, disaster and crisis response	Sources of biological hazards, blood-borne pathogen control protocol, chemical hazards, mutagens/teratogens/carcinogens, exposure limits, routes of entry, acute and chronic exposures, noise, radiation, heat and cold stress, conduct exposure assessment	Environmental hazards awareness, hazardous waste characteristics, water, air, land and conservation, waste elimination/reduction/minimization, hierarchy of conservation, environmental management systems, waste removal, waste treatment, waste disposal, sustainability	Techniques and theory of adult learning, tools for presentations, culture and climate of safety, needs and gap analysis, data collection, feedback, assessing competency	Legal liability, ethical behavior, protection of worker privacy, skill to deal with unethical situations, read and interpret regulations, determine appropriate actions based on knowledge limitations

Modified from from ASP® Exam Blueprint (ASP10), November 10, 2019.

purses, watches, etc. Access to this locker may or may not be allowed depending upon the testing center.

Question What can I take into the exam room?

Answer ID cards are permitted. Everything else must go into personal lockers.

Question What is furnished in the exam cubicle?

Answer One laminated sheet of paper, one marker, and the computer monitor, keyboard, and mouse

Question What is the workstation/cubicle like?

Answer It is generally very nice, although this may vary with different Pearson VUE centers. Cubicles are large, with a desktop about 3' × 4', excellent lighting, in a very quiet setting, with comfortable, padded adjustable chairs. The keyboard and mouse take up all space in front of the monitor, so calculations must be done off to the side.

Question Are there any children in the exam room?

Answer No. The room is for adult testing only. All children's activities are in separate areas of the Pearson VUE center.

Question How many other people are in the room?

Answer There are multiple workstations in the exam room. The number of people varies with time and day. The proctor has a view of the entire room via a glass window and corner mirrors on the ceiling. Testing is also taped by video and audio monitoring.

Question Can I take breaks?

Answer Yes, as many and as often as necessary. However, the clock keeps running and signing out is required each time, along with a fingerprint check.

Question Do I need IDs?

Answer One ID with photo and signature is mandatory. Photograph and a fingerprint are done during sign-in.

Question Do I need my authorization letter with candidate ID number?

Answer This letter is usually not required, but it is advised to take it just in case. The ID number is always needed when scheduling examination appointments.

Question Can I schedule the exam any time?

Answer No. Certain times are designated for professional exams. Book a testing slot several weeks in advance to secure the desired time and day.

Question Is there enough time to finish the exam?

Answer This is very subjective. Most candidates have found there was plenty of time to finish testing and have adequate review time, but other people did not finish in the allotted time. The time per question (1.5 minutes) is the same as the written exam and the authors found the computer not to be a factor in this area.

Question Are there graphs to interpret? How clear are the graphics?

Answer Yes, there are a limited number of graphs to read. They are a little harder to read on the screen, but not significantly. Graphics are quite acceptable.

Question Are the math formulas provided?

Answer If a problem required a formula(s), then they should be provided in the question.

General Comments

The computer exam is a positive, convenient way to take the exam. The Pearson VUE people were friendly and helpful. The cubicles are quiet and well-lit, and the chairs are relatively comfortable. There is adequate table space and the computer was user friendly and nonthreatening.

Conditions may vary considerably between testing locations.

A listing of Pearson VUE center locations is available through the Pearson VUE website. More complete information can be obtained by calling or faxing the Board of Certified Safety Professionals. **Good luck on the exam!**

Applied Study and Testing Techniques

The examination blueprint outlines how the items on an examination are distributed across domains and tasks/topics. Some keys to success include:

1. Analyzing knowledge gaps and identifying strengths and weaknesses

2. Designing a solid examination study plan
3. Developing test-taking strategies

Converting your subject strengths and weaknesses into a study plan is likely to increase your overall examination score. Scoring well in one subject area can compensate for a weaker score in another subject area. However, there may not be enough items in your strong areas to achieve a passing score.

Note that knowledge and understanding are essential in passing the examination. Relying only on simulated examination items is not the best way to increase knowledge and understanding. Use simulated items to provide insight into the areas in which you should engage in additional study.

Knowing how to take the examination will help improve your score. The examination uses multiple-choice items with only one correct answer and three incorrect answers. Remember, the goal is to get as many items correct as possible. There is no penalty for selecting an incorrect answer. However, only correct answers count toward reaching the passing score.

- Read the items carefully.
    - Psychometricians design multiple-choice questions so that all the possible answer choices are plausible. Use deductive and inductive reasoning to eliminate detractor answer choices.
- Understand the problem.
    - Consider the context.
    - What is given? What is wanted?
- Use examination time wisely.
    - Conduct multiple passes, solving the "easy" problems first and saving the challenging problems for the end.
- Complete all items.
    - Blank answers are scored as wrong answers.

While studying resources, identify main thoughts or themes in the literature review. Draw on your experience and on professional and study references and rewrite important ideas in your own words. This helps you remember the concepts in context. Additional references are listed later in the workbook.

In establishing a good study regimen, it is important to find a place conducive to studying. A good study place should meet the following criteria:

- The place should be used exclusively for study. Avoid using a garage, workshop, family room, or other area that represents recreation or other distractions. Find a location that represents a study island, where study is the **only** activity.
- The selected study area should have good lighting and ventilation, and be temperature controlled, comfortable, and quiet.
- A large table or desk to spread necessary readily available study and reference materials is a must. The purpose is to dedicate a comfortable, personal space with minimal interruptions.

Securing a good place to study should eliminate as many external distractions as possible. Also, candidates should consider how to minimize internal distractions. Total elimination of external distractions is often possible; however, total elimination of internal distractions is nearly impossible and can only be minimized through focused thought.

Helpful hints for focusing the mind for studying include the following:

1. Set realistic time limits, determining what to study and keeping with a schedule. Studying a subject too long at one time can lead to daydreaming, which reduces study effectiveness.
2. Personal factors can be distracters and result in additional frustration. All efforts should be made to avoid the intrusion of personal issues. Rescheduling the ASP test date may be a consideration if serious personal problems exist.
3. Minimize dealing with outside details. Having too many obligations and/or responsibilities enables "brain creep." Consider keeping a notebook in the study area and jotting down appointments and details of projects as these brainstorms appear. It's impossible to totally prevent these details from surfacing, but by documenting them, it may free the mind to resume study.
4. Being physically and mentally prepared to study is beneficial. Most of the following suggestions are common sense, but probably deserve repeating.
    - Eat a well-balanced diet. Increase protein intake; a proper level of blood sugar enhances studying effectiveness.
    - Get plenty of sleep. Establish and maintain a regular work/rest cycle.
    - Exercise is beneficial for more than just an exam preparation. Consider choosing a

form of exercise that provides enjoyment and relaxation.
- Avoid mental fatigue. Allocate down time for breaks. The average supervisor should study for the ASP exam for two to four weeks. DO NOT attempt to cram overnight.

The Question-and-Answer Study Method

The ASP exam study workbooks apply a question-and-answer format that allows candidates to concentrate on knowledge gaps and avoid overstudying material in areas where the candidate already possess enough knowledge to pass the exam.

The research has been completed by the authors, who have taken the exam and researched the blueprint areas of interest, developing targeted learning outcomes. This allows candidates to determine if their current level knowledge is adequate, or if a more in-depth understanding is required.

Fundamental to this technique is a good core of questions. The technique is intended to be useful to practitioners who have mastered the skills and tasks necessary to perform in the safety and health arena.

Most adult learners enjoy the process of learning. The difference lies in the ability to retain what is important to the accomplishment of a goal and reject what is not important. Embrace the aspect of professional development while preparing for the ASP examination.

When utilizing this workbook properly, the authors believe candidates can master those areas necessary to achieve the goal of passing the ASP examination with minimum effort on research and actual study. The technique also has some very beneficial side effects. Candidates will also find that the learning process will enhance skill sets in becoming an improved and more proficient safety and health practitioner.

However, the process assumes candidates have the discipline to do the research and study the material where deficiencies may exist. Attempting to study using only the material presented in this workbook brings a risk of not being adequately prepared for the examination.

The steps to using the Q & A method:

1. Dead reckoning: Use existing knowledge, experience, and test-taking strategies; answer the question through logic and reasoning.
2. Process check: Review the results of each practice session, and then study the explanation.
3. Validate knowledge: Was this a known or an unknown concept? Is the answer achieved with the current knowledge base or by an educated guess or dumb luck?

   Note: This is a critical step in the Q&A learning process and determines if one can proceed or must gain more knowledge on the subject. Additionally, is the knowledge base on this subject broad enough to answer questions of similar difficulty on the subject? *"True genius is an uncluttered mind armed with only relevant knowledge."* (John R. Monteith)

4. Filter: Either move on or take notes. When comfortable with knowledge on the subject, move on to the next question. However, if the current level of knowledge on the subject or other aspects of the subject feels inadequate, then research and take additional notes about the information. Write in the workbook margins right next to the question.
5. Enhance deficiencies: Research and study deficient knowledge areas. After completing a set of questions and writing notes on information to study, a knowledge deficiency study plan can be developed. Then research and study the material necessary to enhance the required knowledge. The authors advise focusing on notes in the workbook and staying on subject. It is very easy to wander onto some other interesting subject and lose sight of the desired learning outcome. Keep the goal in mind to pass the test the first time!

Applied Logic: Socratic Method

The following representative question, answer, and explanation illustrate the process.

Question:

Which is the **most** correct statement about the function of an electrical Ground Fault Circuit Interrupter (GFCI)?

A. It is a slow-acting device.
B. It interrupts the electric power within 1/40th of a second.
C. It will detect line-to-line faults.
D. It is not designed for personnel protection.

> **YOUR NAME**
> ASP Exam version
>
> Question: 01 of 200
> Time remaining: 300 min
>
> **Which is the most correct statement about the function of an electrical Ground Fault Circuit Interrupter (GFCI)?**
>
> O A.) It is a slow acting device.
> ● B.) It interrupts the electric power within 1/40th of a second.
> O C.) It will detect line-to-line faults.
> O D.) It is not designed for personnel protection.
>
> FURTHER REVIEW | PREVIOUS | NEXT

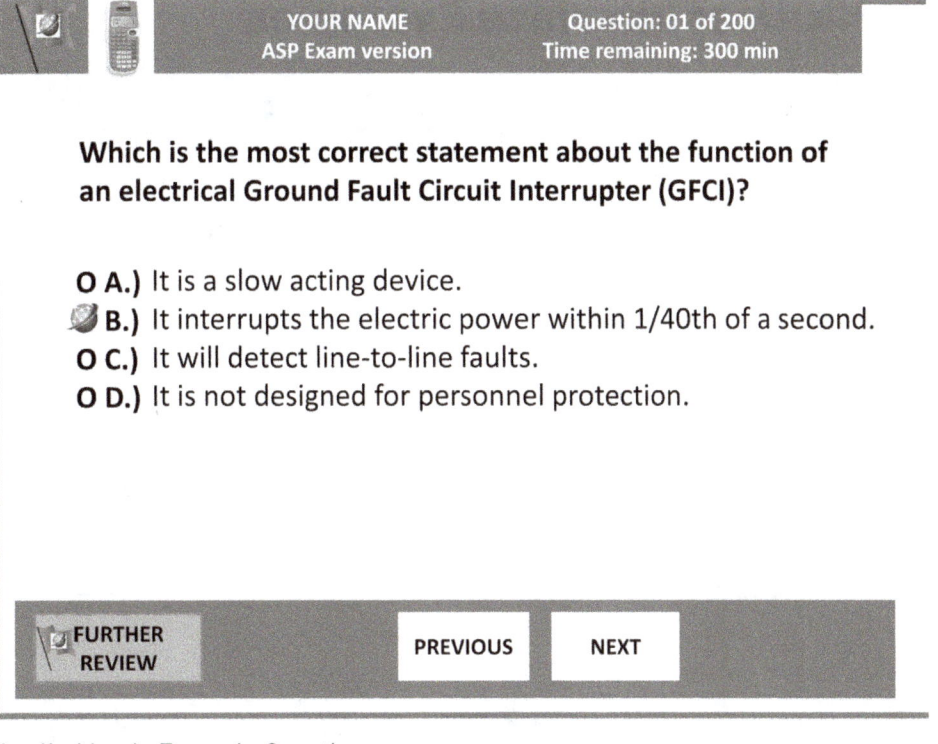

Applied Logic Example Question

Answer: **B**

Explanation: A **GFCI** is specifically designed to **protect people** against electric shock from an electrical system, and it monitors the imbalance of current between the ungrounded (hot) and grounded (neutral) conductor of a given circuit. *These devices will operate on a circuit that does not have an equipment-grounding conductor.* Except for small amounts of leakage, the current returning to the power supply in a typical 2-wire circuit will be equal to the current leaving the power supply. If the difference between the current leaving and returning through the current transformer of the GFCI (leakage) exceeds **5 mA**, the solid-state circuitry opens the switching contacts and de-energizes the circuit. Whenever the amount *going* differs from the amount *returning* by a set trip level, the GFCI interrupts the electric power within **1/40th** of a second.

How much will candidates need to know about the subject of GFCIs? If electrical work represents a strong area, a candidate probably has significant knowledge about the GFCI and is comfortable with this question and the general subject. Another possibility is that one is basically knowledgeable on the subject, but could use some more focused descriptors. Another scenario may be that a candidate knows very little about GFCIs, requiring more focus on concept details and application techniques. How far into the topic does a student need to explore? The level of detail in the example question may serve as a representative indicator. Beyond the basics, another key indicator is the repetition of the workbook question. Content frequently appearing with only minor changes in the question format indicates that the subject matter is important, and authors anticipate the actual exam will have several questions dealing with that subject.

The Q & A method of studying is a proven method. The basic outline is delivered with questions and students can then determine individual levels of subject knowledge. When additional knowledge is required, they can conduct more research and study to develop the required knowledge or skill. This learning technique has proven to be successful for many different levels of adult learners because the **individual** determines what material to study.

Exam Graphic User Interface Examples

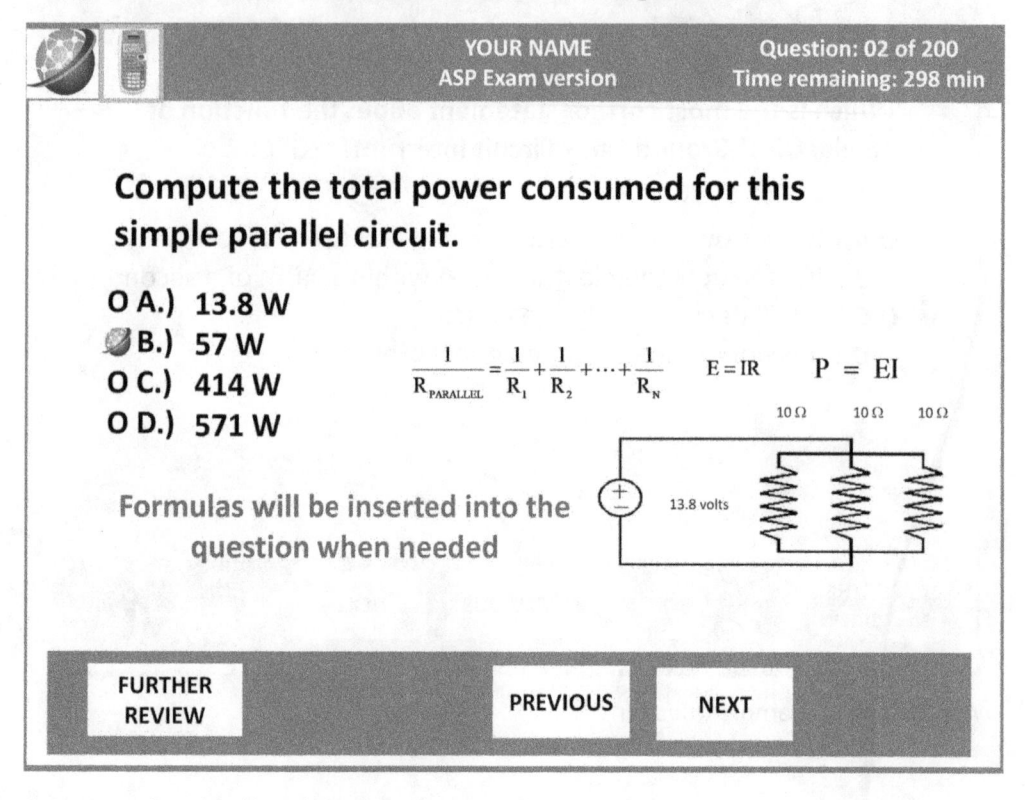

Compute the total power consumed for this simple parallel circuit.

- A.) 13.8 W
- B.) 57 W
- C.) 414 W
- D.) 571 W

$$\frac{1}{R_{PARALLEL}} = \frac{1}{R_1} + \frac{1}{R_2} + \cdots + \frac{1}{R_N} \qquad E = IR \qquad P = EI$$

Formulas will be inserted into the question when needed

Computer Graphic User Interface Example Question 1

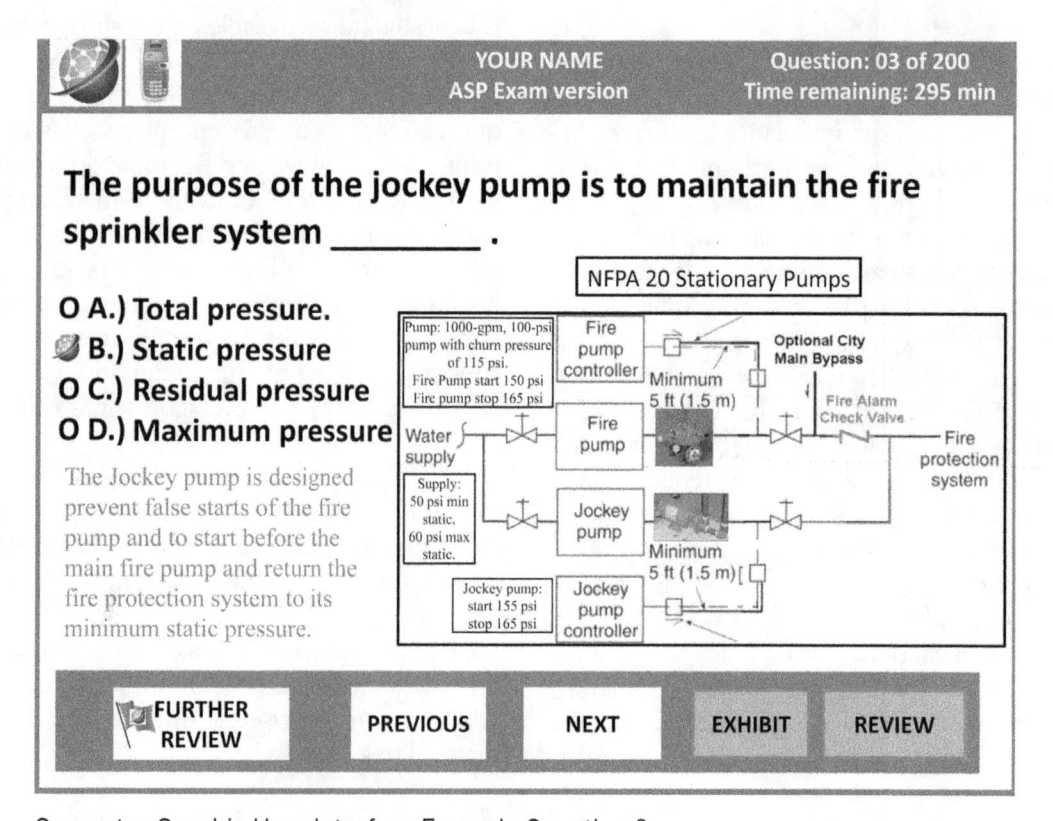

The purpose of the jockey pump is to maintain the fire sprinkler system _____ .

- A.) Total pressure.
- B.) Static pressure
- C.) Residual pressure
- D.) Maximum pressure

The Jockey pump is designed prevent false starts of the fire pump and to start before the main fire pump and return the fire protection system to its minimum static pressure.

Computer Graphic User Interface Example Question 2

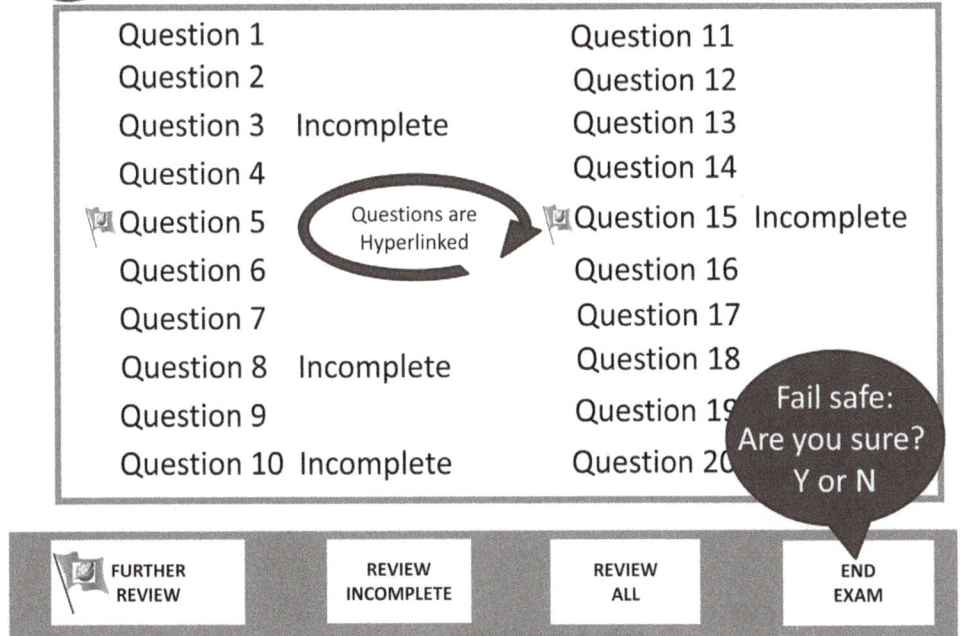

Exam Review Screen

Exam Review Screen Example

Select Study References for the ASP Exam

BCSP maintains a list of examination references for each certification at www.bcsp.org/Sources. Examination items are not necessarily taken directly from these sources. However, BCSP believes these references represent the breadth and depth of coverage of safety, health, and environmental practice. However, it has been the author's experience that *the following references are the ones that have proven to be the most valuable* to safety practitioners studying for this exam.

1. Consensus standards such as ANSI, NFPA, and ISO are also referenced in the exam. The following is a partial list of applicable consensus standards:
   - ANSI-ASSP Z10 Occupational Health & Safety Management Systems
   - ANSI ASSP Z490 Practices and Criteria for Safety & Health Training
   - ~~BSI 18001 Safety & Health Managements~~ ISO 45001 systems
   - ISO 14000 Environmental Managements Systems
   - OSHA VPP
   - ISO 31000 Risk Management Principles
   - ISO 30010 Risk Management Assessment Techniques
   - ISO 19011 Auditing Management Systems
   - ANSI/ASSP Z590.2-2003 Criteria for Establishing the Scope and Functions of the Professional Safety Position
   - ANSI/ Z590.3-2011 Prevention Through Design
   - NFPA 10 Fire Extinguishers
   - NFPA 13 Sprinkler Systems
   - NFPA 30 Flammable Liquids
   - NFPA 70E Electrical
   - NFPA 101 Life Safety Code

2. Snyder, D. *Pocket Guide to Safety Essentials,* 2nd edition. National Safety Council, 2014. This is a quick reference guide to fundamental principles of safety management.
3. BCSP. *Complete Guide to the ASP®.* Champaign, IL: BCSP, 2017.
4. Haight, J. *The Safety Professionals Handbook: Management Applications,* 2nd edition. Des Plaines, IL: American Society of Safety Engineers, 2012.
5. Haight, J. *The Safety Professionals Handbook: Technical Applications,* 2nd edition. Des Plaines, IL: American Society of Safety Engineers, 2012.
6. Peterson, D. *Techniques of Safety Management: A Systems Approach,* 4th edition. Des Plaines, IL: American Society of Safety Engineers, 2003.
7. Brauer, R. *Safety and Health for Engineers,* 2nd edition. Des Plaines, IL: American Society of Safety Engineers, 2006.
8. National Safety Council (NSC). *Accident Prevention Manual for Business and Industry, Administration and Programs,* 13th edition, May 1, 2015.
9. National Safety Council (NSC). *Accident Prevention Manual for Business and Industry, Engineering and Technology,* 13th edition, August 1, 2015.
10. National Safety Council (NSC). *Accident Prevention Manual for Business and Industry, Environmental Management,* 13th edition, September 1, 2000.
11. Hill, D. *Construction Safety Management and Engineering,* 2nd edition. Des Plaines, IL: American Society of Safety Engineers, 2014.
12. Manuele, F. *On the Practice of Safety,* 3rd edition. Hoboken, NJ: John Wiley and Sons, Inc., 2003.
13. Plog, B. *Fundamentals of Industrial Hygiene,* 5th–6th editions. National Safety Council, August 10, 2012.
14. National Fire Protection Association. *Fire Protection Handbook,* 21st edition. The 16th, 17th, 18th, 19th, or 20th editions are acceptable, 2011.
15. *Chemistry of Hazardous Materials,* 2nd–6th editions. Prentice-Hall, Inc. This is a superior text for elementary instruction on applied chemistry in the safety and fire fields, September 24, 2013.
16. Snyder, D. *The Hazardous Materials Management Desk Reference,* 3rd ed. Bethesda, MD: Alliance of Hazardous Materials Professionals, 2013.
17. Hammer, W. *Product Safety Management and Engineering,* 5th edition. American Society of Safety Engineers, March 1, 1993.
18. Yates, D. *Safety Professional's Reference and Study Guide.* CRC Press. A "quick desk reference" for the experienced, practicing safety professional in comprehensive or specialized practice, December 9, 2010.
19. *ACGIH Industrial Ventilation Handbook, Manual of Recommended Practices.* American Conference of Governmental Industrial Hygienists, 2013.
20. *Threshold Limit Values and Biological Exposure Indices.* American Conference of Governmental Industrial Hygienists, 2001.

The purpose of the SPAN™ exam study workbook is to give study effort direction. This workbook effectively narrows down the enormous amount of test material that must be mastered. Knowing what to study is not enough. Candidates must also study the *right* material, specifically the right reference material. Finding the right books from which to study is probably the single most important element in developing a personal study plan.

The latest list of exam references can be found on the BCSP website: https://www.bcsp.org/Portals/0/Assets/DocumentLibrary/ASP10-Blueprint-References.pdf.

Domain 1: Advanced Sciences and Math

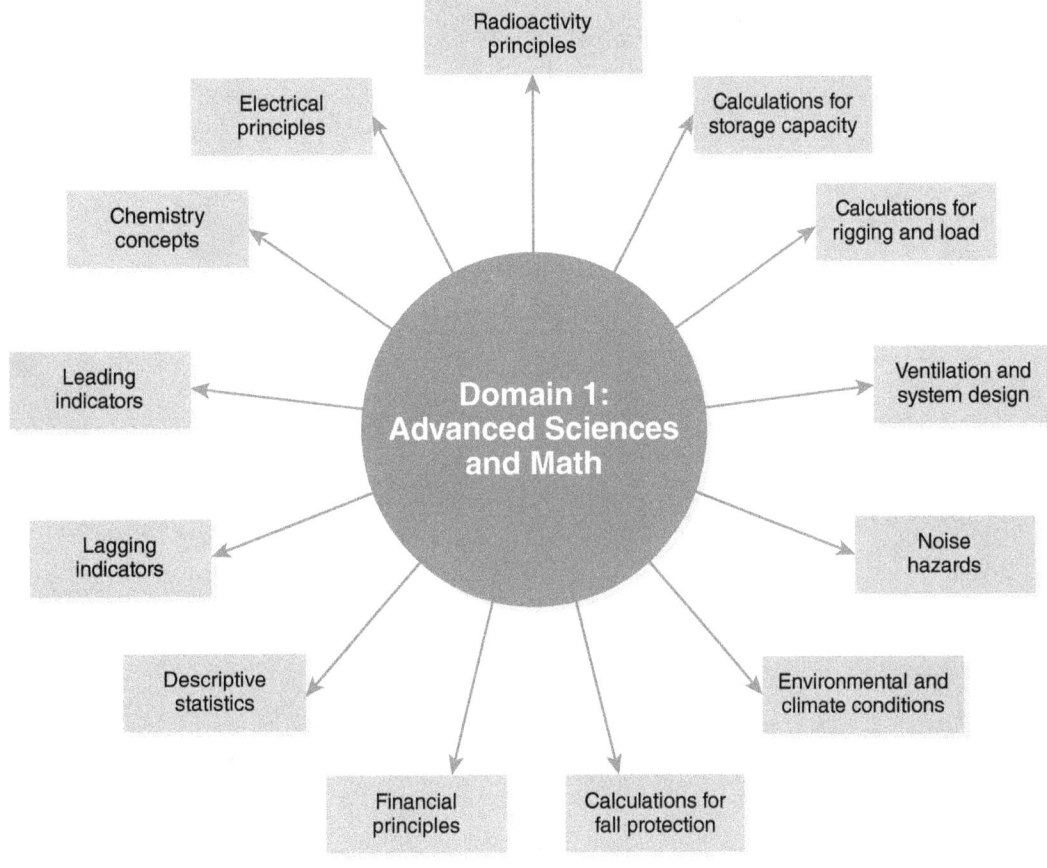

Diagram: Central node "Domain 1: Advanced Sciences and Math" connected to: Radioactivity principles, Calculations for storage capacity, Calculations for rigging and load, Ventilation and system design, Noise hazards, Environmental and climate conditions, Calculations for fall protection, Financial principles, Descriptive statistics, Lagging indicators, Leading indicators, Chemistry concepts, Electrical principles.

Modified from ASP® Exam Blueprint (ASP10), November 10, 2019

ASP Math Equations and Formulas

Concentrations of Vapors and Gases Formulas

$$ppm = \frac{mg/m^3 \times 24.45}{MW}$$

ppm = parts per million in concentration
mg/m³ = milligrams/cubic meter
MW = Molecular Weight of the substance

$$LFL_m = \frac{1}{\frac{f_1}{LFL_1} + \frac{f_2}{LFL_2} + \cdots + \frac{f_n}{LFL_n}}$$

LFL_m = Lower Flammable Limit of a mixture or solvent
f = fraction by weight

$$TWA = \frac{(C_1 \times T_1) + (C_2 \times T_2) + \cdots + (C_n \times T_n)}{(T_1 + T_2 + \cdots + T_n)}$$

TWA = Time Weighted Average
C = Concentration of chemical
T = Time of exposure

$$TLV_m = \frac{1}{\left(\frac{f_1}{TLV_1} + \frac{f_2}{TLV_2} + \cdots + \frac{f_n}{TLV_n}\right)}$$

TLV_m = Threshold Limit Value of a mixture
f = fraction by weight (% expressed as a decimal 0.XX)

$$TLV_{mix} = \frac{C_1}{TLV_1} + \frac{C_2}{TLV_2} + \cdots + \frac{C_n}{TLV_n}$$

Where:
TLV_{mix} = Threshold Limit Value for a mixture of airborne chemicals with additive effects. If the sum is greater than one (1), then an overexposure exists.
C_1 = the measured airborne concentrations of the chemicals.
TLV_1 = published Threshold Limit Value for the respective chemicals.
When two or more hazardous chemicals with similar toxic effects are present in the environment, the combined effect should be evaluated, rather than the individual effect.
NOTE: The units can be either mg/m³ or ppm, but must be consistent in the equation.

Combined Gas Law (Charles and Boyles Laws)

$$\frac{P_1 V_1}{T_1} = \frac{P_2 V_2}{T_2}$$

P = Pressure (expressed in absolute)
  1 atm = 14.7 psi
        = 760 mm Hg
        = 29.92 in Hg
        = 33.90 ft H₂O
        = 760 torr
        = 101.3 kilopascal
V = Volume
T = Temperature (expressed in absolute)

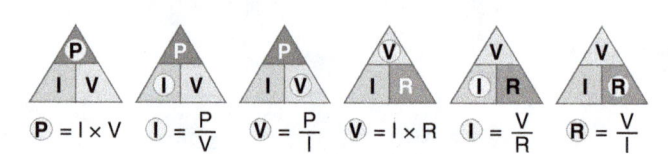

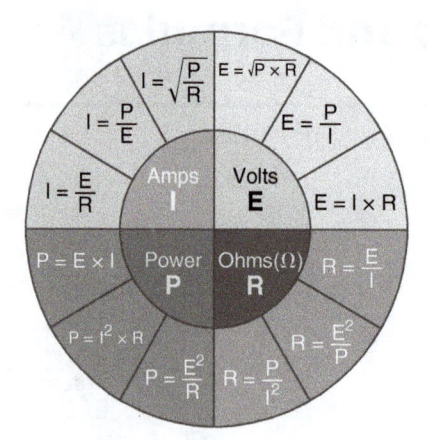

$$t_{°C} = \frac{(t_{°F} - 32)}{1.8}$$

$t_{°K} = t_{°C} + 273$ $\qquad$ $t_{°R} = t_{°F} + 460$

$P = I \times V$ $\quad$ $I = \frac{P}{V}$ $\quad$ $V = \frac{P}{I}$ $\quad$ $V = I \times R$ $\quad$ $I = \frac{V}{R}$ $\quad$ $R = \frac{V}{I}$

Ohm's Law Calculator wheel:
Amps (I): $I = \sqrt{\frac{P}{R}}$, $I = \frac{P}{E}$, $I = \frac{E}{R}$
Volts (E): $E = \sqrt{P \times R}$, $E = \frac{P}{I}$, $E = I \times R$
Ohms (R): $R = \frac{E}{I}$, $R = \frac{E^2}{P}$, $R = \frac{P}{I^2}$
Power (P): $P = E \times I$, $P = I^2 \times R$, $P = \frac{E^2}{R}$

Figure 2 Ohm's Law Calculator

Electrical Formulas

V = IR   or   E = IR
E or V = Voltage
I = Current (Amperage)
R = Resistance (Ohms)

P = VI   or   P = EI
P = Power (Watts)
I = Current (Amperage)
E or V = Voltage

$R_{SERIES} = R_1 + R_2 + \cdots + R_N$
R = Resistance (Ohms)

$\dfrac{1}{R_{PARALLEL}} = \dfrac{1}{R_1} + \dfrac{1}{R_2} + \cdots + \dfrac{1}{R_N}$
R = Resistance (Ohms)

Radiation Formulas

$I_2 = I_1 \dfrac{(d_1)^2}{(d_2)^2}$
I = Intensity
d = distance

$N = N_o e^{-kt}$
N = radioactivity remaining after time t
N_o = radioactivity at a given original time
t = elapsed time
k = disintegration constant
e = second function natural log

$S \cong 6CiEf$
S = Roentgens/hour/foot
Ci = Curie strength (whole curies)
E = Energy in megaelectron volts (MEV)
f = fractional yield

$A = \dfrac{A_o}{e^{\left(\ln 2 \frac{t}{T_{1/2}}\right)}}$
A = radioactivity remaining after time t
A_o = radioactivity at a given original time
t = elapsed time
$T_{1/2}$ = half-life of the radionuclide
ln2 = 0.693 (natural log of 2)

$T_{1/2} = \dfrac{\ln 2}{k}$
$T_{1/2}$ = half-life of the radionuclide
ln2 = 0.693 (natural log of 2)
k = Disintegration constant

TYPE	EFFECTS	SHIELDING
Alpha	Short range; < 4" in air Chemically similar to calcium (can collect in kidneys, bones, liver, lungs, and spleen) Eyes are an internal exposure	Skin, paper, thin film of water
Beta	Secondary release of gamma radiation Higher energies can cause skin burns	Light metals (like aluminum)
Neutron	Secondary release of gamma radiation	Carbon or high hydrogen content (like water)
Gamma and X-ray	Most penetrating Electromagnetic radiation: Gamma (natural); X-ray (man-made)	Heavy metals (like lead)

Structural and Mechanical Calculations

Area and Volume Formulas

Circumference of a circle = $2\pi r$ **or** πd

Area of a circle = πr^2 **or** $\dfrac{\pi d^2}{4}$

Area of a rectangle = length × width

Area of a triangle = ½ × base × height

Volume of a tank = $\pi r^2 h$ **or** $\dfrac{\pi d^2 h}{4}$

Volume of a cube = length × width × height

Trigonometry Functions

$\dfrac{a}{\sin A} = \dfrac{b}{\sin B} = \dfrac{c}{\sin C}$

$\sin A = \dfrac{a}{c}$

$\cos A = \dfrac{b}{c}$

$\tan A = \dfrac{a}{b}$

Angle of a ramp = $\tan^{-1}\left[\dfrac{\text{rise}}{\text{run}}\right]$

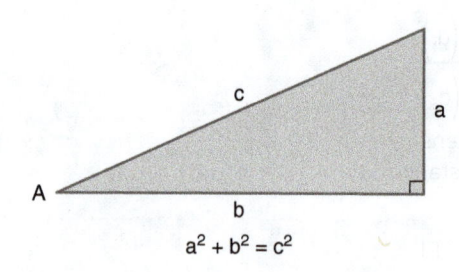

$a^2 + b^2 = c^2$

Figure 3 Pythagorean Theorem

Sling angle and stress rules of thumb:
15° angle = twice the load
30° angle = the load
45° angle = 70% of load
60° angle = 58% load
90° angle = 50% of load
Load ÷ number of slings ÷ sin A = stress on the sling

Engineering Control Calculations

Q = AV Q = the **Volumetric Flow Rate** in the duct, measured in cubic feet/minute = ft³/min [cfm] A = the **Cross-Sectional Area** of the duct under consideration, in square feet [ft²] V = the **Velocity**, or **Duct Velocity**, of the gases moving in the duct, in feet/minute = ft/min [fpm]	$V = 4005\sqrt{VP}$ V = Velocity (lineal feet) VP = Velocity Pressure
$V = 4005 C_e \sqrt{SP_h}$ V = average duct velocity (fpm) 4005 = constant, based on the density of standard air C_e = Coefficient of entry (unitless) SP_h = hood static pressure ("wg)	TP = SP + VP TP = Total Pressure ("wg) SP = Static Pressure ("wg) VP = Velocity Pressure ("wg) Velocity Pressure (VP) is always "positive" downstream of the fan. Static Pressure (SP) is always "negative" upstream of the fan.

Domain 1: Advanced Sciences and Math

$$Q = \frac{G}{TLV} \times 10^6$$

Q = the effective dilution rate (cfm)
G = Generation rate of a gas or vapor (cfm)
10^6 = conversion factor from TLV to ppm
TLV = the acceptable concentration (ppm)

$$Q = \frac{403 \times 10^6 \times SG \times ER \times K}{MW \times C}$$

Q = volumetric flow (cfm)
SG = Specific Gravity
ER = Evaporation Rate (pints/minute)
K = K-factor or dilution ventilation safety factor (3–10 unitless)
MW = Molecular Weight
C = Concentration (TLV)

$$\frac{CFM_1}{CFM_2} = \frac{RPM_1}{RPM_2}$$

CFM_i = the **Air Discharge Volume** of the fan when it is operating at the **i**th set of conditions, in cubic feet per minute [cfm];
RPM_i = the **i**th operating **Rotational Speed** of the fan, in revolutions per minute [rpm].

Hoods WITHOUT Flanges

$$V = \frac{Q}{10x^2 + A}$$

V = the **Capture Velocity**, i.e., the centerline velocity of the air entering the hood under consideration, at a point "**x**" feet directly in front of the face of the hood. This **Capture Velocity** is usually measured in feet per minute [fpm]
Q = the **Volumetric Flow Rate** of the hood, measured in cubic feet per minute [cfm]
x = the **Distance** from the plane of the hood opening to the point directly in front of it where the **Capture Velocity** is to be determined, measured in feet [ft]
A = the **Cross-Sectional Area** of the hood opening, measured in square feet [ft²]

Hoods WITH Flanges

$$V = \frac{4Q}{3[10x^2 + A]}$$

Heat Stress Formulas

Indoor Formula (no solar load)
WBGT = 0.7WB + 0.3GT
WBGT = Wet Bulb Globe Temperature
WB = Wet Bulb temperature
GT = Globe Temperature

Outdoor Formula (with solar load)
WBGT = 0.7 WB + 0.2 GT + 0.1DB
WBGT = Wet Bulb Globe Temperature
WB = Wet Bulb temperature
GT = Globe Temperature
DB = Dry Bulb temperature

Noise Formulas

$$L_w = 10\log_{10}\frac{W}{W_0}$$

L_W = sound power level Watts (dB)
W = acoustic power in watts
W_0 = reference power intensity watts

$$L_p = 20\log_{10}\frac{p}{p_0}$$

L_p = sound pressure level (dB)
P = final sound pressure (Pa)
p_0 = reference sound pressure (Pa) (20 µPa)

$SPL_{Total} = SPL_{Individual} + 10 \log n$

SPL_{Total} = combined dB for all sources
$SPL_{Individual}$ = dB for one source
n = number of noise sources
3-dB rule

$dB_1 = dB_0 + 20 \log_{10}\left(\dfrac{d_0}{d_1}\right)$

dB_1 = noise level at distance d_1 (dB)
dB_0 = noise level at distance d_0 (dB)
d = distance from a noise source (any units of length)
6-dB rule

$T = \dfrac{8}{2^{[(L-90)/5]}}$

T = allowable exposure time
L = exposure (dB)
5-dB rule

$TWA = 16.61 \log_{10}\left[\dfrac{D}{100}\right] + 90$

TWA = Time Weighted Average
D = Dose (%)

$L_{pt} = 10 \log\left[\displaystyle\sum_{i=1}^{N} 10^{\left(\frac{L_{pi}}{10}\right)}\right]$

L_{pt} = total sound pressure level generated by N sources (dB)
L_{pi} = individual sound level of each source (dB)
N = number of sound pressure levels

$L_{pt} = L_{pi} + 10 \log N$

L_{pt} = total sound pressure level generated by N sources (dB)
L_{pi} = individual sound level of each source (dB)
N = number of sound pressure levels

Noise Dose = $\dfrac{C_1}{T_1} + \dfrac{C_2}{T_2} + \cdots + \dfrac{C_n}{T_n}$

C = Calculated exposure time
T = Authorized exposure time

Physics Formulas

Force to Slide	Force to Tip
$F = \mu N$	$F_1 d_1 = F_2 d_2$
F = Force required	F = Force
μ = Coefficient of friction	d = Distance
N = Normal weight	
Force down a ramp (sine function) $N = W \times \sin \angle$	
Force perpendicular to a ramp (cosine function)	
$N = W \times \cos \angle$	

Force	
$F = ma$	$W = mg$
F = Force required	W = Weight
m = mass	m = mass
a = acceleration	g = gravity (acceleration)

$v = v_0 + at$	$s = v_0 t + \dfrac{at^2}{2}$ or $s = v_0 t + \dfrac{1}{2} at^2$
v = final velocity	v_0 = initial velocity
v_0 = initial velocity	s = distance traveled
a = acceleration	a = acceleration
t = time taken	t = time taken

$v^2 = v_0^2 + 2as$
v = final velocity
v_0 = initial velocity
s = distance traveled
a = acceleration

$a = \dfrac{v - v_0}{t}$
a = acceleration
v = final velocity
v_0 = initial velocity
t = time taken

$K.E. = \dfrac{mv^2}{2}$
K.E. = Kinetic Energy
m = mass
v = velocity (ft/sec)

Traffic Formulas

Note: These are the formulas that may be provided on the exam. It is recommended that you memorize the simplified traffic formulas provided in the book.

$V_{kph} = \sqrt{255 \times s \times \mu}$
V_{kph} = Velocity in kilometers per hour
S = distance (length of skid mark)
μ = coefficient of friction

$V_{mph} = \sqrt{30 \times s \times \mu}$
V_{mph} = Velocity in miles per hour
S = distance (length of skid mark)
μ = coefficient of friction

$V_{final} = \sqrt{V_1^2 + V_2^2 + \cdots + V_n^2}$
V_{final} = total velocity over multiple coefficients of friction

$V_{mph} = 5.5\sqrt{\dfrac{K.E.}{W}}$
V_{mph} = Velocity in miles per hour
K.E. = Kinetic Energy
W = Weight

Financial Principles Formulas

$F = P(1 + i)^n$ 	 $P = F(1 + i)^{-n}$

$F = A\left(\dfrac{(1 + i)^n - 1}{i}\right)$ 	 $A = F\left(\dfrac{i}{(1 + i)^n - 1}\right)$

$A = P\left(\dfrac{i(1 + i)^n}{(1 + i)^n - 1}\right)$ 	 $P = A\left(\dfrac{(1 + i)^n - 1}{i(1 + i)^n}\right)$

Where
i = interest rate for a given interest period (remember to divide the interest by 4 to get quarterly interest)
n = number of interest periods (to get quarters, multiply the years by 4)
P = sum of money at the present time
F = future worth of a present sum of money after n interest periods, or the future worth of a series of equal payments
A = a payment or receipt at the end of an interest period in a series of n equal payments or receipts (if the payment is a yearly payment and the question is based on a quarterly deposit, divide by 4)

Statistics Calculations

$t = \dfrac{\bar{X} - \mu}{\hat{s}} \sqrt{n}$

t = t-score
$\bar{X}$ = mean
μ = mean
$\hat{S}$ = standard deviation
n = number of data points

$z = \dfrac{X - \mu}{\sigma}$

z = z-score
X = data point
μ = mean
σ = standard deviation

$P(r) = \dfrac{(\lambda t)^r e^{-\lambda t}}{r!}$

P = Poisson distribution
r = number of observed events or rate
λ = expected number of events or baseline
t = time

$P_f = 1 - R(t)$
P_f = Probability (failure)
$R(t)$ = Reliability (t)

$r = \dfrac{n\sum(XY) - (\sum X)(\sum Y)}{\sqrt{\left[n\sum(X^2) - (\sum X)^2\right]\left[N\sum(Y^2) - (\sum Y)^2\right]}}$

$x = X - \bar{X}$
$y = Y - \bar{Y}$

r = regression (coefficient of correlation)

$R(t) = e^{-\lambda t}$
$R(t)$ = Reliability (t)
e = 2.71828
λ = failure rate (reciprocal of mean time between failure)
t = A specified period of fail-free operation or failure-free operation

$s = \sqrt{\dfrac{\sum(x^2)}{n-1}}$ $\quad (x = X - \bar{X}) \quad$ $\sigma = \sqrt{\dfrac{\sum(x^2)}{n}}$

S = sample standard deviation
σ = population standard deviation
X = data point
$\bar{X}$ = mean

$P^n_k = \dfrac{n!}{(n-k)!} \qquad C^n_k = \dfrac{n!}{k!(n-k)!}$

P^n_k = number of combinations possible when taking n things k at a time
C^n_k = number of combinations possible when taking n things k at a time
n = number of things to sample from
k = number of things taken each time

Hydrostatics and Hydraulics Formulas

$p_v = \dfrac{Q^2}{891d^4}$

P_v = Pressure velocity (psi)
Q = flow rate (gpm)
d = internal diameter in inches

$Q_2 = Q_1 \left[\dfrac{(S - R_2)^{0.54}}{(S - R_1)^{0.54}}\right]$

Q = flow (gpm)
S = Static pressure (psi)
R = Residual pressure (psi)

Domain 1: Advanced Sciences and Math

$$\frac{Q_1}{Q_2} = \frac{\sqrt{P_1}}{\sqrt{P_2}}$$

Q = flow (gpm)
P = Pressure differential (S − R)

$$P_d = \frac{4.52\, Q^{1.85}}{C^{1.85}\, d^{4.87}}$$

P_d = Pressure drop — psi/ft
Q = flow (gpm)
C = Coefficient of roughness (pipe)
d = internal diameter in inches

Unit Conversions

1 kg = 2.2 lbs	1000 mm = 1 m
1 kgm = 9.8 Newtons force	1 in = 2.54 cm
1 pound force = 4.45 Newtons	1 micron = 10^{-4} cm
1000 g = 1 kg	1000 m = 1 km
1 lb = 454 g	1 meter = 3.28 feet
7.48 gal = 1 ft³ *volume in a tank*	1 mile = 1.6 km
16 oz = 454 g	1 ft = 30.48 cm *30.5*
760 mm Hg = 29.92 in Hg	1 mile = 5280 feet
760 mm Hg = 14.7 lb/in²	1 mile = 1609 meters
1 liter = 1.06 qt = 61.02 in³ = 0.03531 ft³ = 0.26 gal 1 gal = 3.78 liters 1 liter = 1000 mL = 1000 cm³ (cc)	1 atmosphere (atm) pressure = 14.7 psi = 760 mm Hg = 29.92 in Hg = 33.90 ft H_2O = 760 torr = 101.3 kilopascal
gram-mole @ 0°C and 1 atm = 22.4 liters @ 25°C and 1 atm = 24.45 liters	1 lumen = 1 candela 1 foot-candle = 10.76 candela/m² 1 foot-candle = 10.76 lux
Water weight density = 62.4 lbs/ft³ = 8.34 lbs/gal	1 rad = 10^{-2} gray 1 rem = 10^{-2} sievert 1 gray = 1 sievert

1 gal = 8.34 lbs

.433 lbs/sq in / per foot of water rise
bottom of a standpipe for
pressure of foot of water

.433 × per ft.³

miles per hour = 1.47 ft./per second

NIOSH Lifting Equation

$$RWL = LC \times HM \times VM \times DM \times AM \times FM \times CM$$

$$RWL(lb) = 51\left(\frac{10}{H}\right)(1 - 0.0075\,|V - 30|)\left(0.82 + \frac{1.8}{D}\right)(1 - (0.0032 \times A))(FM)(CM)$$

$$RWL(kg) = 23\left(\frac{25}{H}\right)(1 - 0.003\,|V - 75|)\left(0.82 + \frac{4.5}{D}\right)(1 - (0.0032 \times A))(FM)(CM)$$

Where
H = Horizontal distance of hands from midpoint between the ankles
V = Vertical distance of the hand from the floor
D = Vertical travel distance between origin and destination
A = Angle of asymmetry, the angular displacement of the load from the sagittal plane in degrees
F = Average frequency of lift in lifts per minute
C = Coupling or grip

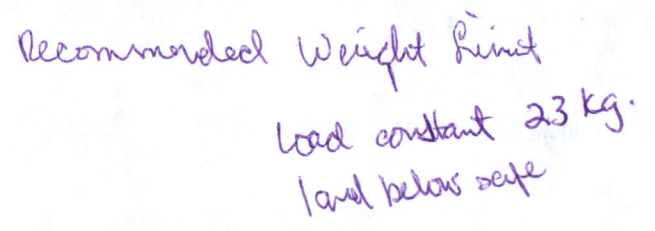

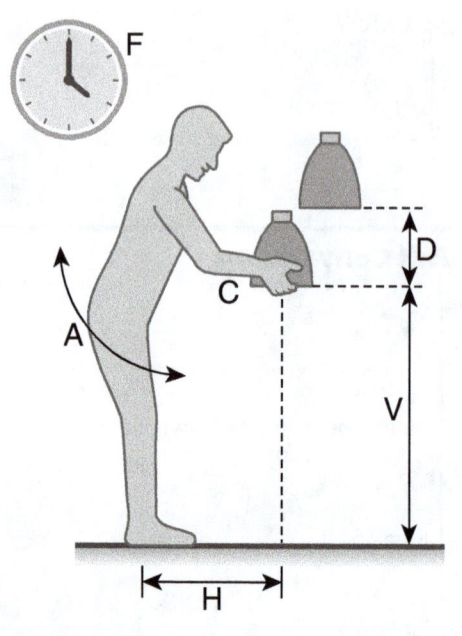

[Handwritten notes: Recommended Weight Limit; load constant 23 kg; load below safe]

Figure 4 NIOSH Lifting Diagram

Notes and Modifications:

H = Must be between 10 and 25 inches
V = Must be between 0 and 70 inches
V = Is an absolute value indicating the absolute deviation from 30 inches; i.e., if V = 36 the absolute value would be 6, likewise if V = 24 the absolute value would also be 6.
D = Must be between 10 inches and (70 − V) inches *if less than 10 inches, D = 10*
F = Must be between 0.2 (one lift every five minutes) and 15 lifts per minute – duration ranges up to 8 hours
A = Must be between 0° and 135° angular displacement

$$RWL = LC \times HM \times VM \times DM \times AM \times FM \times CM$$

$$RWL(lb) = 51\left(\frac{10}{H}\right)(1 - 0.0075\,|V - 30|)\left(0.82 + \frac{1.8}{D}\right)(1 - (0.0032 \times A))(FM)(CM)$$

$$RWL(kg) = 23\left(\frac{25}{H}\right)(1 - 0.003\,|V - 75|)\left(0.82 + \frac{4.5}{D}\right)(1 - (0.0032 \times A))(FM)(CM)$$

	COUPLING MULTIPLIER	
Coupling Type	V < 30 in (75 cm)	V ≥ 30 in (75 cm)
Good	1.00	1.00
Fair	0.95	1.00
Poor	0.90	0.90

FREQUENCY MULTIPLIER

Frequency Lifts/min (F)	≤ 1 hr V < 30	≤ 1 hr V ≥ 30	≤ 2 hr V < 30	≤ 2 hr V ≥ 30	≤ 8 hr V < 30	≤ 8 hr V ≥ 30
≤ 0.2	1.00	1.00	0.95	0.95	0.85	0.85
0.5	0.97	0.97	0.92	0.92	0.81	0.81
1	0.94	0.94	0.88	0.88	0.75	0.75
2	0.91	0.91	0.84	0.84	0.65	0.65
3	0.88	0.88	0.79	0.79	0.55	0.55
4	0.84	0.84	0.72	0.72	0.45	0.45
5	0.80	0.80	0.60	0.60	0.35	0.35
6	0.75	0.75	0.50	0.50	0.27	0.27
7	0.70	0.70	0.42	0.42	0.22	0.22
8	0.60	0.60	0.35	0.35	0.18	0.18
9	0.52	0.52	0.30	0.30	0.00	0.15
10	0.45	0.45	0.26	0.26	0.00	0.13
11	0.41	0.41	0.00	0.23	0.00	0.00
12	0.37	0.37	0.00	0.21	0.00	0.00
13	0.00	0.34	0.00	0.00	0.00	0.00
14	0.00	0.31	0.00	0.00	0.00	0.00
15	0.00	0.28	0.00	0.00	0.00	0.00
> 15	0.00	0.00	0.00	0.00	0.00	0.00

Lifting Index (LI) = a term that provides a relative estimate of the level of physical stress associated with a particular manual lifting task. The estimate of the level of physical stress is defined by the relationship of the weight of the load lifted and the recommended weight limit (RWL).

$$LI = \frac{\text{Load Weight}}{\text{Recommended Weight Limit}} = \frac{L}{RWL}$$

Domain 1 Quiz 1 Questions

1. A direct reading instrument indicates a concentration of 2.5% for a hazardous material that has a Permissible Exposure Limit (PEL) of 250 ppm and an Immediately Dangerous to Life and Health (IDLH) of 2500 ppm and a Lower Explosive Limit (LEL) of 25,000 ppm. If assigned the task of respirator selection for entry into this atmosphere, which of the following statements is most correct?

   A. The instrument shows a reading in excess of the PEL and IDLH.
   B. The instrument shows a reading below the PEL, IDLH and LEL.
   C. The direct reading instrument indicates a concentration below the LEL, but above the IDLH and PEL.
   D. The instrument shows a reading equal to the LEL, which is above the IDLH and PEL.

2. A calibrated hot wire gas detector-type combustible-gas indicator reads 10% for methane, which has a 5.3% LEL. How many parts per million does this represent?

   A. 3500 ppm
   B. 7000 ppm
   C. 5300 ppm
   D. 9200 ppm

3. The balanced equation below shows the complete oxidation of acetylene. If 10 moles of oxygen were consumed in the oxidation process, how many grams of CO_2 (MW = 44) would be produced?

   $2C_2H_2 + 5O_2 \rightarrow 4CO_2 + 2H_2O$

   A. 35.2 grams
   B. 352 grams
   C. 442 grams
   D. 221 grams

4. The best descriptor of the pH scale is:

   A. The pH scale is logarithmic.
   B. The pH scale ranges from 0 to 12.
   C. The pH scale indicates the positive ion concentration of a compound.
   D. The pH scale indicates the number of negative nitrogen ions shown as N_{30+1}.

5. Given a molecular weight of 112, convert 1.6 pounds of a material fully evaporated in a 3000 ft³ confined space to parts per million. Note: The space occupied by a mole of gas at STP (industrial hygiene) is 24.45 liters.

   A. 2465 ppm
   B. 1865 ppm
   C. 1650 ppm
   D. 1112 ppm

   $$ppm = \frac{mg/m^3 \times 24.45}{MW}$$

6. Determine the TWA concentration from the following measurement data: 7:00 a.m. to 10:00 a.m. @ 210 ppm; 10:00 a.m. to 12:00 p.m. @ 195 ppm; 12:00 p.m. to 1:00 p.m. @ 0 ppm; 1:00 p.m. to 2:00 p.m. @ 60 ppm; 2:00 p.m. to 3:00 p.m. @ 300 ppm

   A. 155.0 ppm
   B. 167.8 ppm
   C. 172.5 ppm
   D. 222.6 ppm

   $$TWA = \frac{(C_1 \times T_1) + (C_2 \times T_2) + \cdots + (C_n \times T_n)}{(T_1 + T_2 + \cdots + T_n)}$$

Domain 1: Advanced Sciences and Math

7. If a tank atmosphere contains 76% ambient air and 24% hydrocarbons, what is the oxygen content of the tank?

   A. 16%
   B. 17%
   C. 19%
   D. 21%

8. The pressure in a 5L compressed-gas cylinder has a pressure of 3000 psig at a temperature of 65°F. The cylinder is allowed to heat to 110°F while stored in a commercial transportation van exposed to the sun. What is the new pressure in the gas cylinder?

   A. 5077 psig
   B. 3258 psig
   C. 4372 psig
   D. 3941 psig

   $$\frac{P_1 V_1}{T_1} = \frac{P_2 V_2}{T_2}$$

9. A compound made up of 35% naphtha, 5% toluene, and 60% Stoddard solvent is used to clean parts in a tire repair shop. A review of the SDS for each material yields the following information:

   Naphtha = TLV 1370 mg/m³, MW 110, SG 0.66, FP –40 to 86°F, VP 48.
   Toluene = TLV 377 mg/m³, MW 92, SG 0.87, FP 40°F, VP 22.
   Stoddard solvent = TLV 525 mg/m³, MW 144, SG 0.78, FP 102 to 110°F, VP 2.
   Given the assumption that the percentages indicated are by weight and that the toxicological properties of these solvents are additive, what is the TLV in mg/m³ of the cleaning solution?

   A. 547 mg/m³
   B. 654 mg/m³
   C. 755 mg/m³
   D. 825 mg/m³

   $$TLV_m = \frac{1}{\left(\frac{f_1}{TLV_1} + \frac{f_2}{TLV_2} + \cdots + \frac{f_n}{TLV_n}\right)}$$

10. A compound made up of 35% naphtha, 5% toluene, and 60% Stoddard solvent is used to clean parts in a tire repair shop. A review of the SDS for each material yields the following information:

    Naphtha = TLV 1370 mg/m³, MW 110, SG 0.66, FP –40 to 86°F, VP 48.
    Toluene = TLV 377 mg/m³, MW 92, SG 0.87, FP 40°F, VP 22.
    Stoddard solvent = TLV 525 mg/m³, MW 144, SG 0.78, FP 102 to 110°F, VP 2.
    The TLV of the mixture is 654 mg/m³. Convert the solution TLV into ppm for each individual component.

    A. Naphtha 22.2 ppm, toluene 33.3 ppm, Stoddard 66.6 ppm
    B. Naphtha 44.4 ppm, toluene 22.2 ppm, Stoddard 66.6 ppm
    C. Naphtha 51 ppm, toluene 8.8 ppm, Stoddard 66.6 ppm
    D. Naphtha 33 ppm, toluene 12 ppm, Stoddard 66 ppm

    $$ppm = \frac{mg/m^3 \times 24.45}{MW}$$

11. If the voltage in a DC circuit is 120 volts and the resistance is 9 ohms, what is the current? E = IR

    A. 0.10 amps
    B. 2 amps
    C. 15 amps
    D. 13 amps

12. Compute the total circuit resistance in this simple series circuit.

    $R_{SERIES} = R_1 + R_2 + \cdots + R_N$

    A. 2.15 ohm
    B. 0 ohm
    C. 20 ohm
    D. 40 ohm

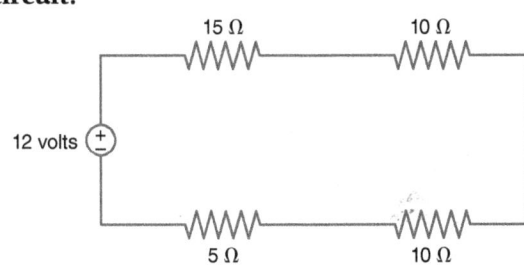

    Figure 5 Simple Series Circuit Example

13. **Compute the total power consumed for this simple parallel circuit.**

$$\frac{1}{R_{PARALLEL}} = \frac{1}{R_1} + \frac{1}{R_2} + \cdots + \frac{1}{R_N} \quad E = IR \quad P = EI$$

   A. 13.8W
   B. 57W
   C. 414W
   D. 571W

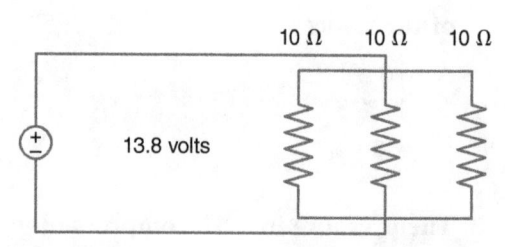

Figure 6 Simple Parallel Circuit Example

14. **What radioactivity would remain from 1 Ci (curie) of Co-60 (5.24 years half-life) after a 20-year period?**

   A. 0.0071
   B. 0.071
   C. 0.71
   D. 7.1

$$A = \frac{A_o}{e^{\left(\ln 2 \frac{t}{T_{1/2}}\right)}}$$

15. **If 0.5 micrograms (µg) of radioactive isotope, $^{131}_{53}I$ is needed at the cancer research facility on January 20 and was created in a lab on January 4, what was the initial amount of the substance? The disintegration constant of $^{131}_{53}I$ is 0.0862 day^{-1}.**

   A. 1.98 µg
   B. 4.28 µg
   C. 3.75 µg
   D. 5.09 µg

$$N = N_o e^{-kt}$$

16. **Ruthenium (Ru) has a half-life of 1 year. How long will it take for a 1600-µCurie source to be reduced to 100 µCurie?**

   A. 1 year
   B. 2 years
   C. 3 years
   D. 4 years

17. **The decay constant for ^{226}Ra is 1.36×10^{-11} Bq per second. What is the half-life?**

   A. 1600 years
   B. 1600 seconds
   C. 5 years
   D. 5.1×10^{11} seconds

$$t_{1/2} = \frac{\ln 2}{k}$$

18. **147 pounds per cubic foot of concrete has a half-value thickness of 2.7 inches for a Cobalt-60 source. How thick does the shielding need to be to reduce an 800-mR source to 200-mR exposure?**

   A. 2.7 inches
   B. 5.4 inches
   C. 10.8 inches
   D. 1.85 inches

19. What radiation reading would result from an unshielded 5-millicurie source of cesium-137 at a distance of one foot, given an MEV of 0.662 and a 0.9 gamma-radiation-per-second disintegration?

   A. 17.8 R/hr/1ft
   B. 0.047 R/hr/1ft
   C. 0.018 R/hr/1ft
   D. 46.8 mR/hr/1ft

   $S \cong 6\ CiEf$

20. Light, radiation, and sound are energy sources that follow the inverse square rule, which states: "The propagation of energy through space is inversely proportional to the square of the distance it must travel." Accordingly, if a radiation source has a reading of 60 at 5 feet, what will the radiation be at 30 feet?

   A. 1.67
   B. 16.7
   C. 0.8
   D. 2.0

   $$I_2 = I_1 \times \frac{(d_1)^2}{(d_2)^2}$$

Domain 1 Quiz 1 Answers

1. Answer: **D**. Convert % to ppm and compare to LEL. From the comparison, the concentration is above both the PEL and the IDLH but equal to the LEL.
   ppm = % × 1,000,000
   ppm = 2.3% × 1,000,000
   ppm = 25,000

   PELs — OSHA Permissible Exposure Limits are time-weighted average (TWA) concentrations that must not be exceeded during any 8-hour work shift of a 40-hour workweek.

   IDLHs — NIOSH definition Immediately Dangerous to Life or Health concentrations represent the maximum concentration from which, in the event of a respirator failure, one could escape within 30 minutes without a respirator and without experiencing any escape-impairing (e.g., severe eye irritation) or irreversible health effects. *[handwritten: inhibit selfrescue]*

   LEL-UEL — Lower Explosive Limit or Lower Flammable Limit. By NFPA definition, lower flammable limit is the minimum concentration of vapor to air below which propagation of a flame will not occur in the presence of an ignition source. The UEL or upper explosive or flammable limit is the maximum vapor-to-air concentration above which propagation of flame will not occur. At or below the UEL means the material can ignite. The area bound by the LEL and the UEL is called the flammability range.

2. Answer: **C**
   Convert to ppm
   0.10 × 0.053 × 1,000,000 = 5300 ppm

3. Answer: **B**
   Step 1 Rebalance the formula using 10 moles of oxygen

   $$2C_2H_2 + 5O_2 \rightarrow 4CO_2 + 2H_2O$$
   becomes
   $$4C_2H_2 + 10O_2 \rightarrow 8CO_2 + 4H_2O$$

   Step 2 Multiply 8 moles × 44 g/mol = 352 g of CO_2.

4. Answer: **A**
The pH scale is logarithmic and is an indicator of the concentration of hydrogen ion dissociation in a solution. The more ionization, the stronger the corrosive.

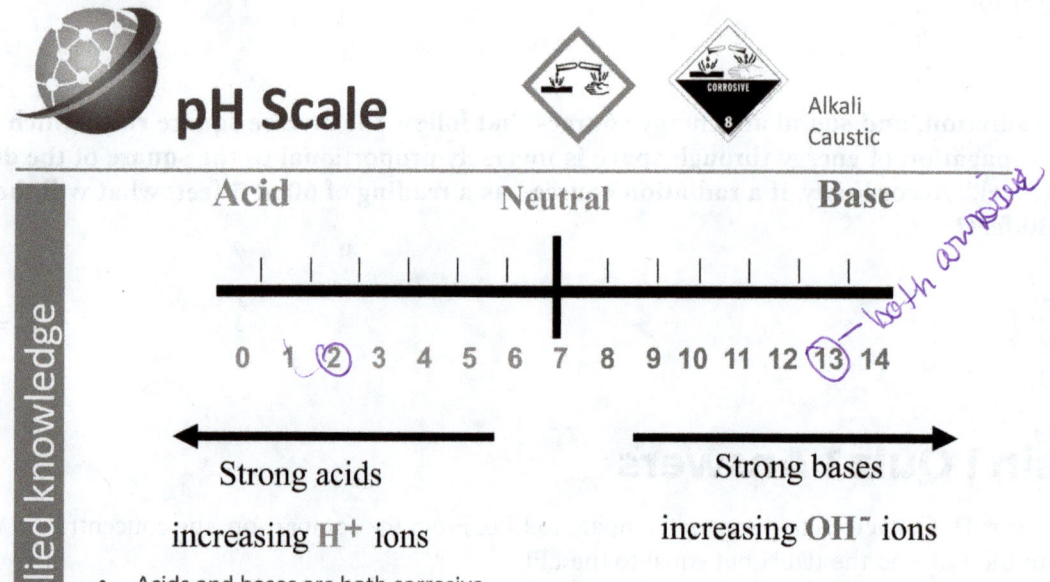

pH Scale

Acid — Neutral — Base

0 1 2 3 4 5 6 7 8 9 10 11 12 13 14

Strong acids — increasing H^+ ions
Strong bases — increasing OH^- ions

Alkali Caustic

- Acids and bases are both corrosive.
- When dissolved in water (the universal solvent) the ions dissociate. The more dissociation the stronger the corrosive.
- Generally corrosives are defined as having a ¼ inch corrosion rate per year on steel.
- Corrosive hazardous wastes are defined by ¼ corrosion rate on steel and a pH of < 2 or >12.5

Figure 7 pH Scale

Strong Acids (highly corrosive)	Weak Acids
Perchloric Acid	Hydrogen Sulfide, H_2S
Sulfuric Acid	Boric Acid
Hydrochloric Acid	Carbonic Acid
Nitric Acid (at high concentrations it is an oxidizer)	Acetic Acid
Phosphoric Acid	Formic Acid

Strong Bases (penetrate skin)	Weak Bases
Sodium Hydroxide (caustic, lye)	Amines
Potassium Hydroxide	(Ammonia NH_3)
Lithium Hydroxide	Ammonium Hydroxide NH_4OH
Strong Bases (neutralize acids, react w/metals, react w/salts)	Pyridine C_5H_5N

Domain 1: Advanced Sciences and Math 35

5. Answer: **B**

   Step 1 Convert lbs to mg.
   $$\frac{1.6 \text{ lbs}}{1} \times \frac{454 \text{ g}}{1 \text{ lb}} \times \frac{1000 \text{ mg}}{1 \text{ g}} = 726,400 \text{ mg}$$

   Step 2 Convert ft³ to m³.
   $$\frac{3000 \text{ ft}^3}{1} \times \frac{1 \text{ m}^3}{(3.28 \text{ ft} \times 3.28 \text{ ft} \times 3.28 \text{ ft})} = 85 \text{ m}^3$$

   Step 3 Apply formula and solve.
   $$\text{ppm} = \frac{\text{mg/m}^3 \times 24.45}{\text{MW}}$$
   $$\text{ppm} = \frac{726,400/85 \times 24.45}{112}$$
   $$\text{ppm} = \frac{8546 \times 24.45}{112} = 1865.6$$

   Alternate Solution

   Step 1 Using the relationship that 1 lb-mole (112 pounds) of commodity will expand to 392 ft³, determine how many ft³ 1.6 pounds will occupy.
   $$\frac{112 \text{ lbs}}{392 \text{ ft}^3} = \frac{1.6 \text{ lbs}}{X \text{ ft}^3}$$
   $$X = \frac{1.6 \times 392}{112} = 5.6 \text{ ft}^3$$

   Step 2 Determine concentration within confined space.
   $$\frac{5.6 \text{ ft}^3}{3000 \text{ ft}^3} = 0.001867$$

   Step 3 Multiply by 1,000,000 to get ppm.
   $$0.001867 \times 1,000,000 = 1867 \text{ ppm}$$

6. Answer: **C**
   $$\text{TWA} = \frac{(C_1 \times T_1) + (C_2 \times T_2) + \cdots + (C_n \times T_n)}{T_1 + T_2 + \cdots + T_n}$$

   $$\text{ppm} = \frac{(C_1 \times T_1) + (C_2 \times T_2) + (C_3 \times T_3) + (C_4 \times T_4)}{T_1 + T_2 + T_3 + T_4}$$

   $$\frac{(210 \times 3) + (195 \times 2) + (0 \times 1) + (60 \times 1) + (300 \times 1)}{3 + 2 + 1 + 1 + 1} = \frac{1380}{8} = 172.5$$

   $3 \times 210 = 630$
   $2 \times 195 = 390$
   $1 \times 0 = 0$
   $1 \times 60 = 60$
   $1 \times 300 = 300$
   $3 + 2 + 1 + 1 + 1 = 8$
   $630 + 390 + 0 + 60 + 300 = 1380$
   $1380 \div 8 = 172.5$

36 ASP Exam Study Workbook

7. Answer: **A**. Normal air contains 21% (20.8%) oxygen by volume. The vessel only contains 76% normal air. Therefore: $0.76 \times 0.21 = 0.1596$ or 16%.

8. Answer **B**. Convert to absolute:
   $T_1 = 65°F + 460 = 525°R$
   $P_1 = 3000$ psig $+ 14.7$ psi (1 Atm pressure) $= 3014.7$ psia
   $T_2 = 110°F + 460 = 570°R$
   $P_2 = ?$

   (1 minute or less)

   $$\frac{P_1 \times V_1}{T_1} = \frac{P_2 \times V_2}{T_2} \qquad \frac{P_1}{T_1} = \frac{P_2}{T_2}$$

   $$\frac{3014.7}{525} = \frac{P_2}{570} \qquad P_2 = \frac{(3014.7 \times 570)}{525} = 3273.1 \text{ psia}$$

   3273.1 psia $- 14.7 = 3258.4$ psig

9. Answer: **B**. When conducting hazard assessments of workplaces using a chemical mixture with similar toxicological properties, it is helpful to calculate the Threshold Limit Value (TLV) of the mixture. This equation for the concentration of gases and vapors describes the method for calculating a TLV for a mixture based on the fractional weights of the individual components and their respective TLVs. The fraction weights must be expressed as a decimal and must be in terms of mass concentration mg/m³.

   TLV_{mix} = Threshold Limit Value of a mixture of chemicals with additive effects (mg/m³)
   $TLV_{1...n}$ = Threshold Limit Value of the contaminant (mg/m³)
   $F_{1...n}$ = weight % of chemical in liquid (unitless decimal)

   $$TLV_{mix} = \frac{1}{\frac{f_1}{TLV_1} + \frac{f_2}{TLV_2} + \cdots + \frac{f_n}{TLV_n}}$$

   $$TLV_{mix} = \frac{1}{\frac{0.35}{1370} + \frac{0.05}{377} + \frac{0.60}{525}}$$

   $$TLV_{mix} = \frac{1}{0.0002555 + 0.0001326 + 0.001143}$$

   $$TLV_{mix} = \frac{1}{0.001531} = 653.2 \text{ mg/m}^3$$

10. Answer: **C**

    Step 1 Determine the fraction of the $TLV_{Solvent}$ for each individual component.
    For naphtha $35\% \times 653.2 = 229$ mg/m³
    For toluene $5\% \times 653.2 = 33$ mg/m³
    For Stoddard $60\% \times 653.2 = 392$ mg/m³

    Step 2 Solve for naphtha.

    $$ppm_{Naphtha} = \frac{mg/m^3 \times 24.45}{MW_{Naphtha}}$$

    $$ppm = \frac{229 \times 24.45}{110} \text{ (molecular weight)}$$

    $$ppm = 51$$

Step 3   Solve for toluene.

$$\text{ppm}_{\text{Toluene}} = \frac{\text{mg/m}^3 \times 24.45}{\text{MW}_{\text{Toluene}}}$$

$$\text{ppm} = \frac{33 \times 24.45}{92}$$

$$\text{ppm} = 8.8$$

Step 4   Solve for Stoddard.

$$\text{ppm}_{\text{Stoddard}} = \frac{\text{mg/m}^3 \times 24.45}{\text{MW}_{\text{Stoddard}}}$$

$$\text{ppm} = \frac{392 \times 24.45}{144} = 66.6$$

11. Answer: **D**

$$E = IR$$

$$I = \frac{E}{R}$$

$$I = \frac{120}{9} = 13.33 \text{ amps}$$

If the energy is 115 volts with a 1.5-amp current, what is the resistance?

$$R = \frac{E}{I}$$

$$R = \frac{115}{1.5} = 76.6 \text{ ohms}$$

12. Answer: **D**. Resistors in a series circuit are added to determine total circuit resistance.
    Total resistance of series components $= 15 + 10 + 10 + 5 = 40 \; \Omega$.

13. Answer: **B**. Select R Parallel formula and solve.

$$\frac{1}{R_{\text{parallel}}} = \frac{1}{R_1} + \frac{1}{R_2} + \cdots + \frac{1}{R_n}$$

$$\frac{1}{R_{\text{parallel}}} = \frac{1}{10} + \frac{1}{10} + \frac{1}{10} = \frac{3}{10}$$

$$\frac{1}{R_{\text{parallel}}} = 0.3$$

$$R_{\text{parallel}} = 3.33 \; \Omega$$

Solve for the current.
Solve for power.
Referencing the formula V = IR, as the total resistance in a circuit increases, the current flowing through the circuit decreases when voltage is held constant.

$E = IR \quad I = \dfrac{E}{R}$

$I = \dfrac{13.8}{3.33} = 4.14$ amps

$P = EI$
$P = 13.8 \times 4.14 = 57.13$ watts

14. Answer: **B**

$$A = \dfrac{A_o}{e^{\left(\ln 2 \dfrac{t}{T_{1/2}}\right)}}$$

$$A = \dfrac{1 \text{ Ci}}{e^{\dfrac{(0.693[20 \text{ yr}])}{5.24 \text{ yr}}}} = \dfrac{1 \text{ Ci}}{e^{2.645}} = \dfrac{1 \text{ Ci}}{14.08} = 0.071 \text{ Ci}$$

A = radioactivity remaining after time t
A_o = radioactivity at a given original time
t = elapsed time
$T_{1/2}$ = half-life of the radionuclide
ln 2 = 0.693 (natural log)

15. Answer: **A**
$N = N_o e^{-kt}$

N = radioactivity remaining after time t = 0.5 µg
N_o = radioactivity at a given original time = ?
t = elapsed time = 16 days
k = disintegration constant = 0.0862
$e^{-kt} = e^{(-0.0862)(16)} = 0.2518$
$0.5 = N_o e^{(-0.0862)(16)}$

$N_o = \dfrac{N}{e^{-kt}}$

$N_o = \dfrac{0.5}{e^{(-0.0862)(16)}}$

$N_o = \dfrac{0.5}{0.2518}$

$N_o = 1.98$ µg

16. Answer: **D**

Strength	Time
1600	now
800	1 year
400	2 years
200	3 years
100	4 years

17. **Answer: A**
    The decay constant for ^{226}Ra is 1.36×10^{-11} Bq per seconds.
    $T_{1/2}$ = half-life of the radionuclide
    ln 2 = 0.693 (natural log of 2)
    k = disintegration constant
    Note: 31,536,000 converts seconds to years (60*60*24*365)

    $$T_{1/2} = \frac{\ln 2}{k}$$

    $$T_{1/2} = \frac{\ln 2}{(1.36 \times 10^{-11} \text{ Bq})\left(\frac{31,536,000 \text{ sec}}{\text{years}}\right)}$$

    $$T_{1/2} = \frac{\ln 2}{(4.2889 \times 10^{-4} /\text{yr})}$$

    $T_{1/2}$ = 1616 years (1600; Answer D is 16,172 yrs)
    On the TI: ln2 / ((1.36 × 10^-11)(31,536,000)) = 1616.14

18. **Answer: B**

Strength	1/2 Value Thickness
800 milliroentgen	0
400 milliroentgen	2.7 inches
200 milliroentgen	5.4 inches

19. **Answer: C**
    S ≅ 6CiEf
    S ≅ 6 × 0.005 × 0.662 × 0.9   *plug and chug*
    S ≅ 0.0018 roentgen/hr/ft

20. **Answer: A**

    $$I_2 = I_1 \times \frac{(d_1)^2}{(d_2)^2}$$

    $$I_2 = 60 \times \frac{(5)^2}{(30)^2}$$

    $$I_2 = 60 \times \frac{25}{900} = 1.67$$

The inverse square law, although found under radiation, can be used for light, radiation, or noise (noise must be in absolute units, not dB). The inverse square formula will work on almost any omni directional energy source. However, it cannot be used for heat calculations.

Domain 1 Quiz 2 Questions

1. A 2000-pound load is lifted with a two-leg sling whose legs are at a 20-degree angle with the load. What is the stress on each leg of the sling?

   A. 588 lbs
   B. 1000 lbs
   C. 2000 lbs
   D. 2925 lbs

2. A 12-foot steel ladder is placed against a building. The base of the ladder is 3 feet from the building. The top of the ladder slips 1 foot down. How far did the bottom of the ladder move?

   A. 2.6 feet
   B. 4.5 feet
   C. 3 feet
   D. 1 foot

3. A small overhead crane is reeved with a block and 10-part line and is being used to lift a load of 20 tons. Discounting the block friction, what is the force required for this pick?

   A. 20 tons
   B. 20,000 pounds
   C. 2 tons
   D. 2000 pounds

4. A load is uniformly distributed over a 10-foot beam that is supported on each end. The load is 40 lbs per foot (400 pounds total weight). What is the moment?

   A. 500 foot-lbs
   B. 1500 foot-lbs
   C. 1800 foot-lbs
   D. 2000 foot-lbs

5. A tank farm is completely diked and contains four fuel storage tanks. Tank 1 is 100 feet in diameter and 35 feet high. Tanks 2 and 3 are 50 feet in diameter and 15 feet high. Tank 4 is 40 feet in diameter and 15 feet high. The area enclosed by the diking is 220 feet by 330 feet. What is the required height for the dike enclosing the tank farm? Assume no slope on dike walls.

   A. 3.9 feet
   B. 4 feet
   C. 4.1 feet
   D. 5.1 feet

6. An exhaust ventilation system in an industrial shop is removing about 3500 cfm from a 10- by 30-foot room with 10-foot ceilings. The shop has no other source of ventilation. What is the air change in this shop?

   A. 2.1 room changes/min
   B. 3.4 room changes/min
   C. 1.16 room changes/min
   D. 11.6 room changes/min

7. It was determined that the air handler that serviced a section of a hospital was not capable of providing an adequate flow of air. To correct this situation, it was decided to change its drive pulley in order to increase its rotational speed from 1450 to 1750 rpm. If its adjusted discharge volume is now 10,500 cfm, what was its discharge volume before the pulley was changed?

   A. 14,500 cfm
   B. 7300 cfm
   C. 8700 cfm
   D. 3280 cfm

   $$\frac{CFM_1}{CFM_2} = \frac{RPM_1}{RPM_2}$$

8. A construction worker is laying stone on an exterior veneer wall. The wet bulb reading is 33°C; the globe temperature 35°C and the dry bulb is 31°C. What is the WBGT in degrees F? Assume outdoor location with solar heat load.

   A. 88°F
   B. 94°F
   C. 102°F
   D. 92°F

   $$t_{°C} = \frac{(t_{°F} - 32)}{1.8}$$
   $$t_{°K} = t_{°C} + 273$$
   $$t_{°R} = t_{°F} + 460$$
   $$WBGT = 0.7\,WB + 0.2\,GT + 0.1\,DB$$

9. Calculate the WBGT index from the following information: indoor globe temperature of 91°F, wet bulb temperature of 87°F.

   A. 112.2°F
   B. 92°F
   C. 88.2°F
   D. 34°C

   $$WBGT = 0.7\,WB + 0.3\,GT$$

10. If the measured noise level of an industrial motor vehicle is 77 dBA at a distance of 60 feet, what is the sound pressure level at 15 feet?

    A. 80
    B. 89
    C. 98
    D. 85

    $$dB_1 = dB_0 + 20\log_{10}\left(\frac{d_0}{d_1}\right)$$

11. An industrial hygienist uses a sound-level meter to determine the noise level in the center of four identical machines. The reading is 79.55 dB. Based upon this reading, determine the sound-level reading of each machine.

    A. 70.3 dB
    B. 72.6 dB
    C. 73.5 dB
    D. 78.0 dB

    $$L_{Pt} = 10\log\left[\sum_{i=1}^{N} 10\left(\frac{L_{Pi}}{10}\right)\right]$$
    $$L_{pt} = L_{pi} + 10\log N$$

12. For a TWA exposure of 97 dBA, what is the allowed exposure time?

    A. 1.5 hours
    B. 6 hours
    C. 3 hours
    D. 5.5 hours

    $$T = \frac{8}{2^{[(L-90)/5]}}$$

PERMISSIBLE NOISE EXPOSURES					
Hrs	dBA	Hrs	dBA	Hrs	dBA
8	90	3	97	1	105
6	92	2	100	0.5	110
4	95	1.5	102	0.25	115

13. Based on the allowable limits in the table, if the noise in a work area was 95 dBA for 3 hours, 90 dBA for 4 hours, and 85 dBA for 1 hour, is the allowable limit exceeded?

    A. No; it is under the limit by > 25%.
    B. Yes; it exceeds the limit by < 50%.
    C. Yes; it exceeds the limit by > 50%.
    D. No; it is under the limit by < 25%.

14. Using the following formula, evaluate the effectiveness of hearing protection provided to an employee who is using an earplug assigned a NRR of 37 combined with muffs (NRR = 21) when exposed to an 8-hour TWA of 115 dBA. Note: When two noise-reduction devices are used, calculate attenuation based on the most effective and add 5 for the second.

    A. Protected TWA = 98.
    B. Protected TWA = 95.
    C. Protected TWA = 85.
    D. Protected TWA = 82.

15. A 25-foot-high, aboveground 10,000-gallon tank filled with 15 feet of water and 5 feet of hydrocarbon with a specific gravity of 0.85 creates _____ total psi at the bottom of the tank.

    A. 8.34 psi
    B. 6.50 psi
    C. 8.66 psi
    D. 10.83 psi

16. Select the list that is in decreasing order of size (largest to smallest).

    A. Deci, milli, nano, pico
    B. Tera, giga, hecto, kilo
    C. Milli, centi, micro, nano
    D. Kilo, deci, milli, peta

17. The evaporation rate of acetone is 0.1 pints per minute. With a safety factor of 5 (this is the K factor), how much dilution ventilation is required to maintain a concentration of 1000 ppm?

    MW = 58.08
    SG = 0.79

    A. 10,963 cfm
    B. 1096 cfm
    C. 5481 cfm
    D. 2741 cfm

    $$Q = \frac{403 \times 10^6 \times SG \times ER \times K}{MW \times C}$$

Domain 1: Advanced Sciences and Math 43

18. Find the velocity pressure in a 1.5-inch (actual diameter) open-ended pipe with 250 gallons per minute of water flowing.

    A. 114 psi
    B. 14 psi
    C. 44 psi
    D. 254 psi

$$P_v = \frac{Q^2}{891d^4}$$

19. Light curtain reaction time plus machine reaction time is 150 ms. The distance from the light curtain to the equipment should be:

    A. 8 inches.
    B. 9.5 inches.
    C. 18.5 inches.
    D. 36 inches.

$$D_s = 63 \text{ inches/second} \times T_s$$

20. You are evaluating a confined space for a specific substance to compare it with the published TLV. You sample the confined space for a period of 7 hours with a flow rate of 1.2 liters per minute. What is your sample volume?

    A. 8.4 L
    B. 73 L
    C. 504 L
    D. 576 L

Domain 1 Quiz 2 Answers

1. Answer: **D**

    $$\sin A = \frac{a}{c}$$

    $$c = \frac{a}{\sin A}$$

    $$c = \frac{1000}{\sin 20} = 2924 \text{ lbs}$$

    a = 1/2 the load = 1000 lbs
    c = stress on the sling
    HINT: Double divided slings are SIN full. Divide the load by the number of sling legs and then divide again by the SIN of the angle. 2000 ÷ 2 ÷ sin 20 = 2924 lbs.

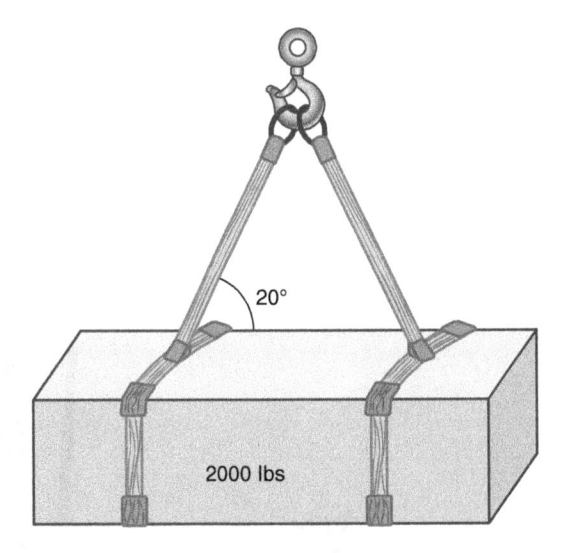

Figure 8 Two Leg Sling Example

2. Answer: **A**. Using the triangle relationship ($a^2 + b^2 = c^2$), you solve for the first situation and find that the ladder is 11.6 feet up on the house. After the ladder slips 1 foot, it is 10.6 feet up on the house and you use the same relationship to solve for the new base.

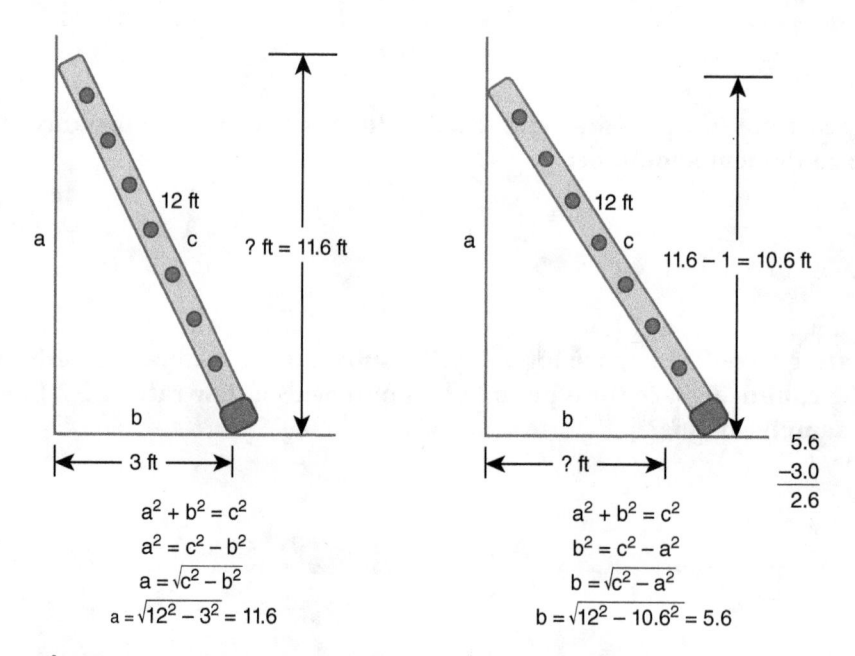

$$a^2 + b^2 = c^2$$
$$a^2 = c^2 - b^2$$
$$a = \sqrt{c^2 - b^2}$$
$$a = \sqrt{12^2 - 3^2} = 11.6$$

$$a^2 + b^2 = c^2$$
$$b^2 = c^2 - a^2$$
$$b = \sqrt{c^2 - a^2}$$
$$b = \sqrt{12^2 - 10.6^2} = 5.6$$

5.6
−3.0
2.6

Figure 9 Ladder Slipping Against Building Schematic

3. Answer: **C**. The ten-part line on the crane referred to in this question provides a mechanical advantage of 10 to 1. 20 tons/10 = 2 tons. Note: 2000 pounds = 1 ton. The term *reeved* refers to the method of routing the wire ropes through the blocks used to develop the mechanical advantage.

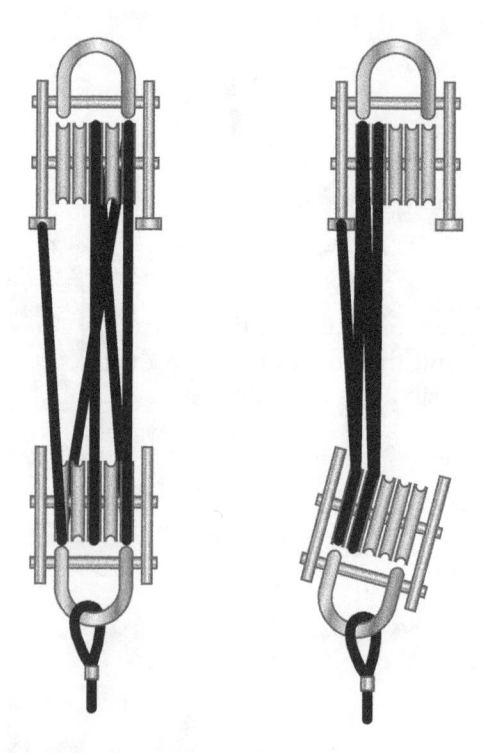

Figure 10 Reeving Methods

4. Answer: **D**. An equally loaded beam represents the same loading as a single load located in the middle of the beam. The moment must be measured from one of the support points.
M = Weight × Distance
M = 400 lbs × 5 ft = 2000 ft-lbs
5. Answer: **C**

   Step 1 Determine the total footage of the diked area.

   $$220 \times 330 = 72{,}600 \text{ sq ft}$$

   Step 2 Determine the footage occupied by tanks 2, 3, and 4.

   Tank #2 and 3

   $$A = \frac{\pi d^2}{4}$$

   $$A = \frac{3.14 \times (50)^2}{4}$$

   A = 1963 sq ft each

   Tank #4

   $$A = \frac{\pi d^2}{4}$$

   $$A = \frac{3.14 \times (40)^2}{4}$$

   A = 1257 sq ft

   TOTAL = 5183 sq ft

   Step 3 Determine the total area not occupied by smaller tanks.

   Total area − Tank area = Area available
   72,600 − 5183 = 67,417

   Step 4 Determine the volume in the largest tank.

   $$V = \frac{\pi d^2 \times h}{4}$$

   $$V = \frac{3.14 \times (100)^2 \times 35}{4}$$

   V = 274,889 cu ft

   Step 5 Divide the volume in the largest tank (cu ft) by total area available (sq ft) to determine the required height of diking.
   $$\frac{274{,}889}{67{,}417} = 4.07 \text{ feet required}$$

   Note: The difference between Answers B and C is about **35,000** gallons of product that would not be contained.

6. Answer: **C**

   Room size = 10 × 10 × 30 = 3000 cubic feet

   $$\frac{3500 \text{ cfm}}{3000 \text{ cf}} = 1.16 \text{ room changes/min}$$

7. Answer: **C**. According to Finucane (2006), this equation relates the Air Discharge Volume being provided by a fan to its Rotational Speed. This is very important whenever one is trying to decide on the relative sizes of the pulleys that will be used (i.e., a pulley on the fan itself, and a second one on the motor that is to serve as the motive force for the fan). This relationship, as well as each of the five that will follow, assumes that the fan being evaluated may well be used under different operating circumstances, but only while handling fluids or gases of the same density.

$$\frac{CFM_1}{CFM_2} = \frac{RPM_1}{RPM_2}$$

CFM_i = the Air Discharge Volume of the fan when it is operating at the set of conditions, in cubic feet per minute [cfm]

RPM_i = the operating Rotational Speed of the fan, in revolutions per minute [rpm]

$RPM_1 = 1450$
$RPM_2 = 1750$
$CFM_2 = 10,500$
$CFM_1 = ?$

$$\frac{CFM_1}{10,500} = \frac{1450}{1750} = \frac{(1450)(10,500)}{1750} = \frac{15,225,000}{1750} = 8700$$

The previous discharge volume of this fan was 8700 cfm.

8. Answer: **D**

$t_{°C} = \frac{(t_{°F} - 32)}{1.8}$

$t_{°C} = t_{°C} + 273$

$t_{°R} = t_{°F} + 460$

WBGT = 0.7 WB + 0.2 GT + 0.1 DB
WBGT = 0.7 × 33°C + 0.2 × 35°C + 0.1 × 31°C
WBGT = 33.2°C
33.2°C = 91.76°F

correct

9. Answer: **C**. Apply indoor formula and solve.

WBGT = 0.7 WB + 0.3 GT
WBGT = (0.7 × 87) + (0.3 × 91)
WBGT = 60.9 + 27.3
WBGT = 88.2°F

Domain 1: Advanced Sciences and Math   47

10. Answer: **B**.
    6-dB Noise Rule:
    If the distance from a noise source is doubled, subtract 6 dB.
    If the distance from a noise source is cut in half, add 6 db.
    As the distance from the source doubles, the noise decreases 6 dB. Since the distance from the source has halved twice, the net change is 12 dB. 77 + 12 = 89 dBA. At 7.5 feet, the level is 89 + 6 = 95 dBA; at 3.75 feet the noise level is 95 + 6 = 101 dBA, and so on.

    $dB_0 = 77$ dB
    $dB_1 = ?$
    $d_0 = 60$ ft
    $d_1 = 15$ ft

    $dB_1 = 77 + 20\log_{10}\left(\dfrac{60}{15}\right)$

    $dB_1 = 77 + 20\log_{10}(4)$

    $dB_1 = 77 + 12.04 = 89$ dB

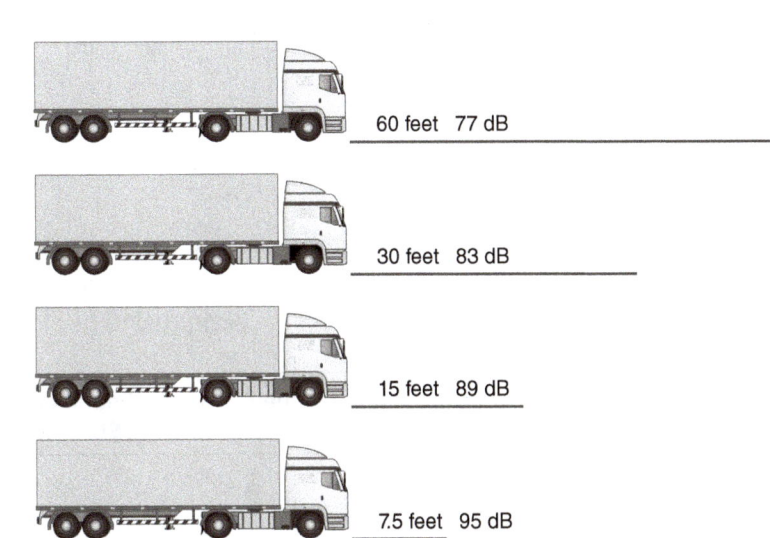

    60 feet   77 dB

    30 feet   83 dB

    15 feet   89 dB

    7.5 feet 95 dB

    Figure 11 Noise Level of Industrial Motor Vehicle

11. Answer: **C**. Decibels are measured using a logarithmic scale, which means decibels cannot be added arithmetically. For example, if two noise sources are each producing 90 dB right next to each other, the combined noise sound level will be 93 dB, as opposed to 180 dB. The following equation should be used to calculate the sum of sound pressure levels, sound intensity levels, or sound power levels:

    $L_{Pt} = 10\log\left[\sum_{i=1}^{N} 10^{\left(\frac{L_{pi}}{10}\right)}\right]$

    $L_{pt} = L_{pi} + 10\log N$

    $L_{pi} = L_{pt} - 10 \times \log 4$

    $L_{pi} = L_{pt} - 6.02$

    $L_{pi} = 79.55 - 6.02$

    $L_{pi} = 73.53$ dB

    L_{Pt} = total sound pressure level generated by N sources (dB)
    L_{Pi} = individual sound level of each source (dB)
    N = number of sound pressure levels
    It is often simplified to the field formula, which will be easier to use in solving this problem.
    $L_{pt} = L_{pi} + 10\log N$

The following table can be used to estimate a sum of various sound levels:

Difference between two levels to be added	Amount to add to higher level to find the sum
0–1 dB	3 dB
2–4 dB	2 dB
5–9 dB	1 dB
10 dB	0 dB

12. Answer: **C**

$$T = \frac{8}{2^{[(L-90)/5]}} = \frac{8}{2^{[(97-90)/5]}} = \frac{8}{2^{[7/5]}} = \frac{8}{2^{1.4}} = \frac{8}{2.639} = 3.03 \text{ hrs}$$

Under OSHA standards, workers are not permitted to be exposed to an 8-hour TWA equal to or greater than 90 dBA. OSHA uses a 5-dBA exchange rate, meaning the noise level doubles with each additional 5 dBA. The following chart shows how long workers are permitted to be exposed to specific noise levels:

Permissible Duration (Hours per Day)	Sound Level (dBA, Slow Response)
16	85
8	90
4	95
2	100
1.5	102
1	105
0.5	110
0.25 or less	115

The values in the chart above are from Table G-16 in the general industry standard, 29 CFR 1910.95.

13. Answer: **B**

$$\frac{C_1}{T_1} + \frac{C_2}{T_2} + \frac{C_3}{T_3} = \text{exposure}$$

$$\frac{3}{4} + \frac{4}{8} = 1.25$$

1.25 is >1 exposure not allowed

14. Answer: **B**

$$A_f = \frac{NRR - 7}{2} + 5$$

$$A_f = \frac{37 - 7}{2} + 5$$

$$A_f = 15 + 5$$

$$A_f = 20$$

Protected TWA = $TWA_8 - A_f$

Protected TWA = 115 − 20

Protected TWA = 95 dBA

When trying to evaluate the impact of high noise levels on the human ear, it is very difficult to determine the effectiveness of hearing protectors. Hearing protectors are evaluated under laboratory conditions specified by ANSI Z24.22 and ANSI S3.19. However, in field conditions, the **Noise Reduction Rating (NRR)** given hearing protectors often is provided a safety factor of 2 or reduced by 50%. This is necessary because field conditions never equal laboratory conditions. Additionally, when two noise reduction devices are properly worn, an additional 5 dB (doubling) of protection is provided. After field attenuation is calculated, it is subtracted from the 8-hour TWA value to obtain the protected TWA (sound level reaching the cochlea). Remember, the exam baseline is the federal OSHA standard of 90 dBA and 85 dBA if the individual has had a threshold shift.

According to the *Fundamentals of Industrial Hygiene*, 6th ed., the most convenient method by which to gauge the adequacy of a hearing protector's attenuation capacity is to check its Noise Reduction Rating (NRR), a rating that was developed by the EPA. According to the EPA regulation, the NRR must be printed on the hearing protector's package. The NRR can be correlated with an individual worker's noise environment to assess the adequacy of the attenuation characteristics of the particular hearing-protective device. Appendix B of 29 CFR 1910.95 describes methods of using the NRR to determine whether a particular hearing-protective device (HPD) provides adequate protection within a given exposure environment. It must be noted, however, that NRRs are based on data obtained under laboratory conditions using trained listeners who are fitted by professionals. Their ratings differ significantly from what is achieved in the real world. In 1998, the National Institute of Safety and Health (NIOSH) published Occupational Noise Exposure, Revised Criteria. Based on studies conducted by numerous researchers of real-world NRRs achieved by 84% of wearers in 20 independent studies, they recommend lowering the manufacturer's NRRs significantly. NIOSH recommended using subject fit data based on ANSI 512.6-1997 to estimate HPD attenuation. If this is not available, they recommend that the labeled NRRs be de-rated as follows:

- Earmuffs: Subtract 25% from the manufacturer's labeled NRR.
- Formable earplugs: Subtract 50% from the manufacturer's NRR.
- All other plugs: Subtract 70% from the manufacturer's NRR (NIOSH, 1998).

Modified from Occupational Noise Exposure, Revised Criteria 1998. DHHS (NIOSH) Publication No. 98-12 https://www.cdc.gov/niosh/docs/98-126/pdfs/98-126.pdf

Noise Reduction Rating (NRR) is a unit of measurement used to determine the effectiveness of hearing-protection devices to decrease sound exposure within a given working environment. The purpose is to calculate the noise attenuation for protecting workers by preventing sensorineural (occupation-induced) hearing loss.

15. Answer: **A**. The weight density of fresh water is 62.4 lbs/ft^3. To convert to inches per foot of rise, divide by 144 (square inches in a foot). 62.4 ÷ (12 × 12) = 0.433 psi/ft of elevation. This equals about 0.433 psi per foot of fresh water with a specific gravity of 1.0.

The five-foot layer of hydrocarbon on the top has a specific gravity of 0.85.

0.433 × 5 × 0.85 = 1.84 psi

The 15-foot layer of fresh water has a specific gravity of 1.0.

0.433 × 15 × 1 = 6.495 psi

Add the two layers to calculate the psi of the column:
6.495 psi water + 1.84 psi hydrocarbon = 8.335 psi
The value of 1 is assigned as the Specific Gravity (SG) of water.

- Liquids with a SG greater than 1 will sink in water.
- Liquids with a SG less than 1 will float in water.

The value of 1 is assigned as the SG of air.

- Vapors with a SG greater than 1 are heavier than air.
- Vapors with a SG less than 1 are lighter than air.

Calculated as the **weight** of a **specific volume** of liquid as compared to an **equal volume** of water:

- Water = 8.34 lb/gal
- Sulfuric acid = 15.33 lb/gal
- SG of H_2SO_4 = $\frac{15.33}{8.34}$ = 1.84

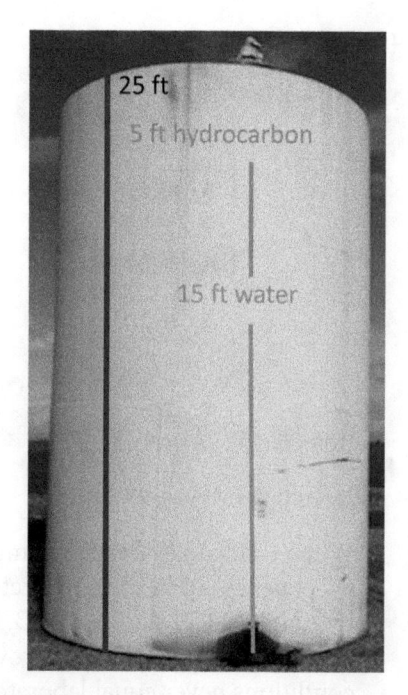

Figure 12 Twenty-five-foot-high above ground 10,000 gallon tank with 15 feet of water, 5 feet of hydrocarbon, and specific gravity of 0.85

16. Answer: **A**
    Unit Conversion Prefixes

Multiplication Factor	Prefix	Symbol
1 000 000 000 000 000 000 = 10^{18}	exa	E
1 000 000 000 000 000 = 10^{15}	peta	P
1 000 000 000 000 = 10^{12}	tera	T
1 000 000 000 = 10^{9}	giga	G
1 000 000 = 10^{6}	mega	M
1 000 = 10^{3}	kilo	k
100 = 10^{2}	hecto	h
10 = 10^{1}	deka	da
1 = 10^{0}		Base
0.1 = 10^{-1}	deci	d
0.01 = 10^{-2}	centi	c
0.001 = 10^{-3}	milli	m
0.000 001 = 10^{-6}	micro	µ
0.000 000 001 = 10^{-9}	nano	n
0.000 000 000 001 = 10^{-12}	pico	p
0.000 000 000 000 001 = 10^{-15}	femto	f
0.000 000 000 000 000 001 = 10^{-18}	atto	a

17. Answer: **D**
    MW = 58.08
    SG = 0.79
    C = 1000 ppm
    ER = 0.1 pints per minute

    $$Q = \frac{403 \times 10^6 \times SG \times ER \times K}{MW \times C}$$

    $$Q = \frac{(403 \times 10^6 \times 0.79 \times 0.1 \times 5)}{(58.08 \times 1000)} = \frac{159{,}185{,}000}{58{,}080} = 2740.8 \text{ cfm}$$

    The K factors are **safety factors** and range from 3 to 10 and depend on:
    1. The toxicity of the material (lower TLV = higher K)
    2. The evolution rate of the contaminant (usually nonuniform)
    3. The effectiveness of ventilation (location in air flows)

    It is anticipated that questions on the professional exams requiring this type of calculation will provide K factors or safety factor; you simply apply the formula. Don't forget the "length of release"; 60 minutes in this problem. The ER must be expressed in pints per minute in the question.

18. Answer: **B**

    $$P_V = \frac{Q^2}{891 d^4}$$

    $$P_V = \frac{250^2}{891 \times 1.5^4}$$

    $$P_V = \frac{62{,}500}{891 \times 5.1}$$

    $$P_V = \frac{62{,}500}{4511} = 13.86 \text{ psi}$$

19. Answer: **B**. The photoelectric (optical) presence-sensing device uses a system of light sources and controls that can interrupt the machine's operating cycle. If the light field is broken, the machine stops and will not cycle. This device must be used only on machines that can be stopped before the worker can reach the danger area. The design and placement of the guard depends upon the time it takes to stop the mechanism and the speed at which the employee's hand can reach across the distance from the guard to the danger zone. The sensing device must be far enough from the danger point to ensure that someone cannot reach into the point of operation faster than the machine can be stopped. OSHA uses the following formula to establish the safe distance, D_s, between sensing point and point of operation.
    (OSHA publication 3067):
    D_s = 63 inches/second × T_s
    D_s is in inches from the point of operation
    63 in/s is an assumed hand speed
    T_s is the stopping time of the machine in seconds

    First, to use the formula, convert 150 milliseconds (ms) to 0.150 seconds.
    D_s = 63 inches/second × 0.150 seconds = 9.45 inches
    Another factor includes the penetration distance (D_{pf}), which is based on the light curtain's MOS (minimum object sensitivity). The following formula is used to compute the minimum safety distance (D_s) on

mechanical power presses to meet the ANSI (American National Standards Institute) B11.1 Press Safety Standard:

$D_s = K \times (T_s + T_c + T_r + T_{bm}) + D_{pf}$

where:

K = Hand speed constant (63 inches/second)
T_s = Stop time of equipment measured at the final control element
T_c = Response time of the control system
T_r = Response time of the presence sensing device and its interface
T_{bm} = Additional time allowed for the brake monitor to compensate for variations in normal stopping time
D_{pf} = The added distance due to the penetration depth factor (MOS).

Note: If the channel-blanking feature is used on light curtains, additional safety distance must be enforced based on the number of channels blanked.

20. Answer: **C**

Time = 7 hours = 420 minutes
Flow rate = 1.2 liters per minute

$$\frac{7 \text{ hours}}{1} \times \frac{60 \text{ minutes}}{1 \text{ hour}} \times \frac{1.2 \text{ liters}}{1 \text{ minute}} = 504 \text{ liters}$$

Domain 1 Quiz 3 Questions

1. A tractor trailer moving with a velocity of 3.02 m/s increases speed at a constant acceleration rate of 2.56 m/s². Determine the time it takes for the tractor trailer to reach a velocity of 28.9 m/s.

   A. 20 seconds
   B. 15 seconds
   C. 25 seconds
   D. 10 seconds

   $t = \frac{v - v_0}{a}$

2. A car is traveling at 70 mph. The operator's reaction time is 0.75 seconds. How far will the car travel during the driver's reaction time?

   A. 48.6 feet
   B. 63 feet
   C. 77 feet
   D. 91.0 feet

3. In a cargo terminal, a cotton bale having a mass of 227 kgm hangs from a device traveling in a straight line. The velocity of the cotton bale increases from 10.0 m/s to 20.0 m/s in 5 seconds. Determine the magnitude of the force acting on the cotton.

   A. 454 N
   B. 325 N
   C. 906 N
   D. 650 N

   $F = ma$

   $a = \frac{v - v_0}{t}$

4. An overhead conveyor system with hanging parts starts from a rest position and moves with a constant acceleration of 0.45 m/s². Determine the velocity of the part at 6 meters from the starting point.

   A. 5.40 m/s
   B. 3.90 m/s
   C. 2.32 m/s
   D. 2.71 m/s

   $v^2 = v_0^2 + 2as$

5. A spacecraft drops an object vertically downward with a velocity of 60 m/s. Assume there is no air resistance and that the acceleration due to gravity is 9.8 m/s². How far will the object fall in 10 seconds?

   A. 650 m
   B. 1090 m
   C. 830 m
   D. 1300 m

$$S = V_0 t + \frac{1}{2} a t^2$$

6. A company has paid $400,000 for workmens compensation over the past ten years. Discounting the value of money and interest, what is the average annual loss?

   A. $20,000
   B. $33,300
   C. $40,000
   D. $50,500

7. In three years, $400,000 will be required for EPA modifications to your plant. How much money should you invest at 10% to have the required amount when needed?

   A. $310,789
   B. $300,526
   C. $287,565
   D. $293,824

$$F = P(1+i)^n \qquad P = F(1+i)^{-n}$$

$$A = P\left(\frac{i(1+i)^n}{(1+i)^n - 1}\right) \qquad P = A\left(\frac{(1+i)^n - 1}{i(1+i)^n}\right)$$

$$F = A\left(\frac{(1+i)^n - 1}{i}\right) \qquad A = F\left(\frac{i}{(1+i)^n - 1}\right)$$

8. Examples of indirect costs of an incident include:

   A. drug testing and ambulance service.
   B. incident review and process delays.
   C. medical treatment and medical treatment supplies.
   D. job accommodations and new equipment.

9. Which of the following correctly evaluates the Boolean expression shown below?

   A. A and not-A or A and B equals A and B.
   B. A plus not-A and A plus B equals A plus B.
   C. A plus A BAR and A plus B equals A plus B.
   D. A or not-A and A or B equals A or B.

$$(A + \overline{A}) \bullet (A + B) = A + B$$

10. A factory has had 30 serious vehicle accidents in the past 10 years, three involving powered industrial trucks. What is the probability that the next serious accident will involve a powered industrial truck (PIT)?

    A. 10%
    B. 8%
    C. 6%
    D. 33%

11. A safety committee is made up of 10 men and two women. What is the probability if making a random selection of two individuals, that both individuals will be female?

    A. 0.045
    B. 0.015
    C. 0.036
    D. 0.005

12. Accident costs and probability for the past year are reflected in the following table. What is the expected value of accident costs?

    A. $6000
    B. $11,500
    C. $9000
    D. $0

Accident Costs	Probability
0	0.1
$5000	0.5
$10,000	0.3
$15,000	0.4

13. A single pump is used to supply hydraulic pressure to a door closer in a regulated biohazard area. The door is closed remotely if an accident should occur. The facility maintenance/engineering staff was concerned about the high probability of failure. The old pump (1×10^{-8}) was replaced with a new dual pump arrangement. With the new dual pump arrangement, either pump can supply enough hydraulic pressure to close the door. Additionally, each pump is a different type and has different probabilities of failure. Pump "A" has a probability of failure of 1×10^{-4} and pump "B" has a failure rate of 1×10^{-3}. Which of the following statements best describes this situation?

    A. Maintenance/engineering should be commended for a good job.
    B. The success of this important safety system has been improved considerably.
    C. The failure rate has increased by a factor of 10.
    D. The failure rate has decreased by a factor of 20.

14. In the following set of numbers, what is the median value?

    8, 8, 10, 12, 13, 15, 19

    A. 12
    B. 8
    C. 12.14
    D. 11

15. The mean plus or minus one standard deviation estimates what percentage of the distribution in a *normal* distribution?

    A. 95.45%
    B. 99.73%
    C. 68%
    D. 50%

16. Given the following numbers, 10, 10, 15, 25, 35, compute the sample standard deviation.

    A. 14.3
    B. 10.8
    C. 16.7
    D. 7.5

    $$S = \sqrt{\frac{\sum (x^2)}{n-1}} \quad (x = X - \bar{X})$$

Domain 1: Advanced Sciences and Math

17. What is the population standard deviation of the following complete set of data points?
    A. 10.36
    B. 12.48
    C. 15.67
    D. 20.25

100 ppm	124 ppm	115 ppm	109 ppm	111 ppm	114 ppm
93 ppm	85 ppm	102 ppm	102 ppm	104 ppm	

18. Exam candidates must pass within one standard deviation of the mean. Given this table of test scores, how many in this sample did not pass the test?
    A. 2
    B. 3
    C. 4
    D. 5

    $$S = \sqrt{\frac{\sum (x^2)}{n-1}} \quad (x = X - \bar{X})$$

100	85	92	73	65	81
62	56	88	87	79	75

19. Which of the following coefficients of correlation best describes the relationships shown in this chart?
    A. +10.90
    B. −0.90
    C. 10.05
    D. −0.05

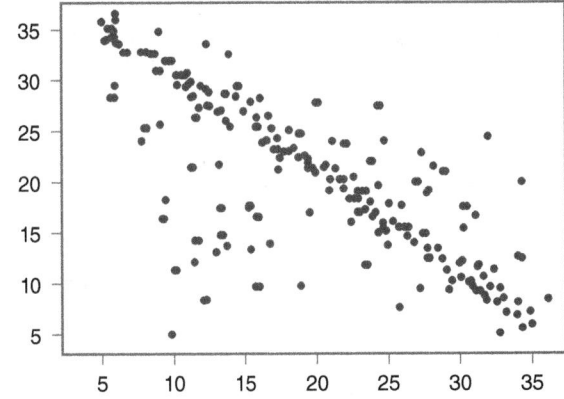

    Figure 13 Scatter Diagram Example

20. A company decides to reflect the worker's compensation losses in terms of profits. The profit margin is 2.5% on each unit sold. What is the gross sales volume needed to offset $90,000 of worker's compensation costs?
    A. $600,000
    B. $3,000,000
    C. $3,600,000
    D. $30,000,000

21. Given the five-year historical data for serious injury and illnesses illustrated in the chart, calculate the lost workday case incident rate for year 4.

Year	Total Serious Injury/Illness Cases	Lost Workdays	Lost Workday Cases	Days Away from Work	Days of Restricted Work Activity	Hours Worked per Year
1	92	1932	67	1565	367	1,398,765
2	88	2002	81	1622	380	1,456,732
3	119	1821	98	1384	137	1,129,565
4	118	1754	90	1316	438	1,623,451
5	122	1234	98	740	494	1,834,225

A. 11.1
B. 21.8
C. 17.4
D. 9.01

22. Given the five-year historical data illustrated in the chart, calculate the combined serious injury and illnesses case incident rate for years three, four, and five.

Year	Total Serious Injury/Illness Cases	Lost Workdays	Lost Workday Cases	Days Away from Work	Days of Restricted Work Activity	Hours Worked per Year
1	92	1932	67	1565	367	1,398,765
2	88	2002	81	1622	380	1,456,732
3	119	1821	98	1384	137	1,129,565
4	118	1754	90	1316	438	1,623,451
5	122	1234	98	740	494	1,834,225

A. 15.7
B. 12.8
C. 21.8
D. 2.76

23. A plant with 1900 full-time employees involved in a straight manufacturing operation has had 22 cases involving lost workdays and 44 cases involving restricted days. The national experience rate for SIC-100 is 6.0. Which of the following statements is correct concerning the rate for this plant?

A. The plant is over the national experience rate.
B. The plant has a rate 1.2 times the national rate.
C. The plant is even with the national rate SIC-100.
D. The plant rate is at 60% of the SIC-100 rate.

24. The average cost of annual injuries that involve two major events is $12,000 each; 10 minor events are at $2500 each. New equipment will cost $56,500 and will eliminate the injuries. Negating the change in value of money over time, in how many months will the new equipment pay for itself?

    A. 12 months
    B. 14 months
    C. 16 months
    D. 11 months

25. Calculate the indirect costs.

    A. $45,000
    B. $33,000
    C. $48,000
    D. $40,000

Increased work comp premiums	$20,000
Incident investigation	$10,000
Medical treatment	$8000
Loss of productivity	$15,000
Therapy	$5000
Cost of hiring	$15,000
Cost of training	$5000

26. Padding the budget is considered a project budgeting method of:

    A. marginalizing.
    B. lowballing.
    C. highballing.
    D. estimating.

Domain 1 Quiz 3 Answers

1. Answer: **D**

   $$t = \frac{v - v_0}{a}$$

   $$t = \frac{28.9 \text{ m/s} - 3.02 \text{ m/s}}{2.56 \text{ m/s}^2}$$

   $$t = \frac{25.88 \text{ m/s}}{2.56 \text{ m/s}^2}$$

   $t = 10.1$ seconds

2. Answer: **C**

   MPH times 1.47 = feet per second
   Distance = Speed × Time

   Use conversion factor of 1.47 :

   $$\frac{1 \text{ mile}}{1 \text{ hour}} \times \frac{5280 \text{ feet}}{1 \text{ mile}} \times \frac{1 \text{ hour}}{60 \text{ min}} \times \frac{1 \text{ min}}{60 \text{ sec}} = 1.47 \text{ fps}$$

   $$70 \text{ mph} \times 1.47 \frac{\text{fps}}{\text{mph}} \times 0.75 \text{ sec} = 77.12 \text{ feet}$$

3. Answer: **A**
The mass of the cotton bail, m, is given as 227 kgm. The initial velocity, v_0, is given as 10.0 m/s. The final velocity, v, is given as 20.0 m/s. The time elapsed, t, is given as 5 seconds.
Step 1 Solve for acceleration.
$$a = \frac{v - v_0}{t}$$
$$a = \frac{20 \text{ m/s} - 10 \text{ m/s}}{5 \text{ s}} = 2 \text{ m/s}^2$$

Step 2 Solve for force.
$$F = ma$$
$$F = (227 \text{ kgm})(2 \text{ m/s}^2) = 454 \text{ N}$$

1-N Force = 1.0 kilogram of mass (kgm) × 1.0 m/s² constant acceleration.

4. Answer: **C**
$$v^2 = v_0^2 + 2as$$
v = Final velocity
v_0 = Initial velocity
s = Distance traveled
a = Acceleration

The initial time, t_0, is 0 second. As the conveyor moves from rest, its initial velocity, v_0, is 0 m/s. The acceleration, a, is constant at 0.45 m/s². The distance, s, is given as 6 m.
$$v^2 = 0 \text{ m/s}^2 + 2(0.45 \text{ m/s}^2)(6 \text{ m})$$
$$v^2 = 0 \text{ m/s}^2 + 5.4 \text{ m}^2/\text{s}^2$$
$$v^2 = 5.4 \text{ m}^2/\text{s}^2$$
$$v = \sqrt{5.4 \text{ m}^2/\text{s}^2}$$
$$v = 2.32 \text{ m/s}$$

5. Answer: **B**
$$s = v_0 t + \frac{1}{2}at^2$$
$$s = (60 \text{ m/s})(10 \text{ s}) + \left(\frac{1}{2}\right)(9.8 \text{ m/s}^2)(10 \text{ s})^2$$
$$s = (600 \text{ m}) + (490 \text{ m})$$
$$s = 1090 \text{ m}$$

6. Answer: **C**
$400,000/10 years = $40,000 per year

Domain 1: Advanced Sciences and Math

7. Answer: **B**

    Future Value

    $i = 0.10 \quad n = 3 \quad F = \$400{,}000 \quad P = ?$

    $P = F(1 + i)^{-n}$ ← *present value*

    $P = 400{,}000 \times (1.1)^{-3}$

    $P = \$300{,}526$

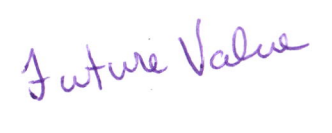

8. Answer: **B**. The term *incident* encompasses first-aid cases, recordable cases, restricted-workday cases, lost-workday cases, permanent disability cases, near misses, and property damage cases. Two basic cost categories are imperative:
    - Direct incident costs represent actual cash outlays attributable to the incident; such outlays would not have been necessary had the incident not occurred.
      Examples of **direct costs** include: Workmens' [ers] compensation; medical treatment; medical treatment supplies; ambulance service; drug testing; job accommodations; and new equipment
    - Indirect incident costs represent costs in terms of time and resources (other than cash) incurred as a result of the incident.
      Examples of **indirect costs** include: Healthcare professional; injured worker; supervisor; return to work; incident review; lost production/productivity; human resources; cost to hire; manager; process delays/interruptions; security; training; and legal *Any thi*

    Thus, total incident costs are the sum of these individual costs.

9. Answer: **D**. When evaluating Boolean logic and applications, the sign + is read "or"; i.e., A + B becomes A or B. The sign "•" is read "and"; thus, A • B is stated A and B. The "A-bar" symbol is read "not-A."

    The expression $(A + \overline{A}) \bullet (A + B) = A + B$ is read:

    A or not-A and A or B equals A or B

    The expression $A \times (B + C) = (A \times B) + (A \times C)$ is also described as a union of one subset with two others that can also be expressed as the union of their intersections.

    Boolean Postulates

A + B = B + A	A + 0 = A
A • B = B • A	A • 1 = A
A(B • C) = (A • B)C	A + A´ = 1
A + (B + C) = (A + B) + C	A • A´ = 0
A(B + C) = (A • B) + (A • C)	A • A = A
A + (B • C) = (A + B) • (A + C)	A + A = A

    Fault tree analysis

Fault tree

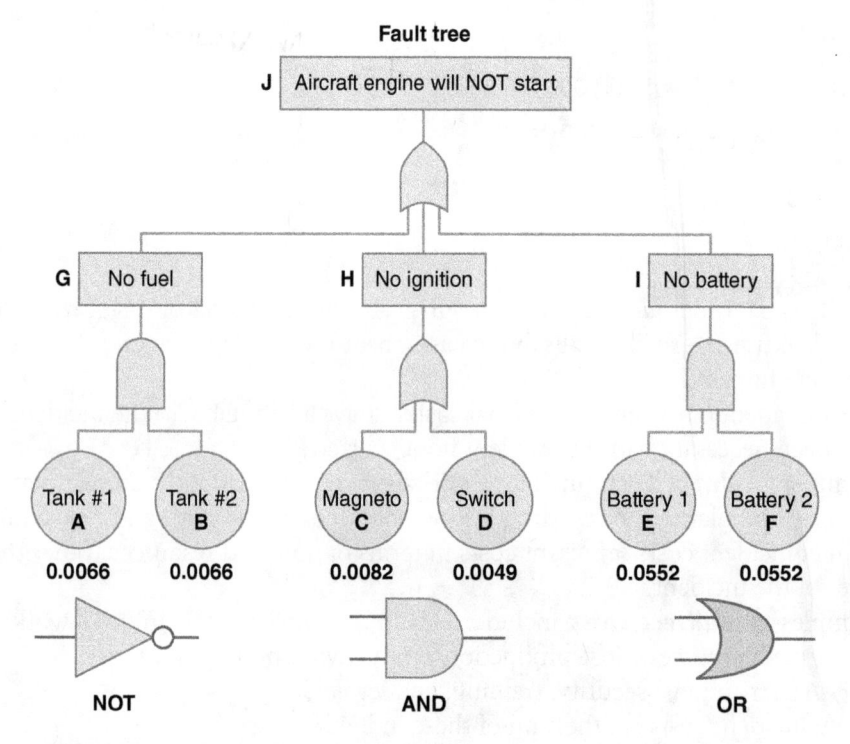

```
J | Aircraft engine will NOT start
```

(OR gate)

- G | No fuel (AND gate)
  - Tank #1 A — 0.0066
  - Tank #2 B — 0.0066
- H | No ignition (OR gate)
  - Magneto C — 0.0082
  - Switch D — 0.0049
- I | No battery (AND gate)
  - Battery 1 E — 0.0552
  - Battery 2 F — 0.0552

Gate symbols: NOT, AND, OR

Figure 14 Fault Tree Analysis Example

How can one qualitatively identify single-point failures on a fault tree? **By locating the OR gates.**

10. Answer: **A**. Probability is the number of fork truck accidents divided by the number of total accidents.

$$P = \frac{3}{30} = 0.1 = 10\%$$

11. Answer: **B**. During the first random selection, there are two chances in 12 of selecting, but in the second selection there is only one chance in 11 in selecting a female.

$$P_{(2\text{Female})} = \frac{2}{12} \times \frac{1}{11} = \frac{2}{132} = \frac{1}{66} = 0.015$$

12. Answer: **B**. The expected value of accident costs is the sum of the costs times the probability of each occurrence.

Accident Cost		Probability		Expected Losses
0	×	0.1	=	$ 0
$5000	×	0.5	=	$ 2500
$10,000	×	0.3	=	$ 3000
$15,000	×	0.4	=	$ 6000
				$11,500

13. Answer: **C**. Since the components are in parallel, the configuration indicates an "AND" gate situation, that is, pump 1 and pump 2 must fail before a hydraulic pump failure occurs. However, the calculation reveals that $(1 \times 10^{-4}) \times (1 \times 10^{-3}) = 1 \times 10^{-7}$, which is 10 times greater than the original pump failure rate. A failure once every 100 million operations is now reduced to a failure for every 10 million operations.

14. Answer: **A**. The median value of a series of numbers is the middle value. The middle or median value is 12 for this set of numbers. The mode is 8, which was selection B. The average value, or the "mean" for the set is 12.14, which was answer C and the range is 11 (19 − 8), which was answer D. The mean is derived by adding up the data points, which is 85, and dividing by the number of data points (7), which equals 12.1429.

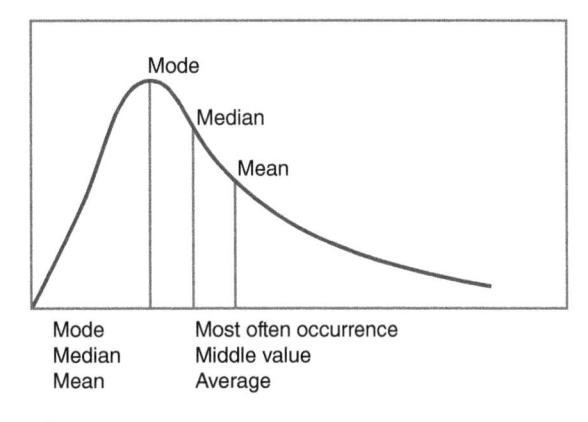

Figure 15 Measurements of Central Tendency

15. Answer: **C** Standard deviation measures the dispersion of the data. The mean plus or minus one standard deviation will estimate the point at which 68% of the observations will fall.

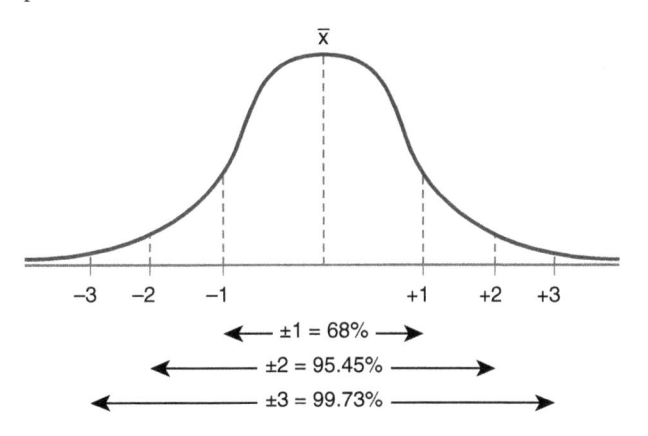

Figure 16 Standard Deviation Definitions

For example, one standard deviation (68%) for 2520 data points = 2520 × 0.68 is 1713.6 data points, which will fall within plus or minus one standard deviation of the mean.

16. Answer: **B**. Build the following table and apply the formula.

TABLE

$\overline{X}$	$\overline{X}$	$X - \overline{X}$	$(X - \overline{X})^2$
10	19	−9	81
10	19	−9	81
15	19	−4	16
25	19	6	36
35	19	16	256
95 = ΣX			$\Sigma(X - \overline{X})^2 = 470$

Formula

$$s = \sqrt{\frac{\Sigma(x^2)}{n-1}} \quad \text{WHERE} \quad (x = X + \overline{X})$$

$$s = \sqrt{\frac{\Sigma(X - \overline{X})}{n-1}} = \sqrt{\frac{470}{5-1}} = 10.839$$

17. Answer: **A**. Build the following table and apply the formula.

TABLE

X	$\overline{X}$	$X - \overline{X}$	$(X - \overline{X})^2$
100	105.4	5.4	29.2
124	105.4	18.6	345.96
115	105.4	9.6	92.16
93	105.4	−12.4	153.76
85	105.4	−20.4	416.16
102	105.4	−3.4	11.56
109	105.4	3.6	12.96
111	105.4	5.6	31.36
114	105.4	8.6	73.96
102	105.4	−3.4	11.56
104	105.4	−1.4	1.96
$\Sigma X = 1159$		$\Sigma(X - \overline{X})^2 = 1181$	

Formula

$$\sigma = \sqrt{\frac{\Sigma(x^2)}{n}} \quad \text{WHERE} \quad (x = X - \overline{X})$$

$$\sigma = \sqrt{\frac{\Sigma(X - \overline{X})^2}{n}} = \sqrt{\frac{1183}{11}} = 10.36$$

18. Answer: **B**
    First calculate the mean = 78.58.
    Calculate the standard deviation = 12.9999.
    Subtract the sample standard deviation (13) from the mean (78.58) to get the minimum passing score out of the set (65.58) and compare to the chart. Three candidates fell below the minimum passing score of 65.58%.

100	85	92
62	56	88
73	65	81
87	79	75

19. Answer: **B**. The statistical term for association between two variables is correlation. The coefficient of correlation is an expression of the correlation as a number between 0 and 1. Thus a perfect coefficient of correlation is 1; on the other hand, 0 represents no correlation. In the scatter diagram shown in this question it is obvious that there is a strong correlation between the Y and X data; however, the correlation is not perfect and there are a number of dots that seem to have no correlation. It is also evident by inspection that the correlation is inverse or negative, that is, with every increase in Y value there is a decrease in X value. The two sets of data are inversely related. The only selection that offers a strong negative correlation is B. If the data had a strong positive correlation, it could be represented by the chart shown here. In that case selection A would be the best choice. Answers C and D show almost no correlation and the scatter diagram depicting that condition would show a very random pattern and would be considered spurious, or unreliable.

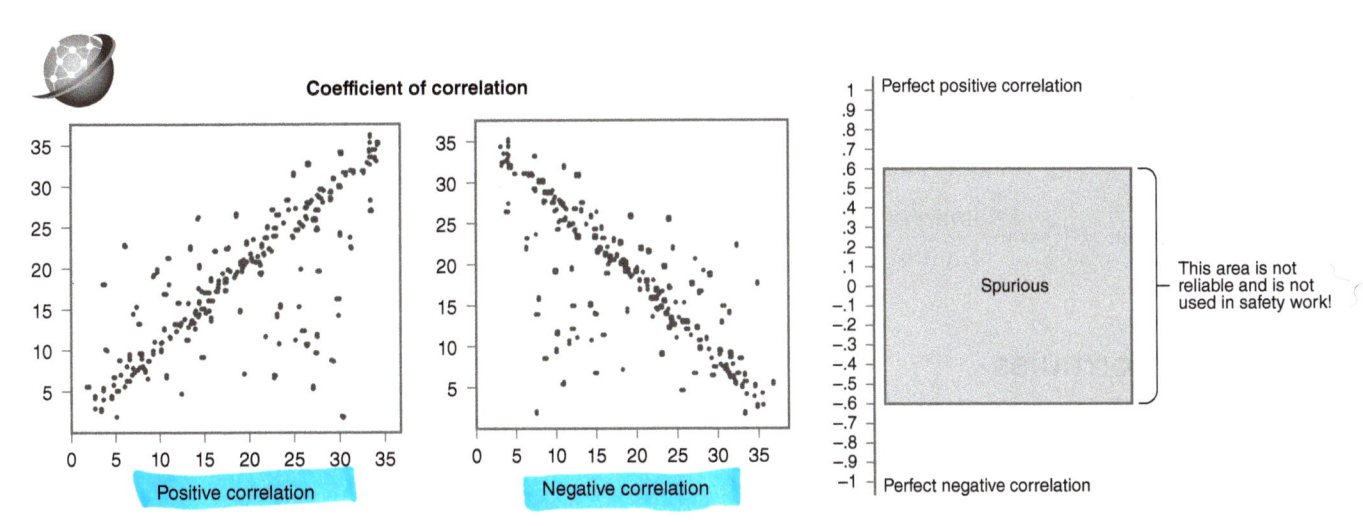

Figure 17 Correlation

Copyright © 2019 by SPAN International Training, LLC

20. Answer: **C**. $3,600,000 in gross sales at 2.5% profit margin is required to offset $90,000 in worker's compensation losses.

    90,000 ÷ 0.025 = 3,600,000

21. Answer: **A**

    $$\text{Rate} = \frac{\text{DART Cases} \times 200,000}{\text{Total hours worked}}$$

    $$\text{Rate} = \frac{90 \times 200,000}{1,623,451}$$

    $$\text{Rate} = \frac{18,000,000}{1,623,451}$$

    Rate = 11.1

The incidence rate for lost-workday cases is the most meaningful performance indicator for a safety program. In the incident rate calculation, 200,000 represents 100 employees, working 50 weeks, 40 hours per week, for 1 year.

Incident rates of various types are used throughout industry. Rates are indications only of past performance (lagging indicators) and are not indications of what will happen in the future performance of the company (leading indicators). Incident rates have been standardized, so that OSHA and other regulatory agencies can compare statistically significant data, and determine where industries may need additional program assistance. OSHA uses the recordable incident rates to determine where different classifications of companies (manufacturing, food processing, textiles, machine shops, etc.) compare to each other with regard to past safety performance. Although OSHA could potentially use this data for enforcement action, unless incident rates are consistently high for a small company over a number of years, OSHA will not normally target particular industries or companies for enforcement action.

OSHA has established specific mathematic calculations that enable any company to report its *recordable incident rates*, *lost time rates*, and *severity rates*, so that they are comparable across any industry or group. The standard base rate for the calculations is based on a rate of 200,000 labor hours. This number (200,000) equates to 100 employees, who work 40 hours per week, and who work 50 weeks per year. Using this standardized base rate, any company can calculate its rate(s) and get a percentage per 100 employees.

Recordable Incident Rate

A mathematical calculation that describes the number of employees per 100 full-time employees that have been involved in a recordable injury or illness.

The OSHA Recordable Incident Rate (or Incident Rate) is calculated by multiplying the number of recordable cases by 200,000, and then dividing that number by the number of labor hours at the company.

$$\text{Incident Rate (IR)} = \frac{\text{Number of OSHA Recordable Cases} \times 200{,}000}{\text{Number of Employee Labor Hours Worked}}$$

Fleet Formulas

$$\text{Fleet Incident Rate} = \frac{\text{\# of Incidents} \times 1{,}000{,}000}{\text{Miles Driven}}$$

$$\text{Fleet Incident Rate} = \frac{\text{\# of Incidents} \times 1{,}600{,}000}{\text{Kilometers Driven}}$$

DART Rate (Days Away/Restricted or Job Transfer Rate)

The DART rate is relatively new to industry. This rate is calculated by adding up the number of incidents that had one or more lost days, one or more restricted days, or that resulted in an employee transferring to a different job within the company, and multiplying that number by 200,000, then dividing that number by the number of employee labor hours at the company.

$$\text{DART Rate} = \frac{\text{\# of DART Incidents} \times 200{,}000}{\text{Total hours worked}}$$

22. Answer: **A**

   Step 1 Total the number of accidents for period in question.

   119
   118
   122
   ___
   359

Step 2 Total the man-hours for the same period.

$$\begin{array}{r}1{,}129{,}565\\1{,}623{,}451\\\underline{1{,}834{,}225}\\4{,}587{,}241\end{array}$$

Step 3 Apply the formula and compute the cumulative accident rate.

$$\text{Rate} = \frac{\text{Total Recordables} \times 200{,}000}{\text{Total hours worked}}$$

$$\text{Rate} = \frac{359 \times 200{,}000}{4{,}587{,}241}$$

$$\text{Rate} = \frac{71{,}800{,}000}{4{,}587{,}241}$$

$$\text{Rate} = 15.7$$

23. **Answer: D**

$$\text{DART Rate} = \frac{\text{Cases} \times 200{,}000}{\text{Total hours worked}}$$

$$\text{DART} = \frac{66 \times 200{,}000}{1{,}900 \times 2{,}000} = \frac{13{,}200{,}000}{3{,}800{,}000} = 3.47$$

$$\frac{3.47}{6.0} = 58\% \text{ of SIC} - 100 \text{ rate}$$

24. **Answer: B**
    $56,500 equipment cost/$49,000 cost of injuries = 1.15 cost/benefit ratio
    1.15(12 months) = 13.8 = 14 months

25. **Answer: A**

Increased work comp premiums	$20,000
Incident investigation	**$10,000**
Medical treatment	$8,000
Loss of productivity	**$15,000**
Therapy	$5,000
Cost of hiring	**$15,000**
Cost of training	**$5,000**
Indirect costs	**$45,000**

26. **Answer: C.** Budgeting:
    - Approaches to estimating
      - Bottom-up—Based on work breakdown
      - Top-down (parametric estimating)—Used when not enough is known about the project to create a work breakdown
    - Highballing (padding)
      - Overestimation of project costs
      - A contingency for unexpected expenditures
      - Projects may not be approved because of higher costs

- Lowballing
  - Underestimating project costs
  - Used to gain approval of questionable projects
  - Often lead to project failures when over budget
- Zero-based budgeting

Instead of assuming each project or manager will receive approximately the budget they had previously, managers and projects are assumed to have no budget until they justify in detail why they should receive any funds at all. According to *The Safety Professionals Handbook* (Haight, 2012), once the decision has been made to pursue a project, the budgeting process should occur. A budget is a financial plan that establishes specific amounts of cash (and sometimes employee hours) that are expected to be spent on specific activities. Decisions about budget allocation should be based on which projects will provide the greatest return on investment to the company. Another dark side of budgeting is that some managers propose excessively large budgets, because the larger the budgets they manage, the more status, power, security, and salary they personally can enjoy.

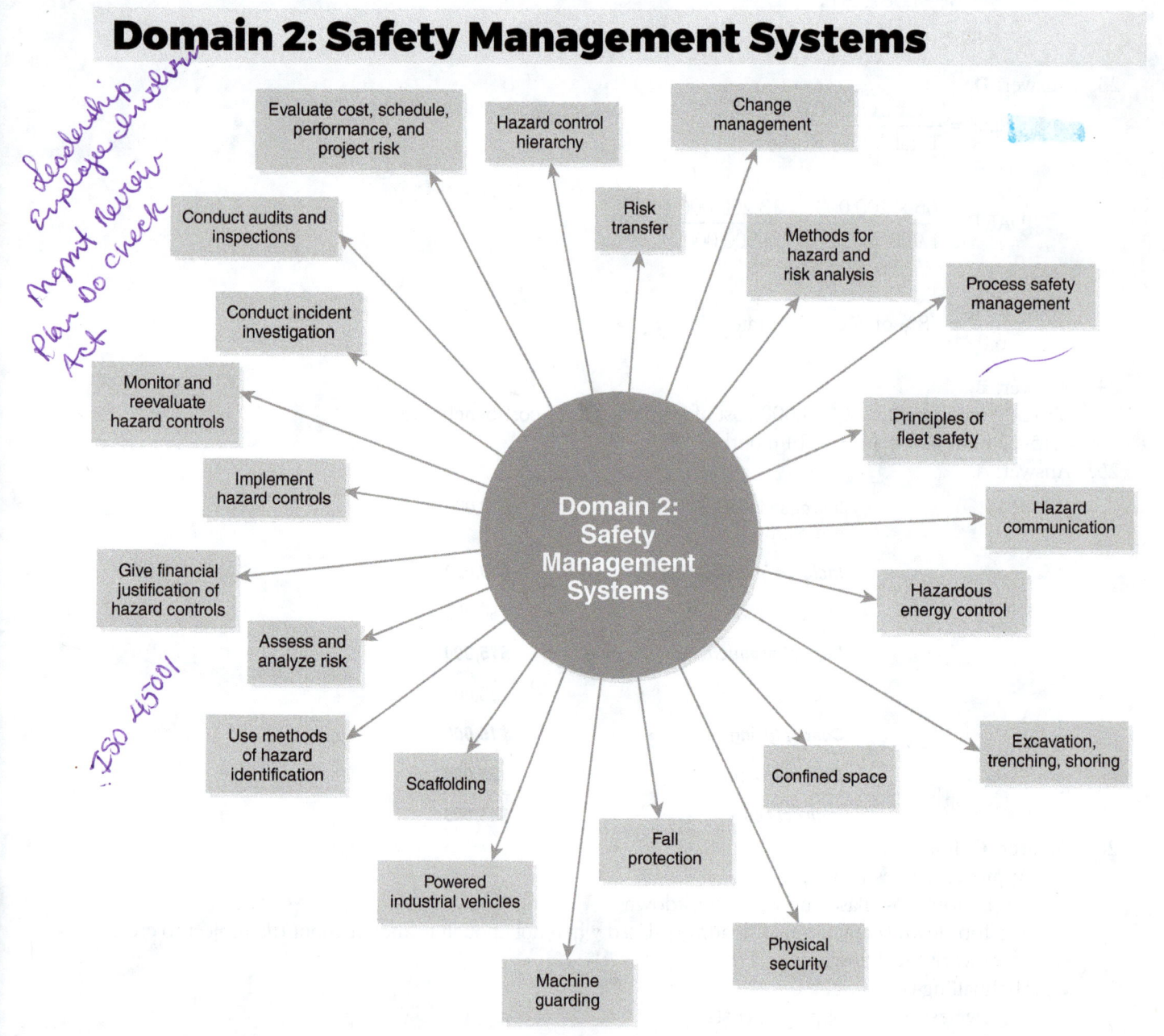

Domain 2: Safety Management Systems

Elements connected to Domain 2: Safety Management Systems:
- Evaluate cost, schedule, performance, and project risk
- Hazard control hierarchy
- Change management
- Conduct audits and inspections
- Risk transfer
- Methods for hazard and risk analysis
- Process safety management
- Conduct incident investigation
- Monitor and reevaluate hazard controls
- Principles of fleet safety
- Implement hazard controls
- Hazard communication
- Give financial justification of hazard controls
- Hazardous energy control
- Assess and analyze risk
- Excavation, trenching, shoring
- Use methods of hazard identification
- Confined space
- Scaffolding
- Fall protection
- Powered industrial vehicles
- Physical security
- Machine guarding

Modified from ASP® Exam Blueprint (ASP10), November 10, 2019

Domain 2 Quiz 1 Questions

1. Which system has as its primary functions to identify hazardous conditions, assess their risk, and establish effective risk control measures?

    A. Risk control
    B. Risk management
    C. Loss control
    D. Loss management

2. When a project has been proposed, it must first go through a preliminary analysis in order to determine whether or not it has a positive net present value using the MARR as the discount rate. The MARR is the target rate for evaluation of the project investment. What is the definition of MARR?

    A. Maximum Attractive Rate of Return
    B. Minimum Attractive Rate of Return
    C. Maximum Alternate Return Rate
    D. Minimum Alternate Return Rate

3. The Z10 is a management system standard compatible and harmonized with quality (ISO 9000 series) and environmental management systems (ISO 14000 series). Which of the following best describes these standards?

    A. Specification standards
    B. Compliance standards
    C. Performance standards
    D. Regulatory standards

4. The first action to be considered in the hierarchy of control is:

    A. training.
    B. elimination of the hazard.
    C. personal protective equipment.
    D. substitution with something less hazardous.

5. Define one type of accident precursor that includes conditions, events, or measures that precede an undesirable event and that have some value in predicting the event arrival, whether it is an accident, incident, near miss, or undesirable safety state.

    A. Leading indicators
    B. Lagging indicators
    C. Loss time frequencies
    D. Workers' compensation losses

6. The risk remaining after preventive measures have been taken is called:

    A. acceptable risk.
    B. tolerable risk.
    C. unacceptable risk.
    D. residual risk.

7. The management term "span of control" refers to:

    A. the breadth of a manager's expertise.
    B. the number of subordinates a manager can supervise.
    C. the number of projects a manager can supervise.
    D. the number of organizations a manager can supervise.

8. Employee motivation or change, a primary behavior model, does not include which of the following?

   A. Specifying objectives and goals
   B. Having the ES&H department write procedures
   C. Giving reinforcement and feedback
   D. Gaining commitment from employees and management

9. Which of the following defines the attributes of employee coaching?

   A. Achievement-oriented, reactive, fault-finding process
   B. Achievement-oriented, proactive, fact-finding process
   C. Achievement-oriented, reactive, fact-finding process
   D. Achievement-oriented, proactive, fault-finding process

10. Management and safety systems built on the principles and processes developed by quality pioneer Edward Deming are known as:

    A. act, do, plan, check.
    B. plan, do, check, act.
    C. plan, act, do, check.
    D. check, plan, do, act.

11. Convincing someone to perform desired behaviors or actions is a part of psychology known as:

    A. attitude.
    B. judgment.
    C. motivation.
    D. discipline.

12. Which of the following is not one of the major provisions of the consensus standard incorporating best practices in OHSMS?

    A. Application of a prescribed hierarchy of controls to achieve acceptable risk levels
    B. Design reviews
    C. Regulatory compliance
    D. Management of change systems

13. What is the most effective method to fix accountability for environmental, safety, and health losses?

    A. Charge the associated cost to each work center.
    B. Compare incident rates with like companies.
    C. Require supervisors to make weekly presentations on their status.
    D. Compare each work center and make an example of the bottom 10%.

14. Measures of a system that are taken after events and assess outcomes and occurrences are called:

    A. leading indicators.
    B. lagging indicators.
    C. measures of behavior.
    D. measures of activities.

15. Safety, environmental, and health performance is best presented to upper management in terms of:

    A. the lost workday incident rate.
    B. total fatalities.
    C. total lost time.
    D. cost relationships.

Domain 2: Safety Management Systems

16. **Risk is a combination of:**
    A. frequency of episodes of an adverse event and probability of occurrence of the adverse event.
    B. probability that an adverse event will occur and consequences of the adverse event.
    C. probability that a hazardous condition exists and consequences of the hazard.
    D. exposure to and consequences of a hazard.

17. **Which question cannot be answered by Pareto charts?**
    A. What are the largest issues facing our team or business?
    B. What 20% of sources are causing 80% of the problems (80/20 rule)?
    C. Where should we focus our efforts to achieve the greatest improvements?
    D. Where are the indirect costs of incidents?

18. **A successful management system, according to OHSAS 18001, should be based on all of the following except:**
    A. a generic occupational health and safety policy.
    B. identification of occupational health and safety risks, along with legal requirements.
    C. objectives, targets, and programs that ensure continual improvements.
    D. management activities that control occupational health and safety risks.

19. **Which of the following best defines a management system audit under ISO 19011?**
    A. A systematic, independent, and documented process for obtaining audit evidence and evaluating it objectively to determine the extent to which the audit criteria are fulfilled
    B. Systematic and independent examination of data, statements, records, operations, and performances (financial or otherwise) of an enterprise for any unstated purpose
    C. Examination of financial statements and formulation of an opinion on the effectiveness of a company's internal control over financial reporting
    D. One that enables organizations to develop their environmental performance through a process of continuous improvement

20. **Auditing is characterized by reliance on many principles. Adherence to these principles is a prerequisite for providing audit conclusions that are relevant and sufficient and for enabling auditors, working independently from one another, to reach similar conclusions in similar circumstances. Which of the following are included in these principles?**
    A. Integrity, confidentiality, due professional care
    B. Confidentiality, conformity, liability
    C. Fair representation, subjective observation, performance in a partial manner
    D. Evidenced based, interdependence, biased

Domain 2 Quiz 1 Answers

1. Answer: **C**.

   Loss control is the proactive measures taken to prevent or reduce **loss** evolving from accident, injury, illness, and property damage. The aim of loss control is to reduce the frequency and severity of losses. Loss control is directly related to human resource management, engineering, and risk management practices.

   Risk is defined as the combination of the severity of a defined exposure with its frequency of occurrence. The technique that effectively decreases a project's schedule risk without increasing the overall risk is to incorporate slack time into the project's critical path schedule early in project planning.

   Hazard: Any real or potential condition that can cause injury, illness, or death to personnel; damage to or loss of a system, equipment, or property; or damage to the environment. It is any potentially unsafe condition resulting from failures, malfunctions, external events, errors, or a combination thereof. It is any condition, set of circumstances, or inherent property damage that can cause injury, illness, or death.

Probability: The likelihood of a hazard causing an incident or exposure that could result in harm or damage for a selected unit of time, events, population, items, or activities being considered

Severity: The extent of harm or damage that could result from a hazard-related incident or exposure

Risk analysis is the process of identifying safety risks. This involves identifying hazards that present mishap risk with an assessment of the risk probability.

Risk assessment is the process of determining the risk presented by the identified hazards. This involves evaluating the identified hazard's causal factors and then characterizing the risk as the product of the hazard severity times the hazard probability.

Processes used to evaluate the level of risk associated with hazards and system issues include:

- Assure management commitment, involvement, and direction (an absolute).
- Select a risk assessment team, including employees with knowledge of jobs and tasks.
- Establish the analysis parameters.
- Select a risk assessment technique.
- Identify the hazards.
- Consider failure modes.
- Assess the severity of consequences.
- Determine the occurrence probability, prominently taking into consideration the exposures.
- Define the initial risk.
- Make risk acceptance or nonacceptance decisions with employee involvement.
- If needed, select and implement hazard avoidance, elimination, reduction, and control measures.
- Address the residual risk.
- Document the results.
- Follow up on the actions taken.

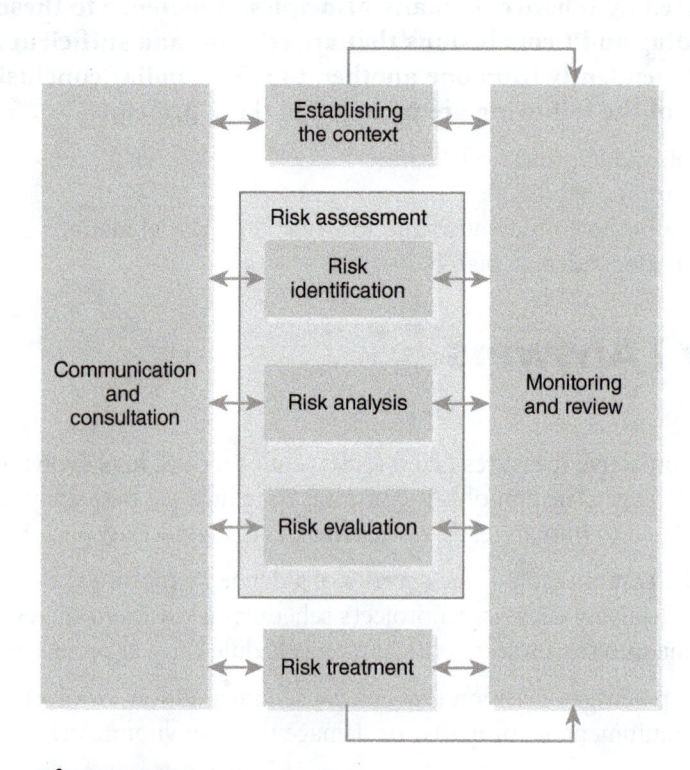

Figure 18 Risk Assessment

Safety is freedom from conditions that can cause death, injury, occupational illness, damage to or loss of equipment or property, or damage to the environment. It is the ability of a system to exclude certain undesired events (i.e., mishaps) during stated operation under stated conditions for a stated time, and the ability of a system or product to operate with a known and accepted level of mishap risk. It is a built-in system characteristic.

Exposure: Contact with or proximity to a hazard, taking into account duration and intensity

Root cause analysis (RCA): The process of identifying the basic lowest level causal factors for an event. Usually the event is an undesired event, such as a hazard or mishap.

Risk communication is the interactive process of exchanging risk information and opinions among stakeholders.

Risk management is the process by which assessed risks are mitigated, minimized, or controlled through engineering, management, or operational means. This involves the optimal allocation of available resources in support of safety, performance, cost, and schedule.

Unacceptable risk: Risk that cannot be tolerated

Acceptable risk: That part of identified mishap risk that is allowed to persist without taking further engineering or management action to eliminate or reduce the risk, based on knowledge and decision-making. The system user is consciously exposed to this risk. It is a risk level achieved after risk reduction measures have been applied, and that is accepted for a given task (hazardous situation) or hazard. For the purpose of this standard, the terms "acceptable risk" and "tolerable risk" are considered synonymous.

Accepted risk: Accepted risk has two parts: (1) risk that is knowingly understood and accepted by the system developer or user and (2) risk that is not known or understood and is accepted by default.

Residual risk: Overall risk remaining after system safety mitigation efforts have been fully implemented. It is, according to MIL-STD-882D, "the remaining mishap risk that exists after all mitigation techniques have been implemented or exhausted, in accordance with the system safety design order of precedence." Residual risk is the sum of all risk after mishap risk management has been applied. This is the total risk passed on to the user.

Mitigation is an action taken to reduce the risk presented by a hazard, by modifying the hazard in order to decrease the mishap probability and/or the mishap severity. Mitigation is generally accomplished through design measures, use of safety devices, warning devices, training, or procedures. It is also referred to as hazard mitigation and risk mitigation.

As low as reasonably practical (ALARP): The level of mishap risk that has been established and is considered as low as reasonably possible and still acceptable. It is based on a set of predefined ALARP conditions and is considered acceptable.

Mishap is an unplanned event or series of events resulting in death, injury, occupational illness, damage to or loss of equipment or property, or damage to the environment.

2. Answer: **B**. This is accomplished by creating a cash flow diagram for the project, and moving all of the transactions on that diagram to the same point, using the MARR as the interest rate. If the resulting value at that point is zero or higher, then the project will move on to the next stage of analysis. Otherwise, it is discarded. The MARR generally increases with increased risk. The **net present worth (NPW)** is the difference between the present worth of all cash inflows and outflows of a project. Since all cash flows are discounted to the present, the NPW method is also known as the **discounted cash flow technique**. This method not only allows the selection of a single project based on the NPW value, but also a selection of the most economical project from a list of alternative projects. To find the NPW of a project, an interest rate is needed to discount future cash flows. The most appropriate value to use for this interest rate is the rate of return that one can obtain from investing the money. Alternatively, it can also be the rate charged if necessary to borrow the money.

The selection of this rate is a policy decision. In engineering economy this interest rate is known as the **minimum attractive rate of return (MARR)**. In business and engineering, the minimum attractive rate of return (MARR), or **hurdle rate,** is the minimum rate of return on a project a manager or company is willing to accept before starting a project, given its risk and opportunity cost of forgoing other projects. A synonymous term seen in many contexts is **minimum acceptable rate of return**. For example, a manager may know that investing in a conservative project, such as a bond investment or another project with no risk, yields a known rate of return. When analyzing a new project, the manager may use the conservative project's rate of return as the MARR. The manager will only implement the new project if its anticipated return exceeds the MARR by at least the new project risk premium.

3. Answer: **C**. The drafters of these standards set out to ensure that it could be easily integrated into any management systems an organization has in place. This flexibility is characteristic of a Performance Oriented Standard. ANSI Z10 adopts from and is in harmony with the International Labor Organization's Guidelines on Occupational Health and Safety Management Systems, ILO-OSH 2001.

Managing safety and health requires planning and setting objectives. According to ANSI Z10 (2012), establishing objectives is fundamental for integrating health and safety into an organization's business plan. The chart below represents the SMART model used to outline key concepts of creating objectives.

Specific	Clearly and operationally define desired outcomes or results by concretely and specifically answering: Who is involved? What do I want to accomplish? Where are you now and where do you want to be? When will it happen? How? Identify requirements and constraints. Why? Specific reasons, purpose, and benefits
Measurable	Establish concrete criteria to measure progress on attaining each objective to help you stay the course, reach target dates, and experience achievement that spurs continued effort required to reach objectives. To determine if an objective is measurable, ask questions such as: How much? How many? How will I know it is accomplished?
Actionable	Create related objectives and actions you can achieve. The objective should be transferable into actionable tasks people can accomplish. Set challenging and purposeful objectives that are realistic.
Realistic	Operationally define objectives in practical and applicable terms, scope of desired performance, and time frames.
Time-oriented	Establish realistic time frames, including start and end dates, deliverables, audit points, and milestones to mobilize stakeholders to achieve objectives.

ANSI/ASSP Z10-2012: American National Standard for Occupational Health and Safety Management Systems

This voluntary consensus standard was published by the American Society of Safety Engineers (ASSP) following American National Standards Institute (ANSI) requirements. It provides management systems requirements and guidelines for improving occupational health and safety. Experts from labor, government, professional organizations, and industry formulated the standard after extensive examination of current national and international standards, guidelines, and practices. For more information: https://www.assp.org/.

OHSAS 18001:2007: Occupational Health and Safety Management Systems Specification—British Standard

This standard specifies requirements for an occupational health and safety management system, to enable an organization to control its risks and improve its performance. The Occupational Health and Safety Assessment Series (OHSAS) Project Group, an international association of government agencies, private industries, and consulting organizations, first published the standard in 1999. Since then, there have been 16,000 certifications to the standard in over 80 countries. The 2007 edition reflects lessons learned from users and increases its compatibility with other international SHMS standards and guidelines. A companion document, OHSAS 18002:2000, serves as a guide to implementing OHSAS 18001. For more information: http://www.bsi-global.com/.

ILO-OSH 2001: International Labor Organization Guidelines on Occupational Safety and Health Management Systems

The International Labor Organization (ILO), a United Nations agency that brings together governments, employers, and workers of its member states, has developed voluntary guidelines on safety and health management systems. The guidelines are designed as an "instrument for the development of a sustainable safety culture within the enterprise and beyond." The key elements of the guidelines are built on the concept of continuous improvement. For more information: http://www.ilo.org/.

OSHA's Voluntary Protection Program (VPP)

The OSHA VPP recognizes and partners with businesses and worksites that demonstrate excellence in occupational safety and health. To qualify for one of the VPPs, applicants must have in place an effective SHMS that meets rigorous performance-based criteria. OSHA verifies qualifications through a comprehensive on-site review process. Using one set of flexible, performance-based criteria, the VPP process emphasizes management accountability for worker safety and health; continual identification and elimination of hazards; and active involvement of employees in their own protection. For more information: http://www.osha.gov/.

The major elements of an effective management system include:

- **Management Leadership**
    - Establish clear safety and health goals for the program and define the actions needed to achieve those goals.
    - Designate one or more individuals with overall responsibility for implementing and maintaining the program.
    - Provide sufficient resources to ensure effective program implementation.
- **Worker Participation**
    - Consult with workers in developing and implementing the program and involve them in updating and evaluating the program.
    - Include workers in workplace inspections and incident investigations.
    - Encourage workers to report concerns, such as hazards, injuries, illnesses, and near misses.
    - Protect the rights of workers who participate in the program.
- **Hazard Identification and Assessment**
    - Identify, assess, and document workplace hazards by soliciting input from workers, inspecting the workplace, and reviewing available information on hazards.
    - Investigate injuries and illnesses to identify hazards that may have caused them.
    - Inform workers of the hazards in the workplace.

4. Answer: **B**. Risks are reduced to an acceptable level through the application of the hierarchy of controls. A hierarchy of controls provides a systematic way of thinking, considering steps in a ranked and sequential order, to choose the most effective means of eliminating or reducing hazards and their associated risks. Acknowledging the premise that risk reduction measures should be considered and taken in a prescribed order represents an important step in the evolution of the practice of safety. These methods are to be applied when new facilities, equipment, and processes are acquired; when existing facilities, equipment, and processes are altered; and when incidents are investigated. In applying a hierarchy of

controls, the desired outcome of actions taken is to achieve an acceptable risk level. Acceptable risk is that risk for which the probability of a hazards-related incident or exposure occurring and the severity of harm or damage that could result are as low as reasonably practicable and tolerable in the situation being considered. That definition requires several factors to be taken into consideration:
- Avoiding, eliminating, or reducing the probability of a hazards-related incident or exposure occurring
- Reducing the severity of harm or damage that may result if an incident or exposure occurs
- The feasibility and effectiveness of risk-reduction measures to be taken, and their costs, in relation to the amount of risk reduction to be achieved
- Six levels of action
- Decision makers should understand that with respect to the six levels of action shown in the following hierarchy of controls, the methods described in the first, second, and third action levels are more effective because they:
    - Are preventive actions that eliminate/reduce risk by design, substitution, and engineering measures
    - Rely the least on the performance of personnel
    - Are less defeatable by supervisors or workers
- Actions described in the fourth, fifth, and sixth levels are contingent actions and rely greatly on the performance of personnel for their effectiveness.

The following are prioritized from most effective to least effective (adapted from ANSI Z10-2012).

CONTROLS	EXAMPLES
Elimination	Design to eliminate hazards: falls, HAZMAT, confined spaces, materials handling, tools and machinery, etc.
Substitution	Substitute for less hazardous materials and equipment, reduce energy, etc.
Engineering Controls	Incorporate safety through design, such as of ventilation systems, enclosures, guarding, interlocks, lift tables, conveyors, etc.
Warnings	Strategically place signs, alarms, enunciators, labels, etc.
Administrative Controls	Implement standard operating procedures (SOPs) such as conduct JSAs, job rotation, inspections, training, mentoring, etc.
Personal Protective Equipment	PPE assessments may result in the use of safety glasses, goggles, face shields, fall protection, protective footwear, gloves, respirators, chemical suits, etc.

Modified from ANSI-Z10.2012

5. Answer: **A**. This defines leading indicators, associated with proactive activities that identify hazards and assess, eliminate, minimize, and control risk. A leading indicator can help predict safety performance. Corrective actions that have been resolved from incident reports are a predictive (leading) measure of safety performance.

6. Answer: **D**. In ANSI Z10, risk is defined as an estimate of the combination of the likelihood of an occurrence of a hazardous event or exposure(s), and the severity of injury or illness that may be caused by the event or exposure(s). According to ANSI/ASSP/ISO Guide 73 (Z690.1-2011), Vocabulary for Risk Management, risk is simply the effect of uncertainty on objectives. Risk tolerance is an organization's readiness to bear the risk after risk treatment in order to achieve its objectives. Risk acceptance is an informed decision to take a particular risk. Acceptable risk is a residual risk level achieved after risk reduction measures have been applied. It is a risk level that is accepted for a given task (hazardous situation) or hazard. The terms "acceptable risk" and "tolerable risk" are considered synonymous. Residual risk is defined as the risk remaining after preventive measures have been taken. No matter how effective the preventive actions, residual risk will always be present if a facility or operation continues to exist.

7. Answer: **B**. The well-known principle of "span of control" is defined as recognizing that a manager cannot effectively supervise more than a half dozen subordinate managers.

8. Answer: **B**. The Organization Behavior Model (OBM) approach to employee motivation or change includes specifying objectives and goals, giving reinforcement and feedback, and gaining commitment from employees and management.
    Goals are frequently incorrectly developed, which makes them likely to fail. They must be attainable, and employees must believe they are relevant and worthwhile.
9. Answer: **B**. A behavior-based approach treats safety as an achievement-oriented process, not outcome based. It also uses fact-finding versus fault-finding and is proactive, not reactive.
10. Answer: **B**. Both quality and EHS management systems are built on the well-known **Plan-Do-Check-Act** process. Briefly stated, the purpose of standards is to provide organizations with an effective tool for continuous improvement in their occupational health and safety management systems to reduce risk of occupational injuries, illnesses, and fatalities.

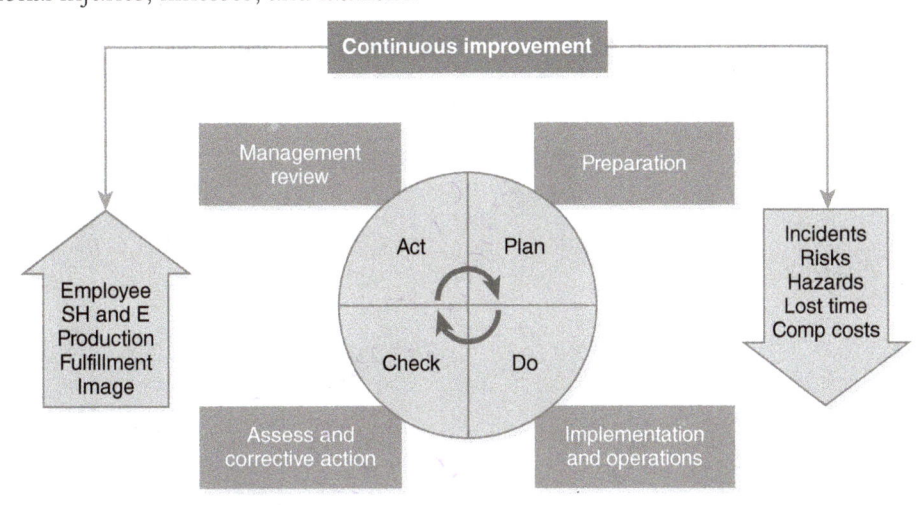

Figure 19 Plan-Do-Check-Act Process

11. Answer: **C**. According to Dr. Roger Brauer (2006), this is the definition of motivation. This includes such areas as overcoming personal deficiencies and increasing safety awareness.
12. Answer: **C**. The ANSI/ASSP Z10 (2012), Occupational Health and Safety Management Systems (OHSMS) consensus standard is applicable to organizations of all sizes. The standard provides safety professionals and senior management with a well-conceived, state-of-the-art concept and action outline to improve safety and health management systems. In crafting Z10, the intent was not only to achieve significant safety and health benefits through its application, but also to favorably impact productivity, financial performance, quality, and other business goals. There is no provision specifically dedicated to regulatory compliance. The key provisions pertain to risk assessment and prioritization, applying a prescribed hierarchy of controls to achieve acceptable levels of risk by designing reviews, managing change systems, having safety specifications in procurement systems, and conducting safety audits.
13. Answer: **A**. According to Dr. Roger Brauer (2006), "Making safety part of a supervisor's appraisal is one means of achieving in an organization. Companies that use cost accounting to encourage safety have the lower accident rates."
14. Answer: **B**. Lagging indicators measure outcomes, which includes the history and overall performance. It is untrue that lagging indicators are poor measures of safety performance, but they are poor predictive measures of safety performance.
15. Answer: **D**. Most experts agree that depicting the bottom-line cost will have the greatest impact on upper-level management. This may be done by comparing losses to budgets or future estimated cost impacts and how they will impact unit costs. **Cost/benefit analysis** is a generic process of evaluating competing courses of action by examining the dollar costs of certain abatement actions versus the dollar value of the benefits received.
    Cost/benefit analysis allows management to understand and prioritize actions to reduce risk of identified financial loss scenarios.

16. Answer: **B**. Risk is defined as the probability that a substance or situation will produce harm under specified conditions. Risk is a combination of two factors: (1) the probability that an adverse event will occur and (2) the consequences of the adverse event (**Table 4**). Risk encompasses impacts on public health and the environment, and arises from exposure and hazard. Risk does not exist if exposure to a harmful substance or situation does not or will not occur. Hazard is determined by whether a particular substance or situation has the potential to cause harmful effects (**Table 5**). Risk is the probability of a specific outcome, generally adverse, given a particular set of conditions (ANSI Z10-2012).

Table 4 Example Risk Assessment Matrix

Likelihood of Occurrence or Exposure	Severity and Consequences			
	NEGLIGIBLE: First aid or minor medical treatment	**MARGINAL:** Minor injury, lost workday	**CRITICAL:** Disability in excess of 3 months	**CATASTROPHIC:** Death or permanent total disability
FREQUENT: Likely to occur repeatedly	MEDIUM	SERIOUS	HIGH	HIGH
PROBABLE: Likely to occur several times	MEDIUM	SERIOUS	HIGH	HIGH
OCCASIONAL: Likely to occur sometime	LOW	MEDIUM	SERIOUS	HIGH
REMOTE: Not likely to occur	LOW	MEDIUM	MEDIUM	SERIOUS
IMPROBABLE: Very unlikely to occur	LOW	LOW	LOW	MEDIUM

Risk Level:
LOW: Risk acceptable or tolerable; remedial action discretionary
MEDIUM: Take remedial action at an appropriate time.
SERIOUS: High-priority remedial action
HIGH: Operation not permissible
These definitions are provided for illustrative purposes and each organization must define these terms as applicable to its own process.

Table 5 Example Prioritizing Scoring Method

Action Item	Frequency (Scale 1–5) 1 = HIGH % SAFE (LESS THAN ONCE A WEEK) 5 = LOW % SAFE (DAILY)	Severity (Scale 1–4) 1 = LEAST (UNLIKELY TO RESULT IN INJURY) 4 = MOST (POTENTIAL FOR FATALITY)	Overall Rating (FREQUENCY) × (SEVERITY) = PRIORITY RATING
Use of Tools	4	4	16
Hearing Protection	3	2	6

17. Answer: **D**. A Pareto chart is used to graphically summarize and display the relative importance of differences between groups of data. The left-side vertical axis of the Pareto chart is labeled Frequency (the number of counts for each category), the right-side vertical axis is the cumulative percentage, and the horizontal axis is labeled with group names of response variables. The number of data points that reside

Domain 2: Safety Management Systems 77

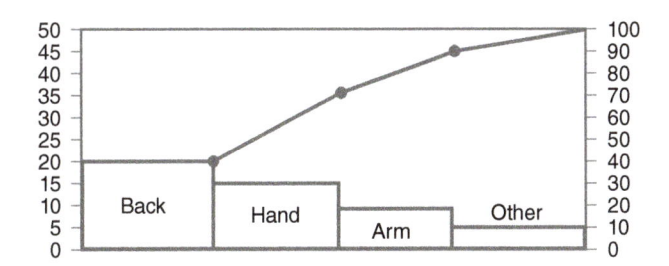

Figure 20 Pareto Chart Example

within each group is determined to construct the Pareto chart. But unlike the bar chart, the Pareto chart is ordered in descending frequency magnitude. Groups are defined by the user.

The Pareto chart answers the following questions:
- What are the largest issues facing our team or business?
- What 20% of sources are causing 80% of the problems (80/20 rule)?
- Where efforts should be focused to achieve the greatest improvements?

To construct a Pareto diagram, the category that accounted for the greatest percentage of cases is placed to the left of the diagram and remaining categories are arranged in descending order of overall percentage of injuries. A line is constructed that indicates the cumulative number of injuries. In this chart, back and hand injuries account for 70%, while back, hand, and arm injuries account for 90%.

18. Answer: **A.** OHSAS 18001 is an *Occupational Health and Safety Assessment Series* for health and safety management systems. It is intended to help an organization control occupational health and safety risks. It was developed in response to widespread demand for a recognized standard against which to be certified and assessed. OHSAS 18001 will measure management systems with regards to several dimensions. The extent of application will depend on such factors as the organization's occupational health and safety policy, the nature of its activities, and the conditions under which it operates.

    A successful management system should be based on these factors:
    - An occupational health and safety policy is appropriate for the company.
    - Identification of occupational health and safety risks is documented, along with legal requirements.
    - Objectives, targets, and programs ensure continual improvements.
    - Management activities control occupational health and safety risks.
    - Monitoring of occupational health and safety system performance is constant.
    - Continual reviews, evaluation, and system improvement are conducted.

19. Answer: **A.** ISO 19011 defines a management system audit as follows:
    "Systematic, independent and documented process for obtaining audit evidence and evaluating it objectively to determine the extent to which the audit criteria are fulfilled" (ISO 19011:2011 3.1).
    Selection B is incorrect, as audits must be for a stated purpose.
    Selection C is the definition of an integrated audit.
    U.S. audits of publicly traded companies are governed by rules laid down by the Public Company Accounting Oversight Board (PCAOB), which was established by Section 404 of the Sarbanes–Oxley Act of 2002. Such an audit is called an integrated audit (**Table 6**), where auditors, in addition to an opinion on the financial statements, must also express an opinion on the effectiveness of a company's internal control over financial reporting, in accordance with PCAOB Auditing Standard No. 5.
    Selection D identifies an **environmental management system**, which enables organizations to develop their environmental performance through a process of continuous improvement.
    ISO 19011 is designed to provide recommendations for **Quality and Environmental Management Systems audits**.
    Audit: A systematic, independent, and documented process for obtaining information and data (audit evidence) and evaluating it objectively to determine the extent to which defined audit criteria are fulfilled.
    Internal audits, sometimes called first-party audits, are conducted by the organization itself, or on its behalf, for management review and other internal purposes (e.g., to confirm the effectiveness of the

management system or to obtain information for the improvement of the management system). Internal audits can form the basis for an organization's self-declaration of conformity. In many cases, particularly in small organizations, independence can be demonstrated by the freedom from responsibility for the activity being audited or freedom from bias and conflict of interest.

External audits include second- and third-party audits. Second-party audits are conducted by parties having an interest in the organization, such as customers, or by other persons on their behalf. Third-party audits are conducted by independent auditing organizations, such as regulators or those providing certification.

A combined audit is when two or more management systems of different disciplines (e.g., quality, environmental, occupational health and safety) are audited together.

A joint audit is when two or more auditing organizations cooperate to audit a single auditee.

Table 6 Document Request for Auditing

Compliance and Management System Auditing	Management System Auditing
Organization chart identifying the names and titles of key personnel	Vision/mission statements and strategic plan
Identification of departments and operating groups with a description of the operations conducted	Environmental manual with ISO 14001 policies and management-level procedures that address the core elements of the EMS
General site-specific information describing number of employees, square feet of building space, location	Current EMS standard operating procedures (SOPs) or work instructions for environmental requirements
Site plot plan showing buildings and setup of processes inside the buildings	Sustainability program and list of long-term sustainability objectives
Environmental policy	Listing of environmental aspects and impacts
Comprehensive list of buildings	Environmental performance metrics and identification of the environmental performance data that is currently collected
Process descriptions and flow charts for those with the greatest environmental risk	Listing of set environmental objectives and targets and the environmental management programs developed to achieve environmental objectives
Lists of raw materials, products, by-products, and waste streams	
Listing of environmental permits	
Listing of environmental plans and best management practices	
Training matrix showing environmental training required for job positions	
Most recent internal and/or external environmental audit reports	

Compliance: Meeting the requirements of local, state, or federal statutes, standards, or regulations

Conformance: Meeting the requirements of the organization's Occupational Health and Safety Management System

Hazard: A condition, set of circumstances, or inherent property that can cause injury, illness, or death

Hazard identification: Process of recognizing that a hazard exists and defining its characteristics

Domain 2: Safety Management Systems

Risk: An estimate of the combination of the likelihood of an occurrence of a hazardous event or exposure(s) and the severity of injury or illness that may be caused by the event of exposures

Acceptable Risk: A risk that has been reduced to a level that can be tolerated by the organization with regard to its legal obligations and its own policy

Risk Assessment: Process(es) used to evaluate the level of risk associated with hazards and system issues. Considering the adequacy of any existing controls and deciding whether or not the risk is acceptable.

Exposure Assessment: The process of measuring or estimating the exposure profiles of workers, including the relevant characteristics of the exposures such as the duration and intensity

Occupational Health Assessment: The collection, analysis, recording, and reporting of biological and other data to identify, evaluate, and track potential or actual health effects that are associated with being in the work environment

Incident: An event in which a work-related injury or illness (regardless of severity) or fatality occurred or could have occurred. This includes close calls and near misses.

Prevention Action: Action taken to reduce the likelihood that an underlying system deficiency or hazard will occur or recur on another similar process. Action taken to fix a potential problem.

Record: A document showing or stating results achieved or providing information or data on activities performed

Validation: The determination that the requirements for a product are sufficiently correct and complete

Verification: Evaluation of an implementation to determine that the applicable requirements are met

20. Answer: **A**. The guidance given in Clauses 5 to 7 of ISO 19011 is based on the six principles outlined below.

Integrity: The foundation of professionalism

Auditors and the person managing an audit program should:
- Perform their work with honesty, diligence, and responsibility
- Observe and comply with any applicable legal requirements
- Demonstrate their competence while performing their work
- Perform their work in an impartial manner (i.e., remain fair and unbiased in all their dealings)
- Be sensitive to any influences that may be exerted on their judgment while carrying out an audit

Fair Presentation: The obligation to report truthfully and accurately. Audit findings, audit conclusions, and audit reports should reflect truthfully and accurately the audit activities. Significant obstacles encountered during the audit and unresolved diverging opinions between the audit team and the auditee should be reported. The communication should be truthful, accurate, objective, timely, clear, and complete.

Due Professional Care: The application of diligence and judgment in auditing. Auditors should exercise due care in accordance with the importance of the task they perform, and the confidence placed in them by the audit client and other interested parties. An important factor in carrying out their work with due professional care is having the ability to make reasoned judgments in all audit situations.

Confidentiality: Security of information. Auditors should exercise discretion in the use and protection of information acquired in the course of their duties. Audit information should not be used inappropriately for personal gain by the auditor or the audit client, or in a manner detrimental to the legitimate interests of the auditee. This concept includes the proper handling of sensitive or confidential information.

Independence: The basis for the impartiality of the audit and objectivity of the audit conclusions. Auditors should be independent of the activity being audited wherever practicable, and should in all cases act in a manner that is free from bias and conflict of interest. For internal audits, auditors should be independent from the operating managers of the function being audited. Auditors should maintain objectivity throughout the audit process to ensure that the audit findings and conclusions are based only on the audit evidence. For small organizations, it may not be possible for internal auditors to be fully independent of the activity being audited, but every effort should be made to remove bias and encourage objectivity.

Evidence-Based Approach: The rational method for reaching reliable and reproducible audit conclusions in a systematic audit process. Audit evidence should be verifiable. It will in general be based on samples of the information available, since an audit is conducted during a finite period of time and with finite resources. An appropriate use of sampling should be applied, since this is closely related to the confidence that can be placed in the audit.

Reproduced from Guidelines for auditing management systems, ISO 19011, © ISO 2011

Domain 2 Quiz 2 Questions

1. When attempting to change safety-related workplace behaviors, the following are all basic steps in the process except:

    A. Identify critical behaviors
    B. Establish a behavior-based safety program
    C. Conduct measurement through observation
    D. Give performance feedback

2. The audit objectives define what is to be accomplished by the individual audit and may include which of the following?

    A. Evaluation of the ineffective monitoring of audit program outcomes
    B. Determination of the extent of nonconformity of activities, processes, and products with the requirements and procedures of the management system
    C. Conformity with audit program procedures
    D. Determination of the extent of conformity of the management system to be audited, or parts of it, with audit criteria

3. Guides and observers (e.g., regulators or other interested parties) may accompany the audit team. Which of the following best describes the roles of these parties?

    A. Guides are appointed by the auditor.
    B. Observers can assist the auditors with suggestions.
    C. Guides ensure that rules concerning location safety and security procedures are known to audit team members.
    D. Observers cannot be denied from taking part in audit activities.

4. Under which category do the following activities belong? A major construction project management team implemented a series of toolbox safety meetings held at the beginning of each shift; housekeeping initiatives; barricade performance for elevated areas; and management walk-through audits to demonstrate leadership and commitment.

    A. Union organizing inhibitors
    B. Leading indicators
    C. Lagging indicators
    D. Cost indicators

5. Regarding collecting and verifying information, all of the following statements are correct except:

    A. Information relevant to the audit objectives, scope, and criteria should be collected by appropriate sampling.
    B. Only verifiable information should be accepted as audit evidence.
    C. Audit findings do not need to be recorded.
    D. The audit team should address any new circumstances that may occur.

Domain 2: Safety Management Systems

6. Which of the following defines a system safety technique that selects an undesired event whose possibility or probability is to be determined and then reviews system requirements, functions, and designs to determine how the top or initial event could occur?

    A. Fault tree analysis
    B. Boolean algebra
    C. Preliminary Hazard Analysis (PHA)
    D. Failure Mode and Effect Analysis (FMEA)

7. To construct an eye in a one-half-inch wire rope, how many clips are required?

    A. 3 clips with U-bolts on live end
    B. 4 clips with U-bolts on live end
    C. 3 clips with U-bolts on dead end
    D. 4 clips with U-bolts on dead end

8. The most correct statement concerning the Failure Mode Effects and Criticality Analysis (FMECA) is:

    A. FMECA is an extension of FMEA.
    B. FMECA is a tool of the nuclear industry.
    C. FMECA is a quality tool, not a system safety tool.
    D. FMECA is reliability, not hazard, based.

9. The best protection when dealing with hoisting and rigging equipment includes having:

    A. chains, slings, and ropes inspected before each job.
    B. hoisting and lifting equipment inspected daily.
    C. a thorough inspection every 18 months of all chains in use.
    D. the use of wire rope bird caged for lifting, if provided with Crosby clamps every six inches.

10. The ISO standard that covers environmental management is:

    A. 9000.
    B. 10,000.
    C. 12,000.
    D. 14,000.

11. What is the design that attempts to ensure that a failure will leave the product unaffected or will convert it to a state in which no injury or damage will occur?

    A. Fail-safe
    B. Fail-secure
    C. Fail-operations
    D. Fail-proof

12. A conveyor belt that runs parallel to a walkway has smooth rods rotating beneath the belt and rods sticking out 3/4 inch past the belt edge. What is the best action to protect workers from this potential hazard?

    A. Do nothing, because 3/4 inch isn't enough for concern.
    B. Place caps over the ends of each rod.
    C. Paint rod ends yellow to warn of possible hazard.
    D. Attach a guard the full length of the conveyor belt that covers rod ends.

13. Which of the following is considered a direct cost when defining hidden costs of an accident?

    A. Time lost from work by injured workers
    B. Time lost by fellow workers
    C. Payment and benefits for lost time
    D. Loss of production

82   ASP Exam Study Workbook

14. What type of manager utilizes an external reward and punishment system to affect performance?
    A. Theory X
    B. Theory Y
    C. MBO
    D. TQM

15. According to Frederick Herzberg's work, which of the following factors is a hygiene factor, as opposed to a motivational factor?
    A. Money
    B. Recognition
    C. Responsibility
    D. Achievement

16. Which of the following factors does not affect how individuals behave pertaining to workplace safety?
    A. Attitudes toward safety
    B. Views regarding team effort
    C. Recognition for personal efforts
    D. Moral standards

17. Which of these terms refers to someone identified with a group or category with oversimplified attributes associated with that person/group?
    A. Selective perception
    B. Stereotype
    C. Halo effect
    D. Projection

18. A company's health and safety management program's audit reveals that the program has failed to accomplish the stated objective of accident prevention. Accident rates are very high, but morale and discipline are low. Varying standards exist throughout the company and supervisors openly defy management authority. What is the best explanation for the safety program management failure?
    A. The safety director neglects to establish an effective program.
    B. Top management fails to support the accident prevention effort.
    C. Management at all levels fails to manage, lead, and direct the workforce.
    D. Procedures to identify correct and safe methods for job accomplishment are ignored.

19. In order to select a system from among three potential safety design candidates, a Safety and Health consultant must recognize that system failure will result in a loss, regardless of choice. An elementary design for each system showing probability of failure is shown below using standard "fault tree" symbols. Which system has the lowest overall failure probability?

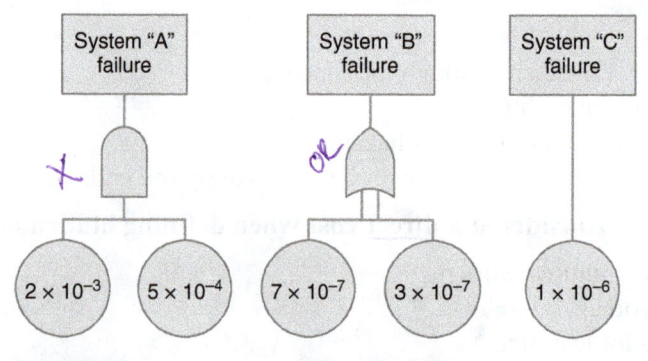

System "A" failure — AND gate — 2×10^{-3}, 5×10^{-4}

System "B" failure — OR gate — 7×10^{-7}, 3×10^{-7}

System "C" failure — 1×10^{-6}

Figure 21 Fault Tree Analysis Example 2

A. System A has lower probability, and offers redundancy.
B. System B has lower probability, but has two potential single-point failures.
C. System C is the simplest and has lowest probability.
D. The probability is the same for all three systems.

20. What is a warning sign's primary purpose?
A. Information for supervisor
B. Information for employees
C. Employees' hazard recognition and comprehension
D. Company protection from OSHA citations and lawsuits

Domain 2 Quiz 2 Answers

1. Answer: **B**. According to the NSC (2015), the three basic steps of the behavior-based safety process are:
   - **Identify Critical Behaviors:** Employers write, in observable terms, what employees should do to properly perform their jobs. The safety and health professional can list a few critical behaviors or a complete inventory, depending on the scope and results desired.
   - **Conduct Measurement through Observations:** Trained observers watch the workplace to determine if listed behaviors are performed safely or unsafely. The total number of observed behaviors is divided into the number of safe behaviors to obtain a percentage figure for safe behaviors.
   - **Give Performance Feedback:** The percentage figure for safe behaviors is shown on a graph displayed in the workplace. At regular intervals, behaviors are again observed and new safe behavior figures are added to the graph. Studies show this critical feedback will improve safety behaviors. Praise and recognition from managers or peer pressure can be effective ways to encourage and reinforce safe behaviors.

   Once data is collected, the data analysis includes:
   - Closing the improvement loop
   - Identifying and correcting equipment and design barriers
   - Establishing procedures and solutions instead of temporary corrections

2. Answer: **D**. Each individual audit should be based on documented audit objectives, scope, and criteria. These should be defined by the person managing the audit program and be consistent with the overall audit program objectives. The audit objectives define what is to be accomplished by the individual audit and may include the following:
   - Determination of the extent of conformity of the management system to be audited, or parts of it, with audit criteria
   - Determination of the extent of conformity of activities, processes, and products with the requirements and procedures of the management system
   - Evaluation of the capability of the management system to ensure compliance with legal and contractual requirements and other requirements to which the organization is committed
   - Evaluation of the effectiveness of the management system in meeting its specified objectives
   - Identification of areas for potential improvement of the management system

   The audit scope should be consistent with the audit program and audit objectives. It includes such factors as physical locations, organizational units, and activities and processes to be audited, as well as the time period covered by the audit.

   The audit criteria are used as a reference against which conformity is determined and may include applicable policies, procedures, standards, legal requirements, management system requirements, contractual requirements, sector codes of conduct, or other planned arrangements.

3. Answer: **C**. They should not influence or interfere with the conduct of the audit. If this cannot be assured, the audit team leader should have the right to deny observers from taking part in certain audit activities. For observers, any obligations in relation to health and safety, security, and confidentiality should be managed between the audit client and the auditee.

    Guides, appointed by the auditee, should assist the audit team and act on the request of the audit team leader. Their responsibilities should include the following:
    - Assisting the auditors in identifying individuals to participate in interviews and confirming timings
    - Arranging access to specific locations of the auditee
    - Ensuring that rules concerning location safety and security procedures are known and respected by the audit team members and observers

    The role of the guide may also include the following:
    - Witnessing the audit on behalf of the auditee
    - Providing clarification or assisting in collecting information

4. Answer: **B**. According to authors Marlowe and Skrabak (2007), the selection of leading indicators is largely judgmental and only time will tell whether the indicators selected are the right ones. It seems logical to suggest that the leading indicators selected should relate directly to opportunities to reduce risk by improving those safety management processes that analysis indicates need improvement, on a prioritized basis. In safety-related literature, the most commonly identified lagging indicators are accidents and cost trends, and sometimes near misses. Toolbox safety meetings held at the beginning of each shift; housekeeping; barricade performance for elevated areas; and management walking around to show leadership and commitment are generally considered examples of leading indicators.

5. Answer: **C**. During the audit, information relevant to the audit objectives, scope, and criteria, including information relating to interfaces between functions, activities, and processes, should be collected by means of appropriate sampling and should be verified. Only information that is verifiable should be accepted as audit evidence. Audit evidence leading to audit findings should be recorded. If, during the collection of evidence, the audit team becomes aware of any new or changed circumstances or risks, the team should address them accordingly.

    NOTE 1: Guidance on sampling is given in Clause B.3 of ISO 19011.

6. Answer: **A**. This is a description of fault tree analysis, which uses deductive analysis involving reasoning from the general to the specific. Most other safety analyses use inductive reasoning and progress from a specific item to the general overall failure.

7. Answer: **C**. Three clips are required, and the U-bolt or U-clip always goes on the dead end. The most common method of making a loop or eye in a wire rope involves the use of cable or "Crosby" clips. The Crosby clip consists of a U-bolt and saddle and if used correctly produces an excellent connection. However, even one loose or incorrectly applied clip reduces the efficiency of the connection by as much as 50%.

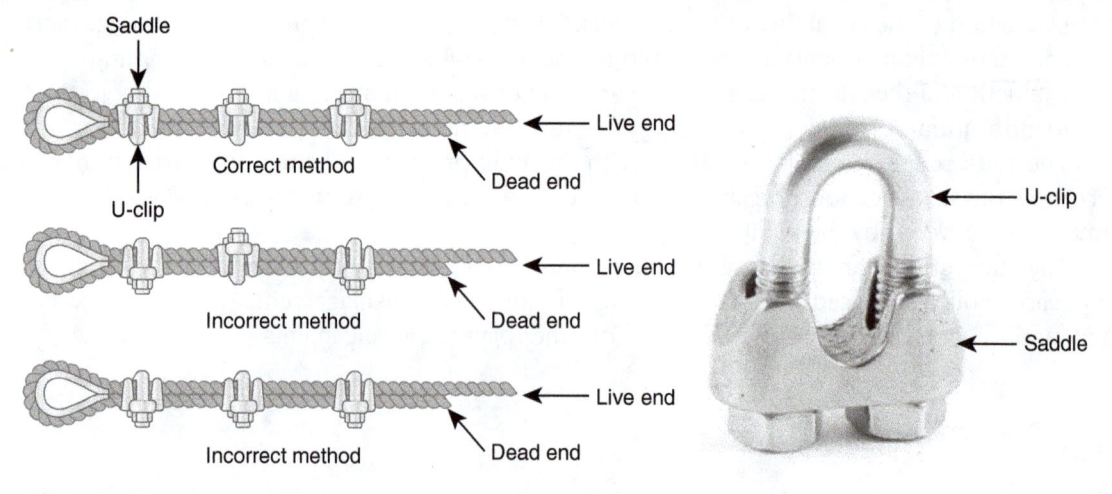

Figure 22 3 Clips with U-bolts on dead end

The U-bolt should always be installed bearing on the dead end of the rope with the saddle bearing on the long or live end of the rope. This is because the U-bolt, when tightened, dents and damages the wire rope. All clips should be installed in the same manner. Additionally, the ridges or corrugation in the saddles must match the lay of the rope (i.e., right lay or left lay). Otherwise the live end of the rope will also be damaged, resulting in broken and cut strands. The number of clips required usually ranges from 3 to 7, depending on material and size of wire rope. One reference is OSHA 1926.251. Hint: Never saddle a *DEAD* horse.

8. Answer: **A**. The Failure Mode and Effects Analysis (FMEA) is generally considered to be a reliability-based analysis. The process provides an exhaustive search for component failure that will affect system operations. The search may uncover failures that will cause hazards or damage, but its main objective is to determine the system reliability. The method can be enlarged to include the "criticality," or critical ranking of components' results in the Failure Mode and Effects Criticality Analysis (FMECA). The FMECA searches for parts or components that will contribute to the system failure and ranks them by their probability to cause a hazard or ability to affect the system safety. The nuclear industry discourages use of the term "FMECA" in favor of "FMEA" because of the nuclear-specific use of the term "criticality," which refers to the amount of radioactive material necessary to sustain a chain reaction (critical mass).

9. Answer: **A**. Inspection of hoisting and rigging equipment before each job provides the greatest protection from use of defective equipment. Selection B is a good practice, but is not as protective as choice A. The frequency on selection C should be dependent on use; however, in no case more than 12 months. Selection D is incorrect; birdcaged wire rope should be removed from service.

10. Answer: **D**. The ISO 9000 ("quality management") and ISO 14000 ("environmental management") families are among ISO's most widely known standards ever. ISO 9000 has become an international reference for quality requirements in business-to-business dealings, and ISO 14000 seems set to achieve at least as much, if not more, in helping organizations meet their environmental challenges. There are similarities between environmental, health, and safety programs and quality assurance programs. They serve common underlying objectives, share common success and failure measures, and use common approaches to achieve objectives.

    The ISO 9000/9001 family addresses "quality management." This means what the organization does to fulfill:
    - Customers' quality requirements
    - Applicable regulatory requirements, while aiming to enhance customer satisfaction
    - Continual improvement of its performance in pursuit of these objectives

    The ISO 14000 family addresses "environmental management," meaning what the organization does to minimize harmful effects on the environment caused by its activities, and to achieve continual improvement of its environmental performance.

11. Answer: **A**. According to Willie Hammer, *Product Safety Management and Engineering*, there are three fail-safe designs:
    - Fail-passive arrangements reduce the system to its lowest energy level.
    - Fail-active design maintains an energized condition that keeps the system in a safe mode until a corrective or overriding action occurs or an alternate system is activated.
    - Fail-operational arrangements allow functions to continue safely until corrective action is possible.

    An example of a fail-active device would be a battery-operated smoke detector that chirps when it is time to replace the battery.

12. Answer: **D**. Answers A and C do not provide sufficient protection from the hazard. Answer B is a possible solution, but not enough information is given as to the size/coverage of the caps and whether they are spinning or not. Answer D may be overkill, but is the best choice available.

13. Answer: **C**. The direct costs are medical and compensation. The indirect or hidden costs are time lost from work by the injured, loss in earning power, economic loss to the injured family, time lost by fellow workers, loss of efficiency due to break-up of crew, lost time by supervision, cost of breaking in a new worker, damage to tools and equipment, time damaged equipment is out of service, spoiled work, loss of production, spoilage, failure to fill orders, overhead costs, and miscellaneous.
14. Answer: **A**. *Theory X* (according to Douglas McGregor's theory) holds that people must be motivated to work by external reward and punishment because they are unmotivated toward work. A *Theory Y* manager assumes all workers are basically interested and motivated to work and therefore have a reduced need for an external reward system. Management by Objectives (*MBO*) is a process of joint objective setting between a superior and a subordinate. It is also known as Management by Results. The managers meet the following performance objectives:
    - Target a key result to be accomplished
    - Identify a date for achieving results
    - Offer a realistic (measurable) and attainable challenge
    - Be as specific and quantitative as possible

    A TQM manager functions and directs operations with an organization-wide commitment to continuous work improvement, product quality, and totally meeting customer needs, by applying them to all operational aspects. Under TQM an employee's initiative to work safely is achieved by instilling a commitment to quality teamwork and continual improvement. These managers include the line manager, who is responsible for activities making direct contributions to the production of the organization's product; the staff manager, who has special technical expertise to advise and support the line manager; and function managers, who are responsible for a support area such as finance, marketing, personnel, etc. Safety professionals can have line authority if they work under the plant manager in an operational extension (extended) capacity.
15. Answer: **A**. Frederick Herzberg in his book *Work and the Nature of Man* develops a motivation-hygiene theory. The theory attempts to explain how persons are satisfied by certain intrinsic job factors while being motivated by other extrinsic factors that are quite peripheral to the job being performed.

Table 7

Satisfaction is influenced by:	Motivation is influenced by:
Money	Achievement
Status	Recognition
Relationships with boss	Enjoyment of work
Company policies	Possibility of promotion
Work rules	Responsibility
Working conditions	Chance for growth

As is shown in the **Table 7**, money is a hygiene or satisfaction factor, as opposed to a motivation factor.

16. Answer: **D**. The safety culture is a group's attitude that everyone in the group will try to behave in a way that protects the safety of each other. Recognition will reinforce their trust in the culture.

    An important factor in developing a safety program is to incorporate concepts of job enrichment, participation, and employee-centered leadership. Management will most likely support a proactive safety effort when prevention of losses relates to achievement of company objectives.
17. Answer: **B**. According to "Management" by John R. Schermerhorn, Jr., this is the definition of stereotype.

18. Answer: **C**. Safety and the responsibility for achieving it rest with management, primarily with the organization's chief executive officer, but in a shared manner with all other managers. There has always been disagreement in management circles about just how to accomplish safety, but there has always been agreement that management of safety, like all other functions, has to start at the top and be supported by subordinate executives and managers. Supervisors, foremen, and workers develop their attitudes about the importance of safety and health from both formal and informal clues.

Management of the safety and health effort is both an art and a science; the Director of Safety and Health is merely the functional steward. When safety is effective, the entire management team deserves credit. Likewise, when it fails, the entire team shares the blame. Good leadership characteristics include building responsibility, educating, setting expectations, and encouraging choices.

19. Answer: **D**. System A is a parallel system; that is, both the first *and* the second components must fail to produce a system failure. To determine probability for a parallel system, individual probabilities are multiplied.

$$(2 \times 10^{-3}) \times (5 \times 10^{-4}) = 1 \times 10^{-6}$$

System B is a series system; that is, if either the first *or* the second components fail, a system failure will occur. For components in series, the total failure rate is the sum of individual components' failure rates.

$$(7 \times 10^{-7}) + (3 \times 10^{-7}) = 1 \times 10^{-6}$$

System C has only one component. Thus, the probability of system failure is the same as single component probability of failure.

$$1 \times 10^{-6}$$

Since the severity and probability for each system is the same, the loss risk is also the same. Given this situation, the selection process would consider overall system cost, deliverability, quality, longevity, human factors, etc.

20. Answer: **C. 1910.145 (extracted)** The word "sign" refers to a surface on prepared for the warning of, or safety instructions of, industrial workers or members of the public who may be exposed to hazards. Excluded from this definition, however, are news releases, displays commonly known as safety posters, and bulletins used for employee education. The wording of any sign should be easily read and concise. The sign should contain sufficient information to be easily understood. The wording should make a positive, rather than a negative, suggestion and should be accurate in fact. "Major message" means that portion of a tag's inscription that is more specific than the signal word and that indicates the specific hazardous condition or the instruction to be communicated to the employee. Examples include:

"High Voltage"
"Close Clearance"
"Do Not Start"
"Do Not Use" or a corresponding pictograph used with a written text or alone
"Signal word" means that portion of a tag's inscription that contains the word or words that are intended to capture an employee's immediate attention.

Domain 2 Quiz 3 Questions

1. To identify the "vital few," whether customers, customer needs, product features, or inputs, this principle helps assure that resources and attention are concentrated where they will do the most good.
    A. Hystograph Principle
    B. Juran Principle
    C. Pareto Principle
    D. KISS Principle

2. The factors that make the greatest impact on whether an employee will or will not work safely are:
   A. strength and endurance.
   B. recognition, attitude, and team spirit.
   C. emotional, moral, and physical factors.
   D. experience and workplace design.

3. The term *incident* encompasses first-aid cases, recordable cases, restricted-workday cases, lost-workday cases, permanent disability cases, near misses, and property damage cases. Which of the following represents an indirect cost?
   A. Incident review
   B. Workers' compensation premiums
   C. Ambulance service
   D. Drug testing

4. Which of the following is the highest safety priority for the typical employee?
   A. Dictated safety standards
   B. Generic safety statement: "Be safe"
   C. Perceived control over the risk
   D. Individual examples that violate safety standards

5. Only a small percentage of car accidents are the result of mechanical failure. How can a company best control the major cause of driver error?
   A. Conducting monthly safety meetings
   B. Requiring substance abuse testing of all drivers
   C. Hiring only drivers under 40 years of age
   D. Implementing a program of driver selection, training, and supervision

6. Should an inspector wish to acquire some structural details for a comprehensive survey, including floor loading at a building site, he/she should:
   A. ask the plant superintendent to relay information from posted floor loading signs in the facility.
   B. have OHST evaluate conditions during an upcoming plant visit.
   C. consult published building plans or have a structural engineer conduct a structural analysis.
   D. obtain a floor load handbook and evaluate any suspicious conditions during a plant visit.

7. What is the term for a neutral or irrelevant event effect in an experiment that is intended to produce the same reaction in a participant as if the event were of importance?
   A. Simple effect
   B. Placebo effect
   C. Hawthorne effect
   D. Theory of negative reward

8. Which of the following are GHS signal words that indicate the relative degree of severity of a hazard?
   A. Warning, Caution
   B. Danger, Warning
   C. Caution, Danger
   D. Hazardous, Dangerous

9. Once a chemical has been classified, the hazard(s) must be communicated to target audiences. The exhibited pictogram represents which hazard class?

   A. Carcinogen
   B. Irritant
   C. Acute Toxicity
   D. Environmental Toxicity

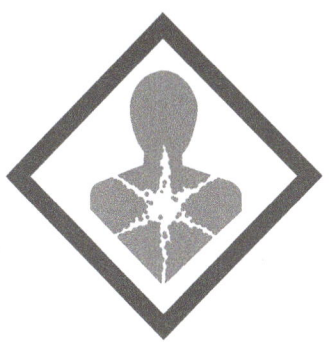

Figure 23 Pictogram

10. Which of the following key label elements are standardized under the Globally Harmonized System (GHS)?

    A. Product identifier, supplier identifier, chemical identity
    B. Hazard pictograms, signal words, hazard statements
    C. Precautionary information, product identifier, hazard statements
    D. Signal words, chemical identity, hazard pictograms

11. Which action, according to current safety philosophy, would have the greatest impact on changing safety behavior?

    A. Posting a sign stating, "Wear Your Eye Protection"
    B. Turning off all machines when finished
    C. Complimenting an employee for wearing eye protection
    D. Providing a free meal for a safe month on the plant floor

12. Which plant leader most influences organizational line management to accept accountability for safety performance?

    A. Supervisor
    B. Staff safety professional
    C. Facility manager
    D. Site engineer

13. Who must be trained on the methods and means necessary for energy isolation and control of hazardous energy?

    A. Area supervisor
    B. Each authorized employee
    C. Each affected employee
    D. All employees whose work operations are or may be in an area where energy control procedures may potentially be used

14. Employees are interviewed randomly to collect accident information concerning near misses, difficulties in operations, and conditions that could have resulted in death, injury, or property loss. This method is described as:

    A. behavior sampling.
    B. critical incident technique.
    C. program quality verification inspection.
    D. unprogrammed process safety management.

15. The integration of hazard analysis and risk assessment methods early in the design and redesign processes and taking the actions necessary so that the risks of injury or damage are at an acceptable level is termed:

    A. severity.
    B. prevention through design.
    C. hazard through design.
    D. hierarchy of controls.

16. Process variations occur because of equipment failures, human errors, and process upsets such as localized chemical reactions. The analysis methodology that implements a systematic way to examine how process variations affect a system is called:

    A. Hazard and Operability (HAZOP).
    B. a checklist.
    C. Fault Tree Analysis (FTA).
    D. Failure Mode and Effects Analysis (FMEA).

17. The hazard analysis method that tabulates the ways in which equipment and components can fail, and the effects of these failures on a system, process, or plant is called:

    A. Hazard and Operability (HAZOP).
    B. Fault Tree Analysis (FTA).
    C. Failure Mode and Effects Analysis (FMEA).
    D. Management Oversight and Risk Tree (MORT).

18. Which of the following methods is a deductive analysis technique that allows the analyst to determine the combinations of failures that are necessary to achieve an event defined as the top or undesired event?

    A. Fault Tree Analysis (FTA)
    B. Failure Mode and Effects Analysis (FMEA)
    C. Hazard and Operability (HAZOP)
    D. Risk Management Plan (RMP)

19. Workplace electrical safety standards are the most often utilized in the industry to perform arc flash hazard analysis. These calculations are based upon:

    A. potential energy.
    B. incident energy.
    C. hazardous energy.
    D. absorbed energy.

20. Which of the following defines observation of worker behaviors at random intervals and classification of these behaviors according to whether they are safe or unsafe?

    A. Critical incident technique
    B. Life safety code
    C. Behavior sampling
    D. Safety orientation

21. Any action that reduces losses incurred, by definition, is:

    A. loss control.
    B. loss transfer.
    C. risk management.
    D. loss reduction.

22. **What is the primary function of a loss control system?**
    A. Assess risk, establish effective risk control measures, and eliminate risk
    B. Establish effective risk control measures for hazardous conditions, establish effective control measures, and eliminate risk
    C. Identify hazardous conditions, assess their risks, and establish effective risk control measures
    D. Assure compliance with applicable regulatory requirements and eliminate residual risk

23. **Which is a financial method for reducing the costs of accidents in an organization?**
    A. Risk transfer
    B. Risk projection
    C. Financial risk management
    D. Hierarchy of loss controls

24. **Which is the best definition of hazard?**
    A. A condition, set of circumstances, or inherent property that can cause injury, illness, or death
    B. An event in which a work-related injury or illness or fatality occurred or could have occurred
    C. A set of interrelated elements that establish and support occupational safety and health objectives
    D. An estimate of the combination of the likelihood of an occurrence of a hazardous event or exposure, and the severity of the injury

Domain 2 Quiz 3 Answers

1. Answer: **C**. This is the definition of the Pareto Principle, sometimes referred to as the 80/20 rule that indicates that 80% of the problems come from 20% of the operations. It is also true that 20% of corrective actions and risk reduction actions can mitigate 80% of the risk, when the risk is understood.
2. Answer: **B**. Many behavior-based safety experts agree that the most critical factors are team spirit, recognition, and attitude. The major factors in work discontent are company policy, interpersonal relationships, and supervision. The best way to reduce injuries and property damage in the future is to systematically reinforce positive employee actions and behavior. The safety culture is a group's attitude that everyone in the group will try to behave in a way that protects the safety of each other. Recognition will reinforce their trust in the culture. An important factor in developing a safety program is to incorporate concepts of job enrichment, participation, and employee-centered leadership. Management will most likely support a proactive safety effort when prevention of losses relates to achievement of company objectives.
3. Answer: **A**

Table 8 Direct Cost

Category	Example
Workers' Compensation	WC premiums
Medical Bills	Treatment by physician, nurse, hospital costs
Medical Treatment Supplies	Bandages, splints, antiseptic
Ambulance Service	Established fees
Drug Testing	Fees for off-site testing
Job Accommodations	Equipment or tool redesign or replacement; ergonomically designed chairs, keyboards
New Equipment	Costs of new equipment/parts purchased as a result of an incident

Table 9 Indirect Cost

Category	Example
Healthcare Professional	Consultation with the victim; treatment time; recordkeeping and filing; follow-up consultation(s)
Injured Worker	All time spent away from the job attributable to the incident. One way to determine this is to ask the nurse or supervisor. Be sure to include travel time to/from the nurse's office, waiting time, treatment and follow-up, and time spent visiting the offsite doctor's office. An important, yet often overlooked, contribution to indirect cost estimates is the percent reduction in efficiency due to restricted work. Often, an injured worker can return to the job at 100%; occasionally, however, the worker is only able to work at 90% until fully recovered. Once the percentage of restricted work has been determined, it can be incorporated into the indirect cost summary. Example: Hourly rate = $10; cumulative time lost due to incident = 2 hours. This yields an initial $20 indirect cost. Restricted work efficiency level = 90% for 8 hours. Since $10 × 0.9 yields work at a level of only $9/hour, there is a $1/hour indirect loss for each hour worked at the restricted level. Therefore, that $1/hour × 8 hours yields an additional $8 loss, which should be added to the original $20 calculation; thus, the ultimate indirect cost is $28.
Supervisor	Consultation with the victim; recordkeeping and filing; follow-up consultation; disciplinary action
Return to Work	Consultation, work process modifications
Lost Production/Productivity	Lost production represents the expected income that would have been received from maintaining production/service that was lost and is attributable to the incident. Often, this cost amounts to the highest of all indirect costs. Also consider the lost productivity of witnesses and colleagues in discussing and investigating the incident.
Incident Review	Sum hourly rates of the incident investigation team, multiply by the average time needed to complete a thorough investigation for each cost category
Human Resources	Managing the case back to 100% duty, consultation, recordkeeping, and filing
Cost to Hire	The cost in terms of all necessary activities to bring in a replacement employee to work while the injured employee recovers
Manager	Consultation with the victim; recordkeeping and filing; follow-up consultation; disciplinary action
Process Delays/Interruptions	Represents lost income expected or lost personnel productivity when a process is delayed or interrupted as the result of an incident
Security	Since security is not involved in all cases, one must first determine the percentage of involvement. Example: Assume 900 cases occur and security is involved in 10 percent (or 90) of them. 90 cases × 1 hour of time devoted × $10/hour = $900 for all cases worked on. If security contributes $900 to the total, the cost for 900 cases = $900/900 = $1 contribution per case.
Training	Include new or retraining efforts, instructor costs, paperwork, recordkeeping, and tracking. For new/retrained employees on a new job, one can also perform an efficiency analysis similar to that of an injured worker (see above).
Legal	Calculate same as security costs

4. Answer: **C**. Motivation in safety is highly situation specific, which means that situational or behavior-specific campaigns (e.g., "don't drink and drive") are more likely to have an impact than general campaigns (e.g., "be safe"). However, behavior change is likely to be short-lived if it is unsupported or sustained by intrinsic beliefs. People are motivated to take risks, as well as to avoid risks, providing they perceive they have personal control over the risk.
5. Answer: **D**. According to the NSC, "Companies can control driver error by introducing a program of driver selection, training, and supervision, while vehicle failure can be reduced by implementing a preventive maintenance program."
6. Answer: **C**. Accurate data is a must when evaluating floor loading in an industrial environment. If data is not readily available from reliable sources, the best choice is to have a competent engineer perform a structural analysis. OSHA 1910.22 states, "In every building or other structure, or part thereof, used for mercantile, business, industrial, or storage purposes, the loads approved by the building official shall be marked on plates of approved design which shall be supplied and securely affixed by the owner of the building, or his duly authorized agent, in a conspicuous place in each space to which they relate." "It shall be unlawful to place, or cause, or permit to be placed, on any floor or roof of a building or other structure a load greater than that for which such floor or roof is approved by the building official."
7. Answer: **C**. An unplanned change in persons taking part in an experiment who know this is called the Hawthorne effect. It was first recognized in a study of worker productivity in the Hawthorne plant of Western Electric Company. A physical change was made to the work area; however, the factor that caused the change was the perception that management was trying to improve the work area.
8. Answer: **B**. The signal word indicates the relative degree of severity of a hazard. The signal words used in the GHS are:
    - "Danger" for the more severe hazards
    - "Warning" for the less severe hazards

    Signal words are standardized and assigned to the hazard categories within endpoints. Some lower-level hazard categories do not use signal words. Only one signal word corresponding to the class of the most severe hazard should be used on each label. The GHS hazard pictograms, signal word, and hazard statements should be located together on the label. The actual label format or layout is not specified in the GHS. National authorities may choose to specify where information should appear on the label or allow supplier discretion.
9. Answer: **A**. The GHS symbols have been incorporated into pictograms for use on the GHS label. Pictograms include the harmonized hazard symbols plus other graphic elements, such as borders, background patterns, or colors that are intended to convey specific information. For transport, pictograms will have the background, symbol, and colors currently used in the UN Recommendations on the Transport of Dangerous Goods, Model Regulations. For other sectors, pictograms will have a black symbol on a white background with a red diamond frame. A black frame may be used for shipments within one country. The GHS pictogram for the same hazard should **not** be located where a transport pictogram appears.
10. Answer: **B**. The GHS Working Group identified about 35 different types of information currently required on labels by different systems. To harmonize, key information elements needed to be identified. Additional harmonization may occur on other elements in time, in particular for precautionary statements.

    The elements are identified below: * = **Standardized**
    - Product identifier
    - Supplier identifier
    - Chemical identity
    - Hazard pictograms*
    - Signal words*
    - Hazard statements*
    - Precautionary information

GHS pictograms and hazard classes

Pictogram	Hazard Classes
(flame over circle)	• Oxidizers
(flame)	• Flammables • Self reactives • Pyrophorics • Self-heating • Emits flammable gas • Organic peroxides
(exploding bomb)	• Explosives • Self reactives • Organic peroxides
(skull and crossbones)	• Acute toxicity (severe)
(corrosion)	• Corrosives
(gas cylinder)	• Gases under pressure
(health hazard)	• Carcinogen • Respiratory sensitizer • Reproductive toxicity • Target organ toxicity
(environment)	• Environmental toxicity
(exclamation mark)	• Irritant • Dermal sensitizer • Acute toxicity (harmful) • Narcotic effects

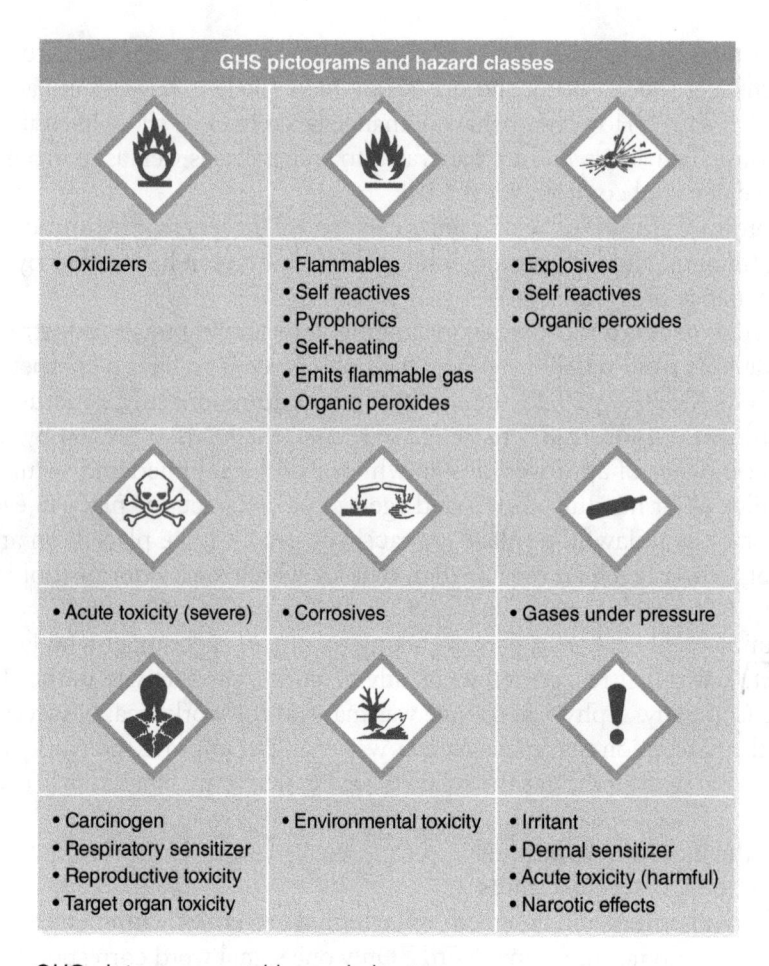

GHS pictograms and hazard classes

Hazard Communication Standard Pictogram, Occupational Safety and Health Administration, Retrieved from https://www.osha.gov/Publications/HazComm_QuickCard_Pictogram.html

11. Answer: **C**. Most experts agree that there are two primary actions that influence behavior change the most: positive reinforcement and reinforcing the behavior as close to action time as possible. The first step in improving behavior in an organization is to establish an ethics program to address organizational culture issues. Safety incentive programs should be designed to influence and change behaviors.

12. Answer: **B**. The role of a staff safety professional is to consult and influence. Because safety should be built into line performance, a key role of a safety professional is to influence line management to accept accountability for safety performance.

13. Answer: **B**. In the OSHA lock-out/tag-out standard (29 CFR 1910.147), an **authorized employee** is one who locks out or tags out the machine or equipment in order to perform servicing or maintenance. An **affected employee** is one whose job requires him/her to operate or use a machine or equipment on which servicing or maintenance is being performed under lock-out/tag-out, or whose job requires him/her to work in an area in which such servicing or maintenance is being performed.

    Authorized employees must receive training in the recognition of hazardous energy sources, the type and magnitude of the energy available in the workplace, and methods and means necessary for energy isolation and control. Affected employees need training in the purpose and use of energy control devices.

    The most significant item in safe operating procedures for equipment maintenance is ensuring that energy at the machine is zero and will remain that way during the repair.

    A review of 29 CFR 1910.147 is recommended if unfamiliar with OSHA's lock-out/tag-out requirements.

14. Answer: **B**. The **critical incident technique** asks those participating to describe any incidents that come to their attention. This technique can be useful in investigating worker–equipment relationships in past or existing systems, evaluating modifications to existing systems, or developing new systems.

    The **behavior sampling** or activity sampling technique involves observation of worker behaviors at random intervals and classifying these behaviors as safe or unsafe.

Safety sampling can be a successful method to verify effectiveness of a safety training program, provided that the technique is adapted to the program, a sound basic accident prevention program is in place, and management is familiar with the technique and its potential.

15. Answer: **B**. **Safety through design** is defined as the integration of hazard analysis and risk assessment methods early in the design and redesign processes and taking the actions necessary so that risks of injury or damage are at an acceptable level. This concept encompasses facilities, hardware, equipment, tools, materials, layout and configuration, energy controls, environmental concerns, and products. **Severity:** The extent of harm or damage that could result from a hazard. **Prevention through design:** Addressing occupational safety and health needs in design and redesign processes to prevent or minimize work-related hazards and risks associated with construction, manufacture, use, maintenance, and disposal of facilities, materials, equipment, and processes. **Hierarchy of controls** is a systematic way of thinking and acting, considering steps in a ranked and sequential order, to choose the most effective means of eliminating or reducing hazards and risks that derive from them. An example is the requirement of suppliers of services to attest that processes have been applied to identify and analyze hazards and to reduce risks deriving from those hazards to an acceptable level. There is precedent for having suppliers attest that risk analyses have been completed. Manufacturers of equipment to be used in the European Union are required by International Organization for Standardization (ISO) standards to certify that they have met applicable standards, including ISO 12100-1 and ISO 14121.

16. Answer: **A**. The Hazard and Operability (HAZOP) analysis methodology is a systematic way to examine how process variations affect a system. Process variations occur as a result of equipment failures, human errors, and process upsets such as localized chemical reactions. The technique can be used for systems with continuous processes as well as batch processes. The use of the HAZOP analysis methodology requires detailed information about the design and operation of the process. The HAZOP methodology is most effective during the design phase of a process or for existing processes. In the HAZOP analysis, a hazard evaluation team composed of experts from different areas systematically examines every part of the process to discover how process design deviations can occur. The hazard evaluation team leader systematically guides the team through the process design, using a fixed set of guide words. These guide words are applied at crucial points or nodes of the process. The guide words include *no, more, less, as well as, part of, reverse,* and *other than*. They are combined with a condition, such as flow or pressure, to define the deviation. For example, "What is the effect of low flow on the process?" Typical deviations include leaks or ruptures, loss of containment, ignition sources, and chemical reactions. The HAZOP analysis should identify hazards and operating problems, and enable the HAZOP team to recommend design or procedural changes that will improve the safety of the process. The results of the HAZOP analysis are documented in a tabular format with a separate table for each segment of the process under study.

17. Answer: **C**. The Failure Mode and Effects Analysis (FMEA) tabulates the ways in which equipment and components can fail, and the effects of these failures on a system, process, or plant. Failure modes describe the ways in which equipment can fail (such as open, closed, on, off, leaks, etc.). The analyst lists all of the components of the system under review and all the failure modes for these components. The FMEA identifies the individual failure modes that can either cause or contribute to an accident. This method of analysis does not address multiple failures. An FMEA analysis should produce a qualitative, systematic list of equipment and components, a list of associated failure modes, and a list of the effects of the failure modes on the system. The list of effects should include a worst-case estimate of the consequences of each failure mode. The information produced by an FMEA analysis can be used to support recommendations for increased equipment and component reliability that would improve safety.

18. Answer: **A**. Fault Tree Analysis (FTA) is a deductive analysis technique that allows the analyst to determine the combinations of failures that are necessary to achieve an event defined as the top or undesired event. FTA is well suited for the analysis of highly redundant systems. The fault tree is a graphic model that displays the various combinations of equipment/component failures and human errors that can give rise to the top event. The FTA provides a means to qualitatively or quantitatively identify the frequency of the top event. It is a deductive technique that employs Boolean logic (the use of AND and OR gate logic) to relate the top event to a combination of basic events that must occur in order for

96 ASP Exam Study Workbook

the top event to happen. The fault tree, once constructed, can be quantified by using the failure rate data for the basic events (i.e., those events at the bottom of the tree). A quantified fault tree projects the rate of occurrence for the top event.

19. Answer: **B**. The arc flash boundary for systems 50 volts and greater shall be the distance at which the incident energy equals 5 J/cm^2 (1.2 cal/cm^2). Determining accurate onset to second-degree burn energy and its significance in computing the arc flash boundary is focused on the prevention of injury to the skin of a human who might be exposed to an arc flash. Different formulas have been proposed to calculate incident energy at an assumed working distance, and the arc flash boundary, in order to determine arc rated personal protective equipment for Qualified Electrical Workers (**Table 10**). The Institute of Electrical and Electronics Engineers (IEEE) Standard P1584 Guide for Performing Arc-Flash Hazard Calculations [*1584 IEEE Guide for Performing Arc-Flash Hazard Calculations. IEEE Industry Applications Society. September 2002*] and formulas provided in Annex D of NFPA 70E [*NFPA 70E Standard for Electrical Safety in the Workplace. 2012.*] and CSA Z462 [*CSA Z462 Workplace Electrical Safety Standards. 2012.*] Workplace electrical safety standards are the most often utilized in the industry to perform arc flash hazard analysis. The formulas are based on incident energy testing performed and calculations conducted for a selected range of prospective fault currents, system voltages, physical configurations, etc.

    The FPB is the distance at which incident energy is 1.2 cal/cm^2, which is the amount of heat needed to cause second-degree burns.

    - **Limited Approach Boundary**
      Entered only by qualified persons or unqualified persons that have been advised and are escorted by a qualified person
    - **Restricted Approach Boundary**
      Entered only by qualified persons required to use shock protection techniques and PPE
    - **Flash Protection Boundary**
      Linear distance to prevent any more than second-degree burns from a potential arc flash (typically 4 feet)

    The purpose of incident energy calculations is to determine the appropriate PPE that will limit the possible thermal energy exposure to critical body parts, such as the face and chest areas. Usually, the calculations give the heat exposure in calories/cm^2 or Joules/cm^2. Once you know the heat exposure level, you can choose the protective clothing to best protect your employees.

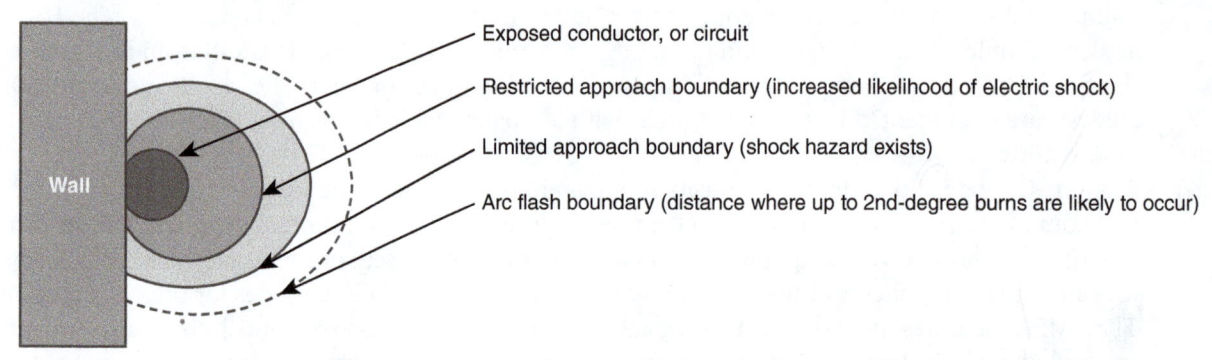

    Figure 24 Arc Flash Boundaries

20. Answer: **C**. Behavior sampling or activity sampling technique involves observation of worker behaviors at random intervals by organizational experts and classification of these natural risk behaviors according to whether they are safe or unsafe. Using this technique, management can apply various components of a safety program (such as safety lectures, posters, brief safety talks, safety inspections, motion picture films, and supervisory training) and immediately note their influence on workers' unsafe behavior.

21. Answer: **D**. **Loss reduction** means any **action** that reduces the losses incurred. The reduction may be by decrease of the physical destruction (as by reducing the amount of material burned or the number of persons injured) or by reducing the operational loss from a given amount of destruction (as having standby equipment or more effective medical care for the injured). It includes the concepts of loss prevention and control as well as the concept of risk avoidance—the refusal to accept a given risk.

Table 10 Personal Protective Equipment for Qualified Electrical Workers

Hazard Category	Range of Calculated Incident Energy	Minimum Arc Rating of PPE, cal/cm^2	Clothing Description	Clothing Required
1	> 1.2 to 4 cal/cm^2	4 cal/cm^2	Arc rated clothing, minimum arc rating of 4 cal/cm^2	Fire-resistant (FR) fabric shirt and pants or coveralls
2	> 4 to 8 cal/cm^2	8 cal/cm^2	Arc rated clothing, minimum arc rating of 8 cal/cm^2	Cotton underclothing plus FR shirt and pants
3	> 8 to 25 cal/cm^2	25 cal/cm^2	Arc rated clothing selected so that the system rating meets the required minimum arc rating of 25 cal/cm^2	Cotton underclothing plus FR shirt, pants, coveralls, or equivalent
4	> 25 to 40 cal/cm^2	40 cal/cm^2	Arc rated clothing selected so that the system rating meets the required minimum arc rating of 40 cal/cm^2	Cotton underclothing plus FR shirt, pants, plus a multi-layer flash suit

Protective Clothing Characteristics Based on Source: NFPA 70E. (All details in the NFPA table have not been reproduced.)
Modified from NFPA 70E Standard for Electrical Safety Requirements for Employee Workplaces, Reytrieved from https://www.csulb.edu/sites/default/files/groups/college-of-engineering/electrical_safety.pdf

Planning actions are not generally considered part of loss reduction. The four steps required in an effective loss control program are problem identification, selection of corrective measures, implementation, and feedback and control.

There are five stages in risk analysis and management: identification, estimation, evaluation, response, and monitoring.

22. **Answer: C.** As described in *Assurance Technologies*, a loss control system must be able to identify the hazardous conditions as well as understand the real risks associated with those hazardous conditions. A loss control system is incomplete if it solely identifies hazardous conditions and does not take action to understand the risks. Effective risk control measures are relative to the risks associated with the hazardous conditions.

23. **Answer: A.** Several control techniques available are for treating loss exposures. The two categories for reducing the costs of accidents in an organization are prevention (loss control) and financial (cost reduction). Loss control techniques include engineering, administrative controls, and personal protective equipment to deal with losses. Engineering controls include building a ventilation system to reduce explosive vapor levels, whereas administrative controls might limit exposures to toxic materials. Issuing personal protective equipment (PPE) such as respirators is the last line of defense against hazards in the workplace. Sprinkler systems and distance to a means of egress are examples of loss reduction, not loss prevention. A company might try to avoid the loss altogether. Organizations can reduce exposure by substitution. Instead of mixing methylene chloride as a solvent ingredient in a commercial aerosol product, a company could substitute a "safer" solvent to reduce the likelihood of a worker being exposed. **Risk transfer** assigns the liability to another party, rather than run the risk of loss itself. If methylene chloride mixing could not be accomplished safely in the plant, the company may choose to have the product shipped to a contractor who would mix the ingredient. If the contractor's workers are overcome by vapors from the solvent mixing, then the contractor would typically hold the liability. Another form of risk transfer is insurance. **Insurance** is designed to permit the company to shift the financial consequences of the risk to an insurance company. By paying the insurance company's **premiums**, the organization can expect specified **benefits** in the event of loss. With large numbers of insureds, insurance companies can more accurately estimate their own losses. Organizations may retain their loss exposures without dealing with them. This may be a result of ignorance or choice. Organizations that retain their own exposures may ignore them, or attempt to

reduce them, or they may, in fact, self-insure. Ignoring the risks may make the owners more confident, but dealing with the risks will make them more prepared for loss. Self-insurance is simply no insurance; the company retains the loss exposure. It should only be undertaken by companies with the financial resources necessary to absorb potential losses (Friend & Kohn, 2007).

Identification techniques include individual consultation and group discussion. Individual consultations are one-on-one meetings arranged as a preliminary exercise to initially identify the risks. This process involves key participants in the project in question. The purpose of this stage is to allow the interviewee to contemplate what he/she thinks are the main risks attached to the project as a whole, or as individual stages of the project, or both. As the participants are from different disciplines, their viewpoints about the project are influenced by the specialized nature of their field. Group discussion is a process by which potential sources of risk are identified with a clear set of rules and a timetable. This technique should be carried out with the project team. One person should be the coordinator who chairs the meetings. The discussion process should have two distinct stages, a creative stage and an assessment stage. The creative stage permits any member of the team, one at a time, to suggest potential risks or sources of risk. Individual team members are not restricted to their own knowledge domain and outlandish ideas are encouraged. The assessment stage then follows. Estimation includes interviewing and brainstorming with personal and corporate experience. The analysis and/or estimation stage is more extensive than the identification stage. All the ideas are analyzed individually and a final draft of the risks is assembled. The idea of the analysis stage is to categorize or rank the risks by using the one-on-one situation in interviewing, or the group discussions from brainstorming. Therefore, the end result from this stage is to prioritize the risks so as to know which of them are to be forwarded to the quantitative analysis. At this point, a threshold level or cut-off point must also be decided, the notion being that risks below this level, and thus those not to be analyzed quantitatively, are covered by project contingent reserves. The ones above would thus not require further analysis.

Personal and corporate experience is an important factor. If there are employees with experience, then this property should be utilized. Experience enables the main risks in a project to be identified. Obviously, one looks at the more senior officers to excel in this department. However, there is always a chance that certain risks never encountered before are overlooked. If the project is not equivalent to a previous project, then the policies of the company, or engineering judgment, decides on a contingency percentage. Factors of safety are used extensively in the construction industry and are based on this method.

Response strategies include:

Risk Avoidance
- Avoiding risk can be as simple as a contractor not placing a bid or even the owner not proceeding with project funding. Other methods are tendering a very high bid, placing conditions on the bid, and not bidding on the high-risk portion of the contract.

Risk Transfer
Risk transfer can take two basic forms:
- The property or activity responsible for the risk may be transferred, such as hiring a subcontractor to work on a hazardous process
- The property or activity may be retained, but the financial risk transferred, such as to insurance or by having the client take the costs of risk by contract

Risk Retention
- This is the method of responding to risks by the body that controls them. The risks, foreseen or unforeseen, are controlled and financed by the company or contractor that is fulfilling the terms of the contract. There are two retention methods, active and passive. Active retention, sometimes referred to as self-insurance, is a deliberate management strategy after a conscious evaluation of the possible losses and costs of alternative ways of handling risks. Passive retention, on the other hand (sometimes called noninsurance), occurs through neglect, ignorance, or absence of decision, such as when a risk has not been identified and responding to the consequences of that risk must be borne by the contractor performing the work.

Risk Reduction
- Loss prevention is one of the ways of risk reduction. Loss prevention can be classified into four basic categories:
  - Preconditions for a loss (e.g., faults in the premises such as badly insulated wire)
  - Prevention of loss; devices designed to prevent preconditions for loss (e.g., cut-off switches)
  - Early discovery of loss-producing events (e.g., sprinkler systems)
  - Limitation of loss (e.g., fire doors, compartmentalization)

24. Answer: **A**
    - **Hazard:** A condition, set of circumstances, or inherent property that can cause injury, illness, or death
    - **Incident:** An event in which a work-related injury or illness or fatality occurred or could have occurred
    - **Occupational Health and Safety Management System (OHSMS)**: A set of interrelated elements that establish and support occupational safety and health objectives
    - **Risk:** An estimate of the combination of the likelihood of occurrence of a hazardous event or exposure, and the severity of the injury

Domain 3: Ergonomics

Domain 3: Ergonomics
- Fitness for duty
- Stressors
- Risk factors
- Work design
- Material handling
- Work practice controls
- Use qualitative and quantitative analysis methods

Modified from ASP® Exam Blueprint (ASP10), November 10, 2019

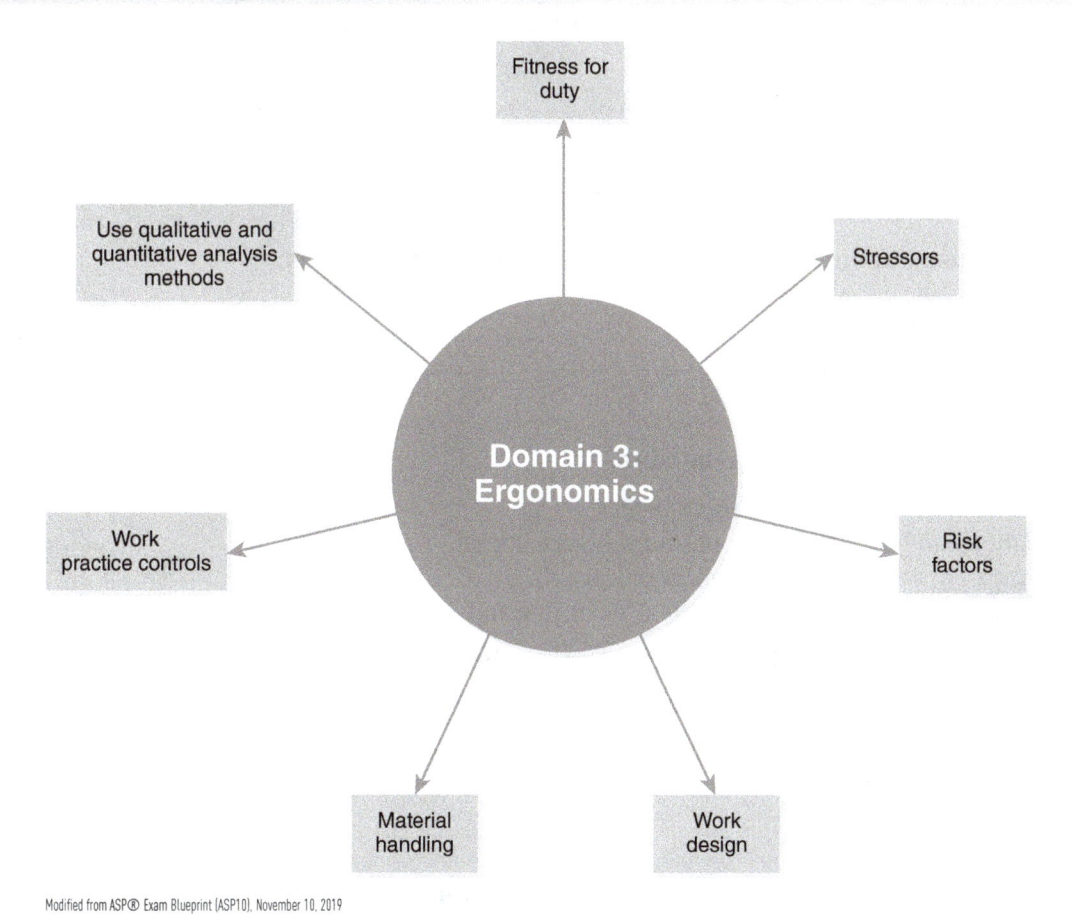

Domain 3 Quiz 1 Questions

1. Which is the best design for continuous input with precision for operator control?
   A. Toggle switch
   B. Knob
   C. Limit switch
   D. Push button

2. What would be an example of an engineering control?
   A. Design the job to fit the worker.
   B. Assign workers to specific jobs.
   C. Implement a job rotation schedule.
   D. Provide customized fitted gloves.

3. Back belts (braces) used for support:
   A. are recommended by NIOSH and required by OSHA if back strain is possible.
   B. are considered a form of personal protective equipment for prevention of back injuries.
   C. have not been shown to lessen the risk of back injury among uninjured workers.
   D. must be provided at no cost to employees who request them.

4. What is the Lifting Index for an operator to lift a 12-kg weight and a recommended weight limit of 12.1 kg?
   A. 0.526
   B. 0.992
   C. 1.008
   D. 1.901

5. The term *CLI* used in the professional practice of ergonomics means:
   A. Composite Lifting Index.
   B. Controlled Lifting Indices.
   C. Coordinated Lifting Indicator.
   D. Coupling Lifting Index.

6. The term *psychophysical* is most related to:
   A. isotonic dynamic muscle force development.
   B. the relationship between sensations and physical stimuli.
   C. the study of how our emotions impact our health.
   D. the study of biological indicators such as heart rate and energy expenditure.

7. Compression of nerves and blood vessels between the clavicle and first and second ribs is a disease known as:
   A. polymorphous light eruption.
   B. pneumothorax.
   C. atelectasis.
   D. thoracic outlet syndrome.

8. What are two primary situations where biomechanics analysis should be performed?
   A. During manual lifting and to evaluate the effects of body postures
   B. During manual lifting and to evaluate the effects of work rest cycles
   C. During manual lifting and to evaluate the effects of dynamic loads
   D. During manual lifting and to evaluate the effects of static loads

9. **To reduce eye strain while transposing data from a paper to a computer, it is best to:**
   A. place the paper next to computer screen.
   B. place paper above the computer screen.
   C. place paper on the desk.
   D. place the paper below the computer screen.

10. **What is the term for a postural analysis system sensitive to musculoskeletal risk in a variety of jobs that is based on body segment–specific ratings within specific movement planes, using a scoring system for muscle activity including static, dynamic, rapidly changing, or unstable postures, and that provides a benchmark for urgency of action?**
    A. Rapid Upper Limb Assessment
    B. Rodger's Muscle Fatigue Assessment
    C. Strain Index
    D. Rapid Entire Body Assessment

11. **Which of the following best describes carpal tunnel syndrome?**
    A. Elbow and shoulder swelling and inflammation
    B. Inflammation of ligaments in the wrist
    C. Raynaud's syndrome of the hand and wrist
    D. Numbness of the lower legs

12. **For double-handled pinching, gripping, or cutting tools, select a tool with handles that:**
    A. are designed with a grip span that is at least 1/2 inch when fully closed.
    B. are spring-loaded to return the handles to the open position.
    C. have finger grooves.
    D. are bent when the force is applied vertically.

13. **To reduce the chance of injury, work tasks should be designed to limit exposure to ergonomic risk factors. Which of the following represents an administrative control?**
    A. Use diverging conveyors off a main line so that tasks are less repetitive.
    B. Use padding to reduce direct contact with any hard, sharp, or vibrating surface.
    C. Staff "floaters" to provide periodic breaks between scheduled breaks.
    D. Install diverters on conveyors to direct materials toward the worker to eliminate excessive leaning or reaching.

14. **Excessive leaning and reaching is required to access material on the far side of a conveyor or slide in a poultry processing plant. Which of the following is the best solution?**
    A. Design a diverter mechanism.
    B. Create a chute.
    C. Add a tilt or dumper.
    D. Install stationary seating.

15. **A cooperative nursing home patient who weighs 150 pounds cannot bear his own weight and needs to be moved. Which is the best method to eliminate manual lifting?**
    A. Use a stand-and-pivot technique.
    B. Use a friction-reducing device.
    C. Use a lateral sliding aid.
    D. Use a portable lift device.

16. **Truck drivers and equipment operators are most likely to suffer from which of the following occupational diseases?**
    A. Carpal tunnel syndrome from repetitive forceful tasks
    B. Back disability from whole-body vibration
    C. Rotator cuff tendinitis
    D. De Quervain syndrome from gripping

102 ASP Exam Study Workbook

17. Three approaches for evaluating manual material-handling tasks and implementing acceptable workload criteria are:

    A. anthropometric, psychological, and physical.
    B. physiological, cardiovascular, and psychological.
    C. anthropometric, physiological, and ergonomic.
    D. biomechanical, physiological, and psychophysical.

18. A generally accepted practice for use of a video display terminal is to locate the VDT slightly below the operator's horizontal line of sight (HLOS). The recommended angle suggested is:

    A. 5° below the horizontal line of sight.
    B. 5° to 35° below the horizontal line of sight.
    C. 15° to 35° below the horizontal line of sight.
    D. 15° to 25° below the horizontal line of sight.

19. The science of measuring the human body for differences in various physical characteristics is:

    A. kinesiology.
    B. anthropometry.
    C. physiology.
    D. ergonomics.

20. Disorders that affect the muscles, nerves, blood vessels, ligaments, and tendons are called:

    A. chronic wasting disease (CWD).
    B. musculoskeletal disorders (MSDs).
    C. cumulative trauma disorders (CTDs).
    D. soft tissue diseases (STDs).

21. Which of the following is not a design parameter that could affect performance with foot controls?

    A. Whether the controls require a thrust with or without ankle action
    B. The location of the fulcrum (if the pedal is hinged)
    C. The color and brightness of the foot control pedal
    D. The load or force that is required to activate the foot pedal

22. The movement of a body segment in a lateral plane away from the midline of the body is:

    A. abduction.
    B. adduction.
    C. flexion.
    D. extension.

23. Which of the following pass through the carpal tunnel?

    A. Medial nerve and radial artery
    B. Ulnar nerve and ulnar artery
    C. Ulnar nerve and flexor tendons
    D. Median nerve and flexor tendons

Domain 3 Quiz 1 Answers

1. Answer: **B**. **Toggle switches** are easily seen and reliable in operation. They should preferably have only two positions: "on" and "off." **Knobs** without click stops are suitable for fine and precise regulation over a wide range. **Limit switches** are operated by the motion of a machine part or presence of an object. They are used for controlling machinery as part of a control system, as a safety interlocks, or to count objects passing a point. **Push buttons** are to be operated by the pressure of either finger or hand and operate similarly to a switch.

2. Answer: **A**. One of the best ways to prevent and control occupational injuries, illnesses, and fatalities is to "design out" or minimize hazards and risks. NIOSH leads a national initiative called Prevention through Design (PtD). PtD's purpose is to promote this concept and highlight its importance in all business

decisions. The mission of the Prevention through Design National initiative is to prevent or reduce occupational injuries, illnesses, and fatalities through the inclusion of prevention considerations in all designs that impact workers. The mission can be achieved by:
- Eliminating hazards and controlling risks to workers to an acceptable level "at the source" or as early as possible in the life cycle of items or workplaces
- Including design, redesign, and retrofit of new and existing work premises, structures, tools, facilities, equipment, machinery, products, substances, work processes, and the organization of work
- Enhancing the work environment through the inclusion of prevention methods in all designs that impact workers and others on the premises

PtD encompasses all of the efforts to anticipate and design out hazards to workers in facilities, work methods and operations, processes, equipment, tools, products, new technologies, and the organization of work. The focus of PtD is on workers who execute the designs or have to work with the products of the design. The initiative has been developed to support designing out hazards, the most reliable and effective type of prevention.

3. Answer: **C**. The use of lifting belts for professional material handling does not seem to be an effective way of preventing overexertion injuries. When preparing to lift or lower a load, we instinctively develop intra-abdominal pressure within the trunk cavity. The pressure is believed to help support the curvature of the spine during the lifting or lowering effort. An external wrapping around the abdominal region might help to maintain the internal pressure because it makes the walls of the pressure column stiffer. A large number of studies have been performed, summarized, and reviewed by McGill (1999), Lavender et al. (1998), and Thoumier et al. (1998). Their conclusions neither summarily support nor condemn the wearing of support belts in industrial jobs.

4. Answer: **B**. Lifting Index (LI) is a term that provides a relative estimate of the level of physical stress associated with a particular manual lifting task. The estimate of the level of physical stress is defined by the relationship of the weight of the load (L) lifted and the recommended weight limit (RWL). An LI greater than 1 is considered a hazardous lift.

$$LI = \frac{L}{RWL}$$

$$LI = \frac{12}{12.1} = 0.992$$

$$LI = \frac{\text{Load Weight}}{\text{Recommended Weight Limit}} = \frac{L}{RWL}$$

5. Answer: **A**. The Composite Lifting Index (CLI) is the term used in the revised NIOSH Lifting Equation to denote the overall lifting index for a multitask manual lifting job. The multitask procedure is quite complicated and involves calculation of the Frequency-Independent Recommended Weight Limit (FIRWL), the Single-Task Recommended Weight Limit (STRWL), the Frequency-Independent Lifting Index (FILI) and the Single-Task Lifting Index (STLI) for each task.

6. Answer: **B**. Psychophysical methods are used to study acceptable weights for manual lifting. The worker can adjust the weight of the lift to match his or her own personal feelings of fatigue or perception of what can be sustained for several hours.

7. Answer: **D**. Thoracic outlet syndrome is defined as a disorder resulting from compression of nerves and blood vessels between the clavicle and first and second ribs at the brachial plexus. It can be caused by typing, keying, carrying heavy loads, or keeping the head, arms, and/or shoulders in an unnatural position.

8. Answer: **A**. Body postures are an important consideration when performing biomechanical analyses.

9. Answer: **A**. The name for eye problems caused by computer use is computer vision syndrome (CVS). CVS is not one specific eye problem. Instead, the term encompasses a whole range of eyestrain and pain experienced by computer users. Working at a computer requires that the eyes continuously focus, move back and forth, and align with what you are seeing. Working at a computer gets even more difficult as you get older. That's because the lens of your eye becomes less flexible. The ability to focus on near and far objects starts to diminish after about age 40—a condition called presbyopia. To reduce eyestrain, papers should be placed next to the computer screen at eye level.

10. Answer: **D**. The purpose of Rapid Entire Body Assessment (REBA) is to develop a postural analysis system sensitive to musculoskeletal risk in a variety of jobs that is based on body segment–specific ratings

within specific movement planes, using a scoring system for muscle activity including static, dynamic, rapidly changing, or unstable postures, and provide a benchmark for urgency of action. Rapid Upper Limb Assessment (RULA) is used to investigate the exposure to risk factors for upper limb disorders and provide a method of screening the work population quickly so that results can go into a wider, more versatile ergonomic assessment, while eliminating the need for assessment equipment. Rodger's Muscle Fatigue Assessment provides a method of evaluating the physiological demands of a task against published criteria of acceptable levels of oxygen consumption for whole-body or upper-body work. A strain index provides a relatively simple risk assessment method designed to evaluate a job's level of risk for developing a disorder of the distal upper extremities such as hands, wrists, forearms, and elbows.

11. Answer: **B**. According to NIOSH, carpal tunnel syndrome occurs when the median nerve, which runs from the forearm into the palm of the hand, becomes pressed or squeezed at the wrist. The median nerve controls sensations to the palm side of the thumb and fingers (although not the little finger), as well as impulses to some small muscles in the hand that allow the fingers and thumb to move. The carpal tunnel—a narrow, rigid passageway of ligament and bones at the base of the hand—houses the median nerve and tendons. Sometimes, thickening from irritated tendons or other swelling narrows the tunnel and causes the median nerve to be compressed. The result may be pain, weakness, or numbness in the hand and wrist, radiating up the arm. This injury is common among repetitive motion workers. The median nerve is compressed, resulting in numbness, tingling, and sometimes pain in the fingers and wrist.

    Symptoms usually start gradually, with frequent burning, tingling, or itching numbness in the palm of the hand and the fingers, especially the thumb and the index and middle fingers. Some carpal tunnel sufferers say their fingers feel useless and swollen, even though little or no swelling is apparent. The symptoms often first appear in one or both hands during the night, since many people sleep with flexed wrists. A person with carpal tunnel syndrome may wake up feeling the need to "shake out" the hand or wrist. As symptoms worsen, people might feel tingling during the day. Decreased grip strength may make it difficult to form a fist, grasp small objects, or perform other manual tasks. In chronic and/or untreated cases, the muscles at the base of the thumb may waste away. Some people are unable to tell between hot and cold by touch.

12. Answer: **B**. Tools used for power require high force. Tools used for precision or accuracy require low force.
    - For double-handled tools (plier-like) used for power tasks: Select a tool with a grip span that is at least 2 inches when fully closed and no more than 3½ inches when fully open. When continuous force is required, consider using a clamp, a grip, or locking pliers.
    - For double-handled tools (plier-like) used for precision tasks: Select a tool with a grip span that is not less than 1 inch when fully closed and no more than 3 inches when fully open.
    - For double-handled pinching, gripping, or cutting tools: Select a tool with handles that are spring-loaded to return the handles to the open position.
    - Select a tool without sharp edges or finger grooves on the handle.
    - Tools with bent handles are better than those with straight handles when the force is applied horizontally (in the same direction as your straight forearm and wrist).
    - Tools with straight handles are better than those with bent handles when the force is applied vertically.
    - Select a tool that can be used with your dominant hand or with either hand.

    DHHS (NIOSH) Publication No. 2004-164. *Easy Ergonomics: A Guide to Selecting Non-Powered Hand Tools*. Retrieved 1/29/2015 http://www.cdc.gov/niosh/docs/2004-164/pdfs/2004-164.pdf

13. Answer: **C**

Type of Control

Type of Control	Workplace Examples
Engineering Controls (implement physical change to the workplace, which eliminates/reduces the hazard on the job/task)	• Use a device to lift and reposition heavy objects to limit force exertion • Reduce the weight of a load to limit force exertion • Reposition a work table to eliminate a long/excessive reach and enable working in neutral postures • Use diverging conveyors off a main line so that tasks are less repetitive • Install diverters on conveyors to direct materials toward the worker to eliminate excessive leaning or reaching • Redesign tools to enable neutral postures

Type of Control	Workplace Examples
Administrative and Work Practice Controls (establish efficient processes or procedures)	• Require that heavy loads are to be lifted by two people, to limit force exertion • Establish systems so workers are rotated away from tasks to minimize the duration of continual exertion, repetitive motions, and awkward postures • Design a job rotation system in which employees rotate between jobs that use different muscle groups • Staff "floaters" to provide periodic breaks between scheduled breaks • Properly use and maintain pneumatic and power tools
Personal Protective Equipment (use protection to reduce exposure to ergonomics-related risk factors)	• Use padding to reduce direct contact with hard, sharp, or vibrating surfaces • Wear well-fitting thermal gloves to help with cold conditions while maintaining the ability to grasp items easily

Solutions to Control Hazards, U.S Department of Labor, Retrieved from https://www.osha.gov/SLTC/ergonomics/controlhazards.html

14. Answer: **A**. Diverters are mechanical barriers that direct the materials on a conveyor or slide to the workers. Diverters are used where excessive leaning or reaching is required to access material on the far side of a conveyor or slide. Delivering and placing parts closer to the worker minimizes reaching and bending. Maximum reach should not exceed arm's length with the torso upright. This can be adjusted to split poultry parts delivery onto either side of a conveyor, slide, or work area so that employees can work on both sides of the line.

15. Answer: **D**. The engineering control of a portable lifting device is the best answer choice in this case. OSHA (2009).

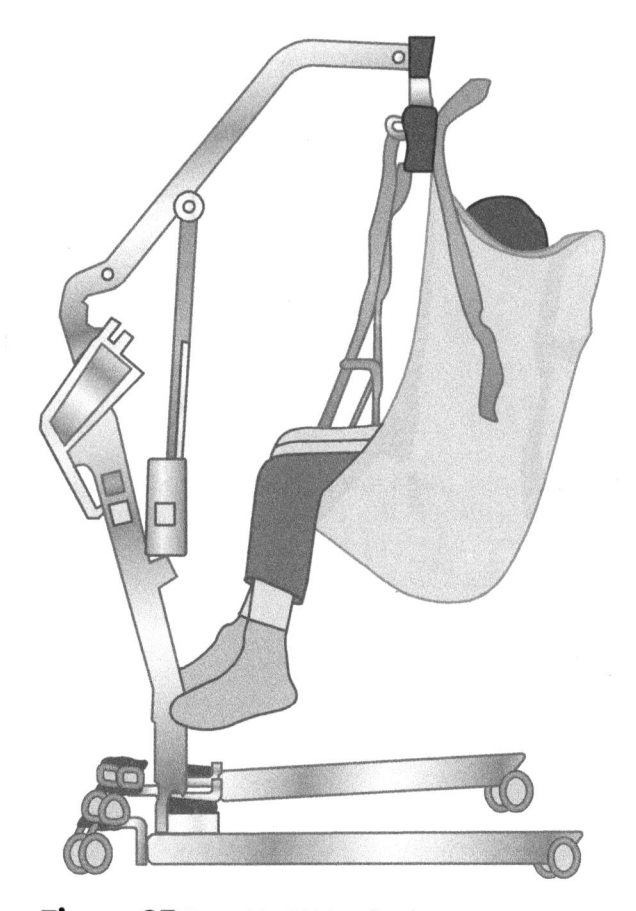

Figure 25 Portable Lifting Device

OSHA Publication 3182 (2009) Guidelines for Nursing Homes Ergonomics for the Prevention of Muscular Skeletal Disorders.

16. Answer: **B**. Musculoskeletal disorder (MSD) risk factors:
    - Force
    - Repetition
    - Awkward postures
    - Static postures
    - Quick motions
    - Compression or contact stress
    - Vibration
    - Cold temperatures

    OSHA (2000)

Table 11 Examples of Musculoskeletal Disorders

Body Parts Affected	Symptoms	Possible Causes	Workers Affected	Disease Name
thumbs	pain at the base of the thumbs	twisting and gripping	butchers, housekeepers, packers, seamstresses, cutters	de Quervain syndrome
fingers	difficulty moving finger; snapping and jerking movements	repeatedly using the index fingers	meatpackers, poultry workers, carpenters, electronic assemblers	trigger finger
shoulders	pain, stiffness	working with the hands above the head	power press operators, welders, painters, assembly line workers	rotator cuff tendinitis
hands, wrists	pain, swelling	repetitive or forceful hand and wrist motions	coremaking, poultry processing, meatpacking	tenosynovitis
fingers, hands	Numbness, tingling; ashen skin; loss of feeling and control	exposure to vibration	chain saw, pneumatic hammer, and gasoline-powered tool operators	Raynaud's syndrome (white finger)
fingers, wrists	tingling, numbness, severe pain; loss of strength, sensation in the thumbs, index, or middle or half of the ring fingers	repetitive and forceful manual tasks without time to recover	meat and poultry and garment workers, upholsterers, assemblers, VDT operators, cashiers	carpal tunnel syndrome
back	low back pain, shooting pain or numbness in the upper legs	whole-body vibration	truck and bus drivers; tractor and subway operators; warehouse workers; nurse's aides; grocery cashiers; baggage handlers	back disability

17. Answer: **D**

    Biomechanical: Calculation of compressive forces at the L5/S1 lumbosacral disc from internal forces of the back-extensor muscles and intra-abdominal pressure used to resist the load moments of lifting

    Physiological: Measures the effect of tasks on body functions (i.e., heart rate, oxygen uptake, etc.)

    Psychophysical: Holds all but one variable constant and allows workers to adjust the variable to their preference

18. Answer: **D**. Although there is not complete agreement on this design principle, most references, including the NSC *Accident Prevention Manual*, suggest that 15° to 25° below horizontal line of sight is the proper placement for video display terminals. This allows the operator to assume a normal head position that develops a slightly lowered sight or viewing angle. This means the video monitor top is placed at eye level to allow proper head and neck position.

19. Answer: **B**

    Anthropometry refers to the measurement of the human individual. Anthropometry involves the systematic measurement of the physical properties of the human body, primarily dimensional descriptors of body size and shape. Today, anthropometry plays an important role in industrial design, clothing design, ergonomics, and architecture, where statistical data about the distribution of body dimensions in the population are used to optimize products. Changes in lifestyles, nutrition, and ethnic composition of populations lead to changes in the distribution of body dimensions (e.g., the obesity epidemic), and require regular updating of anthropometric data collections.

    Kinesiology is a scientific study of human or nonhuman body movement. Kinesiology addresses physiological, biomechanical, and psychological mechanisms of movement. Applications of kinesiology to human health (i.e., **human kinesiology**) include biomechanics and orthopedics; strength and conditioning; sport psychology; methods of rehabilitation, such as physical and occupational therapy; and sport and exercise. Studies of human and animal motion include measures from motion-tracking systems, electrophysiology of muscle and brain activity, various methods for monitoring physiological function, and other behavioral and cognitive research techniques.

    Physiology is the scientific study of the normal function in living systems. A subdiscipline of biology, its focus is how organisms, organ systems, organs, cells, and biomolecules carry out the chemical or physical functions that exist in a living system.

    Ergonomics (human factors), also known as comfort design, functional design, and systems, is the practice of designing products, systems, or processes to take proper account of the interaction between them and the people who use them. It also includes the study of people's efficiency in their working environment. The field has seen contributions from numerous disciplines, such as psychology, engineering, biomechanics, industrial design, physiology, and anthropometry. In essence, it is the study of designing equipment, devices, and processes that fit the human body and its physical and cognitive abilities. The terms *human factors* and *ergonomics* are essentially synonymous.

20. Answer: **B. Musculoskeletal disorders (MSDs)** affect the muscles, nerves, blood vessels, ligaments, and tendons (**Table 11**). Workers in many different industries and occupations can be exposed to risk factors at work, such as lifting heavy items, bending, reaching overhead, pushing and pulling heavy loads, working in awkward body postures, and performing the same or similar tasks repetitively. Exposure to these known risk factors for MSDs increases a worker's risk of injury.

    MSDs are very difficult to define within traditional disease classifications. These disorders have received many names, such as:
    - Repetitive motion injuries
    - Repetitive strain injuries
    - Cumulative trauma disorders
    - Occupational cervicobrachial disorders
    - Overuse syndrome
    - Regional musculoskeletal disorders
    - Soft tissue disorders

    Most of the names do not accurately describe the disorders. For example, the term *repetitive strain injuries* suggests that repetition causes these disorders, but awkward postures also contribute. These terms are used synonymously, but *MSD* is the term is used in current literature.

Work-related MSDs can be prevented. Ergonomics—fitting a job to a person—helps lessen muscle fatigue, increases productivity, and reduces the number and severity of work-related MSDs. Examples of musculoskeletal disorders (MSDs) are:

- Carpal tunnel syndrome
- Tendinitis
- Rotator cuff injuries (affects the shoulder)
- Epicondylitis (affects the elbow)
- Trigger finger
- Muscle strains and low back injuries

The Bureau of Labor Statistics (BLS) defines musculoskeletal disorders (MSDs) to include cases where the nature of the injury or illness is pinched nerve; herniated disc; meniscus tear; sprains, strains, tears; hernia (traumatic and nontraumatic); pain, swelling, and numbness; carpal or tarsal tunnel syndrome; Raynaud's syndrome or phenomenon; musculoskeletal system and connective tissue diseases and disorders, when the event or exposure leading to the injury or illness is overexertion and bodily reaction, unspecified; overexertion involving outside sources; repetitive motion involving microtasks; other and multiple exertions or bodily reactions; and body parts being rubbed, abraded, or jarred by vibration.

The risk of MSD injury depends on work positions and postures, how often the task is performed, the level of required effort, and how long the task lasts. Risk factors that may lead to the development of MSDs include:

- **Exerting excessive force**. Lifting heavy objects or people, pushing or pulling heavy loads, manually pouring materials, or maintaining control of equipment or tools
- **Performing the same or similar tasks repetitively**. Performing the same motion or series of motions continually or frequently for an extended period of time
- **Working in awkward postures or being in the same posture for long periods of time**. Using positions that place stress on the body, such as prolonged or repetitive reaching above shoulder height, kneeling, squatting, leaning over a counter, using a knife with wrists bent, or twisting the torso while lifting
- **Localized pressure into the body part**. Pressing the body or part of the body (such as the hand) against hard or sharp edges, or using the hand as a hammer
- **Cold temperatures**. In combination with any one of the above risk factors, cold temperatures may also increase the potential for MSDs to develop. For example, many of the operations in meatpacking and poultry processing occur with a chilled product or in a cold environment.
- **Vibration**. Vibration, both whole body and in the hand and/or arm, can cause a number of health effects. Hand/arm vibration can damage small capillaries that supply nutrients and can make hand tools more difficult to control. Hand/arm vibration may cause a worker to lose feeling in the hands and arms, resulting in increased force exertion to control hand-powered tools (e.g., hammer drills, portable grinders, chainsaws), in much the same way that gloves limit feeling in the hands. The effects of vibration can damage the body and greatly increase the force that must be exerted for a task.
- **Combined exposure to several risk factors**. May place workers at a higher risk for MSDs than does exposure to any one risk factor

To reduce the chance of injury, work tasks should be designed to limit exposure to ergonomic risk factors. Engineering controls are the most desirable, where possible. Administrative or work practice controls may be appropriate in cases in which engineering controls cannot be implemented, or when different procedures are needed after implementation of the new engineering controls. Personal protection solutions have only limited effectiveness when dealing with ergonomic hazards. **Chronic wasting disease (CWD)** is a transmissible spongiform encephalopathy (TSE) of mule deer, white-tailed deer, elk, and moose. As of 2016, CWD had only been found in members of the deer family. CWD is typified by chronic weight loss leading to death. No relationship is known between CWD and any other TSE of animals or people. Although reports in the popular press have been made of humans being affected by CWD, a study by the Centers for Disease Control and Prevention suggests, "[m]ore epidemiologic and laboratory studies are needed to monitor the possibility of such transmissions." The epidemiological study further concluded, "[a]s a precaution, hunters should avoid eating deer and elk tissues known to harbor the CWD agent (e.g., brain, spinal cord, eyes, spleen, tonsils, lymph nodes) from areas where CWD has been identified."

21. Answer: **C**. Hand controls are far more widely used than foot controls. Generally, the feet are slower and less accurate. Although color may help an operator identify the correct foot pedal in some cases, the color would not affect the performance. Another factor would be the placement of the control relative to the user.

22. Answer: **A**. **Abduction** is defined as movement away from the central axis of the body—away from the median plane. **Flexion** is movement that decreases the angle between two adjacent bones. **Extension** is movement that increases the angle between two adjacent bones. **Adduction** is defined as movement toward the central axis or midline; it is the opposite of abduction.

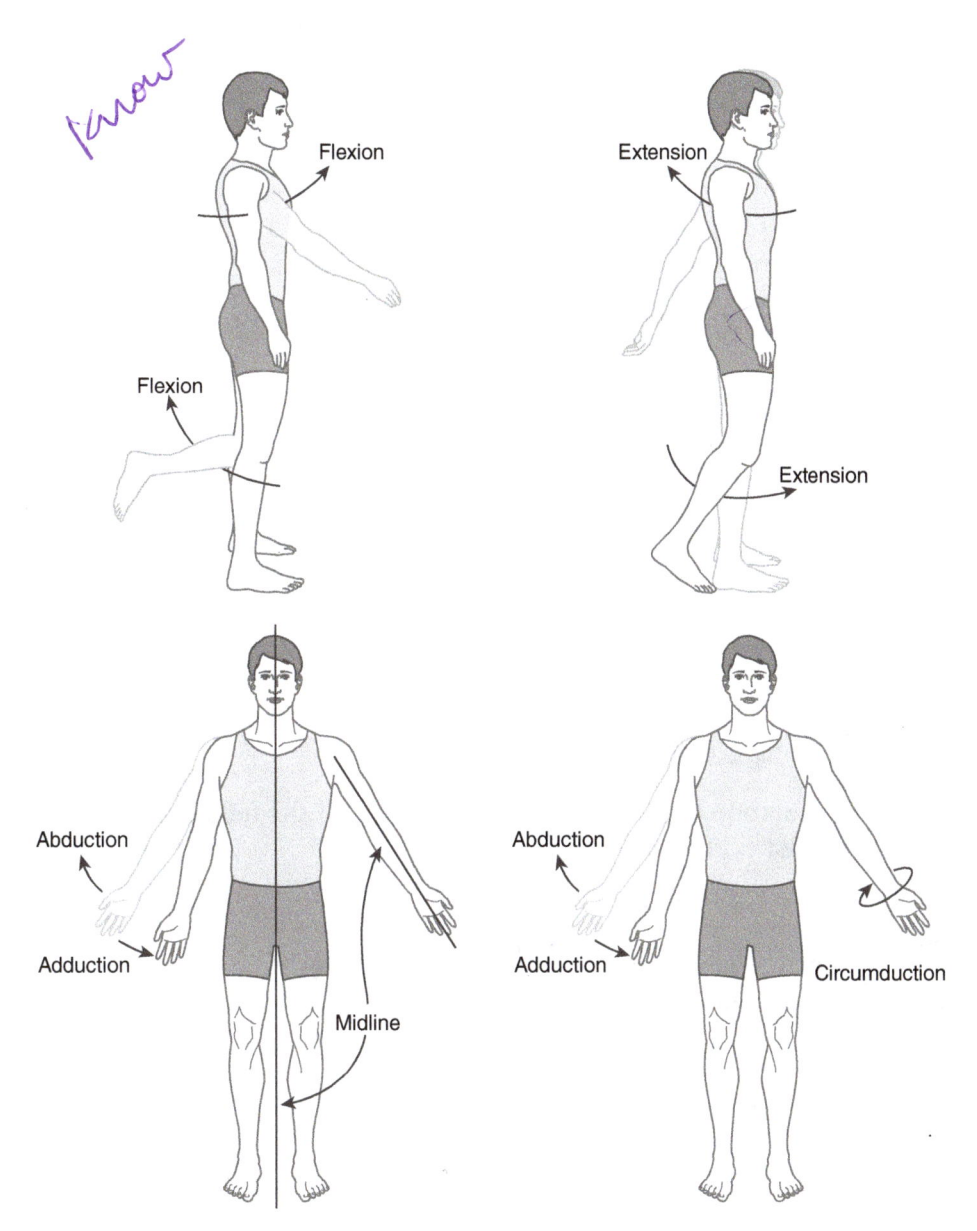

Figure 26 Defining Movement

23. Answer: **D**. The carpal tunnel, or carpal canal, is the passageway on the palmar side of the wrist that connects the forearm to the middle compartment of the palm. The tunnel consists of bones and connective tissue. Several tendons and the median nerve pass through it.

Domain 4: Fire Prevention and Protection

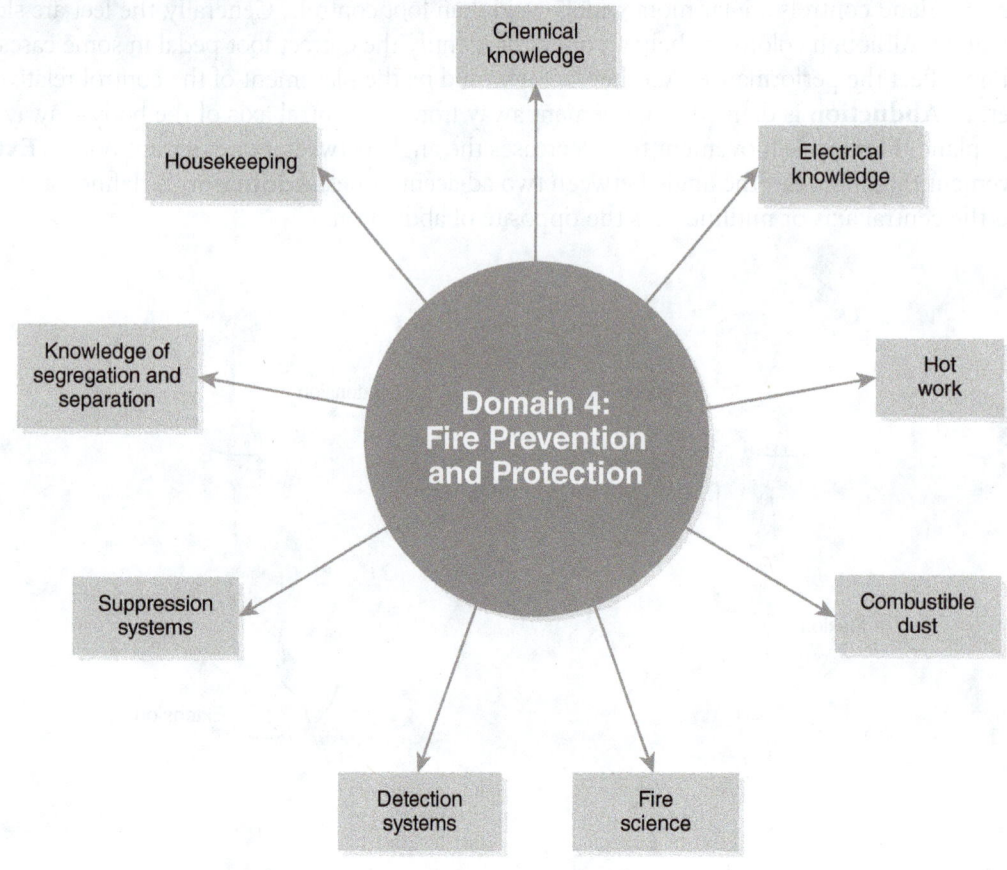

Modified from ASP® Exam Blueprint (ASP10), November 10, 2019

Domain 4 Quiz 1 Questions

1. During a workplace evaluation for combustible dust, which of the following is of least importance in the prevention of a dust explosion?

    A. A documented process hazard analysis and operator training
    B. Physical and chemical properties that establish hazardous characteristics of materials used in a facility
    C. Housekeeping and predictive/preventative maintenance programs
    D. Properly installed and operational sprinkler systems

2. Which term best describes a subsonic explosion?

    A. Propagation
    B. Detonation
    C. Deflagration
    D. Auto ignition

3. In coal mining, overexposure to respirable coal mine dust can lead to coal workers' pneumoconiosis (CWP), a lung disease that can be disabling—and fatal in its most severe form. The best protective measure to control respirable coal dust during long-wall mining shearer operations is:

    A. face ventilation.
    B. drum-mounted water sprays.
    C. cutting drum bit maintenance.
    D. directional water spray systems.

4. A type of protective signaling (fire alarm) system that does not notify the local fire department in the event of an alarm condition is:

   A. auxiliary.
   B. remote.
   C. local.
   D. proprietary.

5. A paint spray booth operation, according to OSHA, should provide enough dilution air to reduce the vapor of flammable materials to ____ of the lower explosive limit.

   A. 10%
   B. 15%
   C. 20%
   D. 25%

6. When welding immovable objects in an area with a fire hazard, which action is least appropriate?

   A. Suitable fire-extinguishing equipment shall be maintained nearby in a state of readiness.
   B. All movable objects must be covered with a fire-resistive material.
   C. Whenever there are floor openings or cracks in flooring that cannot be closed, precautions shall be taken so that no readily combustible materials on the floor below shall be exposed to sparks potentially dropping through the floor.
   D. Before cutting or welding is permitted, the area shall be inspected by the individual responsible for authorizing cutting and welding operations by means of a written permit.

7. Flammable inside storage locations must be provided with all of the following except:

   A. a clear aisle at least 22 inches wide.
   B. a raised 4-inch sill.
   C. self-closing fire doors.
   D. either a gravity or a mechanical exhaust system.

8. An overcurrent device is best defined as a/an:

   A. electrical capacitor, with discharge resistor.
   B. step-up transformer.
   C. pendant push-button control station, with metal messenger.
   D. expulsion fuse.

9. Which of the following is not an oxidizer?

   A. Fluorine
   B. Hydrazine
   C. Potassium permanganate
   D. Hydrogen peroxide

10. Water is immediately available in sprinkler piping in a wet pipe system in the event of fire. The sprinkler head fuse is melted by heat from the fire and water is delivered to control or extinguish the ensuing fire. In a pre-action fire sprinkler system:

    A. air under pressure is maintained in the system piping.
    B. piping includes open sprinklers.
    C. the building occupant manually opens a deluge valve.
    D. sprinkler heads are connected to a rate-of-rise detector that assures a dual fault tolerance.

112 ASP Exam Study Workbook

11. **The NFPA identifies a combustible liquid as one having a flash point:**
    A. at or above 140°F.
    B. at or above 100°F.
    C. at or above 200°F.
    D. at or below 70°F.

12. **An inspector checklist for a dry pipe sprinkler system requires opening the inspector test valve and timing the delay between valve opening and water discharge. NFPA 13 requires that dry systems must deliver water to the inspector test pipe outlet within:**
    A. 3 minutes.
    B. 15 seconds.
    C. 1 minute.
    D. 30 seconds.

13. **The three distinct parts of a "means of egress" include:**
    A. exit access, exit, and exit discharge.
    B. door, passageway, and ramps.
    C. door opening device, door, and exit light.
    D. horizontal exits, stairs, and ramps.

14. **NFPA 101, *Life Safety Code*, requires emergency lighting to illuminate the means of egress in some occupancies (places of assembly, educational buildings, healthcare facilities, etc.). When required, these lights must provide not less than 1 foot-candle for a period of 1½ hours if the normal lighting fails. What are the periodic testing requirements for these lights?**
    A. A 30-second functional test every 30 days and a 1½-hour test annually
    B. A 30-second functional test monthly
    C. A 5-minute functional test every 30 days and a 1½-hour test annually
    D. A 1½-hour functional test annually

15. **Building sprinklers systems often do not pass the inspection criteria due to:**
    A. broken water pipes.
    B. a closed post-indicator valve (PIV).
    C. electrical failure.
    D. lack of pressure.

16. **One example of a "Class A" incident includes a fire involving:**
    A. ordinary combustibles.
    B. flammable liquids.
    C. combustible metals.
    D. live electrical equipment.

17. **The forklift truck primarily recommended for use in an area that contains a flammable vapor is one with fuel that is:**
    A. electric.
    B. diesel.
    C. LP gas.
    D. gasoline.

18. What should SH&E professionals consider when evaluating ignition sources such as lift trucks and information technology equipment?
    A. Electrical machines
    B. Dust-producing processes
    C. Class IV forklifts
    D. Several potential ignition sources

19. What provides the best protection when transferring an extremely flammable liquid from a 55-gallon drum via a hand pump to a small metal safety can?
    A. Ground both containers.
    B. Bond containers together.
    C. Bond containers together and ground each to a separate low-resistance ground.
    D. Ground each container to a single low-resistance ground and then bond them to each other.

20. Fuel and oxygen cylinders in storage locations must be separated by a minimum distance, or a firewall must be provided. If a firewall is provided, the fire-resistance rating of the wall must be at least:
    A. ½ hour.
    B. 1 hour.
    C. 2 hours.
    D. 3 hours.

Domain 4 Quiz 1 Answers

1. Answer: **D**. Sprinkler systems and distance to a means of egress are examples of loss reduction, not loss prevention. A dust explosion involves determining the actual hazard, as well as the manufacturing process that led to high dust concentration levels. Safety professionals should be thoroughly familiar with processes and facilities that handle combustible particulate solids in a facility. They also should be familiar with physical and chemical properties that establish hazardous characteristics of materials used in a facility. The facility should have a documented process hazard analysis, and SH&E professionals should be familiar with hazards identified in the study. A management of change program should be implemented. Also, SH&E professionals should be familiar with the NFPA standards that apply to a facility. One obvious item to assess is housekeeping. Poor housekeeping may lead to accumulations of dust on machinery and building structural members. SH&E professionals should also identify hidden areas that may not be obvious while standing at the floor level. Other areas, such as spaces above drop ceilings and around ductwork junctions and gates, should be inspected. Dust can accumulate on elevated building and equipment members. In the event of an initial ignition, the shock wave may shake this accumulation, creating another dust cloud and another potentially greater ignition that can shake even more dust from the elevated members, setting up a chain reaction. Process equipment should be designed for the operation in which it is used. Typically, initial installation of a process incorporates several features to help mitigate a fire or deflagration. These may include explosion vents on machines and/or buildings. It may be a fast-acting explosion suppression system. Gates and dampers may be installed inside of ductwork or equipment. Each device should be inspected and tested regularly, with documentation created to record and verify its condition. Conductive components should be grounded and bonded. Training is another important aspect of a dust hazard mitigation program. Operators should be trained on the equipment's operation and maintenance and on emergency plans to follow. Initial as well as refresher training should be provided, and training records should be maintained.

    According to **Hazard Communication Guidance for Combustible Dusts** OSHA 3371-08 200, Five elements are necessary to initiate a dust explosion, often referred to as the "Dust Explosion Pentagon."[2] The first three elements are those needed for a fire (i.e., the familiar "fire triangle"):
    1. Combustible dust (fuel);
    2. Ignition source (heat); and

3. Oxygen in air (oxidizer).

   An additional two elements must be present for a combustible dust explosion:
4. Dispersion of dust particles in sufficient quantity and concentration; and
5. Confinement of the dust cloud.

   If one of the above five elements is missing, an explosion cannot occur.

2. Answer: **C**. *Deflagration* is a term describing subsonic combustion propagating through heat transfer; hot burning material heats the next layer of cold material and ignites it. Most "fire" found in daily life, from flames to explosions, is deflagration. Deflagration is a rapid, high-energy-release combustion event that propagates through a gas or an explosive material at subsonic speeds, driven by the transfer of heat. Deflagration is different from detonation, which is supersonic and propagates through shock. Deflagration to detonation transition refers to a phenomenon in ignitable mixtures of a flammable gas and air (or oxygen) when a sudden transition takes place from a deflagration type of combustion to a detonation type of combustion. In its most benign form, a deflagration may simply be a flash fire. In contrast, detonation is characterized by supersonic flame propagation velocities, perhaps up to 2000 m/s, and substantial overpressures, up to 20 bars. Under certain conditions, mainly in terms of geometrical conditions such as partial confinement and many obstacles in the flame path that cause turbulent flame eddy currents, a subsonic flame may accelerate to supersonic speed, transitioning from deflagration to detonation.

3. Answer: **A**. Historically, longwall operations have had difficulty in maintaining consistent compliance with the federal dust standard of 2.0 mg/m^3. On most longwall faces, the shearer cutting action is the primary dust source and the largest contributor to respirable dust exposure of face personnel.

   Face ventilation: As with all mining methods, ventilation is the primary means to dilute liberated methane to safe levels. It is also the principal method of controlling respirable dust on the longwall face. Providing adequate amounts of air to dilute and carry airborne dust down the face and prevent it from migrating into the walkway has been and continues to be a goal for longwall operators.

   Drum-mounted water sprays: Drum-mounted water sprays apply water for dust suppression directly at the point of coal fracture and add moisture to the product to minimize dust liberation during coal transport. Although very effective at minimizing dust generation at the point of coal fracture, shearer drum water sprays can actually increase airborne respirable dust levels if operated at water pressures that are too high.

   Cutting drum bit maintenance: Previous research has shown that bits with large carbide inserts and a smooth transition between the steel shank and the carbide reduce dust levels. Prompt replacement of damaged, worn, or missing bits is crucial. A dull bit rubs against the coal, which results in an ineffective use of available cutting force and the inability to penetrate the coal at designed rates. This results in shallow cutting, which greatly increases dust generation.

   Directional water spray systems: Water sprays can be very efficient air movers and, if applied properly, can be used to augment the primary airflow and reduce the amount of shearer-generated dust that migrates into the walkway near the shearer. Water sprays mounted on the shearer body act very much like small fans, moving air and entraining dust in the direction of their orientation. Poorly designed shearer-mounted spray systems with nozzles directed upwind at the cutting drums actually force dust away from the face, where it mixes with clean intake air and is carried out into the walkway over shearer operators.

4. Answer: **C**. The *local* fire alarm system is intended to warn local residents and usually only sounds an evacuation alarm. It does not normally ring in the fire protection service. The *auxiliary* system is a local alarm with the added feature of a circuit to the municipal fire alarm system (usually through a local master alarm box). The *remote* alarm system sends a signal to a remote location (usually staffed 24 hours per day) that in turn notifies the local fire protection agency. The *proprietary* system is widely used in commercial occupancies. The term *proprietary* indicates that the alarm is received by someone with proprietary interest in the property as well as by the fire department. This system, coupled with a central alarm, can allow on-site activation of protections such as closing of doors, adjusting vents for smoke control, control of elevators, start-up of ventilators, etc.

5. Answer: **D**. OSHA at 1910.94(c)(6)(ii) states "The total air volume exhausted through a spray booth shall be such as to dilute solvent vapor to at least 25% of the lower explosive limit of the solvent being sprayed." The standard gives an example of calculation for a typical solvent.
6. Answer: **B**. According to 1910.252, if an object to be welded or cut cannot be readily moved, all movable fire hazards in the vicinity shall be taken to a safe place.
7. Answer: **A**. Storage within inside storage rooms must normally comply with NFPA 30, which requires that every inside storage room be equipped with one clear aisle at least 3 feet wide, not 22 inches as specified in answer selection A. The standard also requires a raised 4-inch sill to prevent runoff of any spilled material, self-closing fire doors, and some type of exhaust system.

    The minimum width of an exit access in most new business construction is 36 inches.
8. Answer: **D**. The basic overcurrent devices are the fuse and circuit breaker. They should be installed in every circuit to interrupt the current flow when it exceeds the safe capacity of the conductors. Expulsion fuses are intended for use in central distribution stations, in generation plants, or on overhead lines, and are designed such that when they blow, the gases generated aid in quenching the arc.
9. Answer: **B**. Oxidizing agents generally are recognizable by their structures or names. They tend to have a high oxygen ratio in their structures and sometimes release oxygen as a result of thermal decomposition. Oxidizing agents often have *per* prefixes (perchlorate, peroxides, and permanganate) and end in *-ate* (chromate, nitrate, chlorate). Strong oxidizers have more potential incompatibilities than perhaps any other chemical group (with the possible exception of water-reactive substances). Oxidizers should not be stored or mixed with any other material except under carefully controlled conditions. Storing oxidizing and reducing agents where they could mix can be a recipe for disaster. Common oxidizing agents listed in decreasing order of oxidizing strength include:
    - Fluorine
    - Chlorine
    - Ozone
    - Sulfuric acid (concentrated)
    - Hydrogen peroxide
    - Oxygen
    - Perchloric acid (concentrated)
    - Hypochlorous acid
    - Metallic iodates
    - Metal chlorates
    - Bromine
    - Lead dioxide
    - Ferric (iron +3) salts
    - Metallic permanganates
    - Iodine
    - Metallic dichromates
    - Sulfur
    - Nitric acid (concentrated)
    - Stannic (tin +4) salts
10. Answer: **A**. In a pre-action fire sprinkler system, system piping is pressurized. The piping is charged through the activation of supplemental detection systems located in the same area as the sprinklers. Water is then free to flow through the piping to sprinkler heads. If a sprinkler head has fused (through heat from a fire), water will be delivered to the fire. Pre-action systems are used when there is a danger of serious water damage to the protected area. Calcium carbide combines with water to create the corrosive calcium hydroxide and liberates acetylene (ethyne). Therefore, it is not recommended to use a water system with calcium carbide.

11. Answer: **B**

FLAMMABLE		
CLASS	Boiling Point	Flash Point
I		below 100°F
IA	below 100°F	below 73°F
IB	at or above 100°F	below 73°F
IC		at or above 73°F and below 100°F

COMBUSTIBLE		
II		at or above 100°F and below 140°F
III		at or above 140°F
IIIA		at or above 140°F and below 200°F
IIIB		at or above 200°F

12. Answer: **C**. NFPA 13 establishes the maximum size for dry pipe systems at 500 gallons for gridded systems and 750 gallons for nongridded systems. However, these maximums can be exceeded if delivery of water to inspectors' test pipe does not exceed 60 seconds. Many times, to ensure rapid delivery of water, *quick opening* devices are installed. These devices generally consist of accelerators, which cause the deluge or dry pipe valve to cycle more rapidly, or exhausters, which dump air more rapidly.

13. Answer: **A**. NFPA 101, Life Safety Code, states, "A means of egress is a continuous and unobstructed way of exit travel from any point in a building or structure to a public way and consists of three separate and distinct parts: (a) the exit access, (b) the exit, and (c) the exit discharge. A means of egress comprises the vertical and horizontal travel and shall include intervening room spaces, doorways, hallways, corridors, passageways, balconies, ramps, stairs, enclosures, lobbies, escalators, horizontal exits, courts, and yards."

14. Answer: **A**. NFPA 101, Chapter 31, states that a functional test shall be conducted on every required emergency lighting system at 30-day intervals for a minimum of 30 seconds. An annual test shall be conducted for the 1½-hour duration. Equipment shall be fully operational for the duration of the test. Written records of visual inspections and tests shall be kept by the owner for inspection by the authority having jurisdiction.

    Exception:
    Self-testing/self-diagnostic, battery-operated emergency lighting equipment that automatically performs a minimum 30-second test and diagnostic routine at least once every 30 days and indicates failure by a status indicator shall be exempt from the 30-day functional test, provided a visual inspection is performed at 30-day intervals.

15. Answer: **B**. The most common cause of building sprinkler system failure is that someone has closed the post-indicator valve (PIV) and failed to reopen it.

16. Answer: **A**. Class A fires involve ordinary combustibles. Class B fires involve flammable or combustible liquids. Class C fires involve live electrical equipment. Class D fires involve combustible metals. Examples of Class A extinguishing agents are monoammonium phosphate and ammonium phosphate.

17. Answer: **A**. According to 29CFR1910.178, the electric forklift is the only forklift truck authorized in certain flammable atmospheres.

18. Answer: **D**. Several ignition sources can cause a dust explosion or deflagration. Primary sources of ignition include electrical sparking from tramp metals or broken equipment pieces; heat from bearings, belts, and

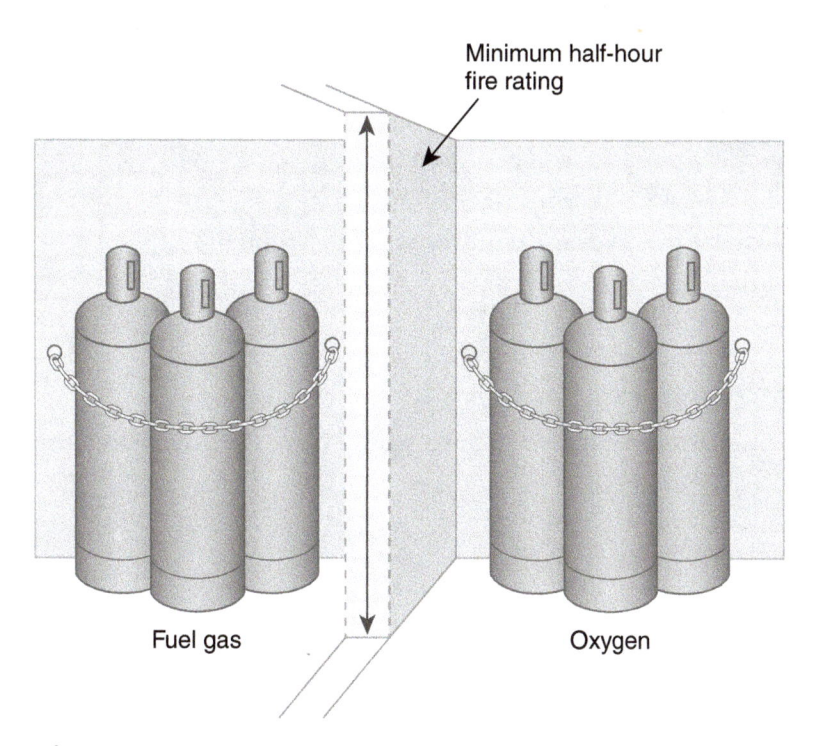

Figure 27 Fire resistance rating of a firewall

misaligned buckets; improperly prepared maintenance and hot work operations; forklifts and vehicles; and natural causes, such as lightning.

First, identify the electrical classification of the area or room volume. NFPA 70, the National Electrical Code (NEC), Chapter 5, Special Occupancies, addresses hazardous locations. It defines the classification of several special occupancies, such as flammable liquids, gases, and vapors; combustible dusts; and other materials. It is meant to integrate with other NFPA standards that more fully address the particular occupancy.

For electrical issues, the NEC defines what electrical devices are permitted in a given area. This section defines terms such as dust ignition-proof, dust tight, purged, and pressurized.

19. Answer: **D**. *Bonding* is the process of connecting two or more conductive objects together by means of a conductor to minimize the potential electrical difference between them. *Grounding* is the process of connecting the conductive object to the ground, and is a specific type of bonding. A conductive object may also be grounded by bonding it to another conductive object that is already connected to the ground. Bonding minimizes potential differences between conductive objects. Grounding minimizes potential differences between conductive objects and the ground. The purpose of grounding or bonding in this question is to ensure that there are no potential differences between the containers and earth ground; therefore, all objects must be connected to the same grounding point and bonded together. Alternatively, the same objective could be accomplished by insulating the drum and can from earth ground and then bonding the drum to the can.

20. Answer: **A**. Firewalls separating fuel and oxygen cylinders must have at least a 30-minute rating and be at least 5 feet high. Fuel and oxidizers can also be segregated by 20 feet as per OSHA and NFPA.

Domain 4 Quiz 2 Questions

1. An electrical conduit that is very warm to the touch is discovered during an industrial safety inspection. Which of the following descriptions best fits this condition?

   A. The conduit is hot with electric energy due to a ground fault.
   B. Conduits are always warm to the touch.
   C. The conduit is likely absorbing radiant heat from the furnace.
   D. The conduit likely contains overloaded electrical wiring.

2. Flow testing an industrial fire hydrant requires what instrument?

   A. Pitot tube with gauge
   B. Aneroid with gauge
   C. Magnehelic gauge
   D. Burdon gauge with pickup tube

3. Which of the following groups of hydrocarbons would have the greatest chance of not being flammable?

   A. Aliphatic hydrocarbons
   B. Aromatic hydrocarbons
   C. Halogenated hydrocarbons
   D. Ethers

4. Flash point is defined as the _____ temperature that will produce a vapor concentration high enough to propagate a flame when a source of ignition is present.

   A. lowest
   B. highest
   C. normal
   D. absolute

5. The term *dry chemical* fire-extinguishing agent is associated with flammable liquids. What material is the term *dry powder* associated with?

   A. Electrical insulation
   B. Exotic chemicals
   C. Metals
   D. Fibers

6. Which will not leave a residue?

   A. CO_2 extinguisher
   B. Chemical extinguisher
   C. AFFF
   D. Dry chemical

7. Responders to a fire involving a propane tank would want to prevent a BLEVE, which is an acronym for:

   A. Burning Liquid Expanding Vapor Explosion.
   B. Boiling Liquid Expanding Vapor Explosion.
   C. Burning Liquid Elevated Volume Expansion.
   D. Boiling Liquid Exacerbated Volume Expansion.

8. Which is not a particulate?

   A. Fume
   B. Mist
   C. Gas
   D. Smoke

9. Static electricity is best described as:

   A. low current with low voltage.
   B. low voltage with high current.
   C. high voltage with low current.
   D. high voltage with high current.

10. GFCI operates on sensing leakage of:

    A. resistance.
    B. current.
    C. ohms.
    D. watts.

11. Which is an example of panic hardware?

    A. Emergency escape windows from a high-rise building
    B. Delayed egress locks
    C. Magnetic deadbolts
    D. Breakaway bars on doors

12. The fire tetrahedron states that combustion requires an oxidizer, fuel, heat, and which of the following?

    A. Confinement
    B. Surface area
    C. A chain reaction
    D. Deflagration

13. The five (5) categories of Weapons of Mass Destruction (WMD) are commonly referred to as CBRNE, which is an acronym for:

    A. chemical, biological, radiological, nuclear, and explosive.
    B. corrosive, bacterial, reflexive, nuclear, and energetic.
    C. chemical, bacterial, respiratory, neurological, and explosive.
    D. corrosive, biological, radiation, neurological, and explosive.

14. A chemical explosion requires an oxidizer, fuel, an ignition source, and which of the following?

    A. Overpressure
    B. Confinement
    C. Reduction
    D. Detonation

15. The characterization of a Class II, Division 2 location, according to the National Electrical Code, is:

    A. a site where flammable or combustible vapors may be present in sufficient quantities to be hazardous.
    B. a place where combustible dust is normally present in adequate quantities to be hazardous.
    C. a scene where flammable or combustible vapors are not normally present, but could be, due to atypical or intermittent operations.
    D. a location where combustible dust is not normally present, but has the potential to be, due to abnormal or periodic operations.

Domain 4 Quiz 2 Answers

1. Answer: **D**. One of the most common causes of electrically created fires is overheated wiring because of overloading. Many factors contribute to a safe installation. The wire must be sized (correct gauge) properly to handle the current. Overcurrent protection (fuses or circuit breakers) must also be correctly sized and function properly. Additionally, electrical raceways must not be overloaded with electrical wiring. The sizing of wiring and the amount of wiring allowed for a given size of raceway is strictly regulated in the National Electrical Code. Generally, conduit will not feel hot to the touch even under severe circuit loading if installed according to code.
2. Answer: **A**. A pitot tube equipped with a gauge could be used for flow testing water.
3. Answer: **C**. *Hydrocarbons* are compounds that contain atoms of carbon and hydrogen only. They are broadly classified into two types: aliphatic and aromatic. *Aliphatic hydrocarbons* are subdivided into saturated and unsaturated compounds and include the alkanes: methane, ethane, propane, and butane. *Aromatic hydrocarbons* are derivative of the parent compound benzene. *Ethers* are members of a class of organic compounds in which an oxygen atom has bridged between two hydrocarbon groups. Aliphatic ethers are highly volatile and extremely flammable. Hydrocarbons that have been partially halogenated burn, but generally with much less ease than their nonhalogenated analogs. The fully *halogenated* derivatives such as carbon tetrachloride are noncombustible.
4. Answer: **A**. The flash point of a liquid corresponds roughly to the lowest temperature at which the vapor pressure of the liquid is just sufficient to produce a flammable mixture at the lower limit of flammability. (Reference: National Fire Protection Association, *Fire Protection Handbook*.)
5. Answer: **C**. The designation "dry powder" has been especially chosen to indicate an agent's suitability for use on Class D (combustible metal) fires. The term "dry chemical" is reserved for agents effective on A:B:C or B:C fires.
6. Answer: **A**
   - **Halons, halon-replacement clean agents,** and **carbon dioxide agents** extinguish fire by displacing oxygen (CO_2 or inert gases), removing heat from the combustion zone, or inhibiting the chemical chain reaction (halons). They are referred to as clean agents because they do not leave any residue after discharge, which is ideal for protecting sensitive electronics, aircraft, armored vehicles, archival storage, museums, and valuable documents.
     - Halons are gaseous agents that inhibit the chemical reaction of the fire in Classes B:C and A:B:C, depending on the type. Halon gases were banned from new production under the Montreal Protocol as of January 1, 1994, as their properties contribute to ozone depletion and they have a long atmospheric lifetime, usually 400 years. The industry has moved to halon alternatives. Nevertheless, halon 1211 is still vital to certain military and industrial users, so there is a need for it.
     - Halocarbon replacements, HCFCs, were approved by the FAA for use in aircraft cabins in 2010. Considerations for halon replacement include human toxicity when used in confined spaces, ozone-depleting potential, and greenhouse warming potential.
     - Carbon dioxide (CO_2) is a clean gaseous agent that displaces oxygen to extinguish Class B:C fires. It is not intended for Class A fires, as the high-pressure cloud of gas can scatter burning materials. CO_2 is not suitable for use on fires containing their own oxygen source, metals, or cooking media.
   - **Dry powder** constitutes several available Class D fire extinguisher agents; some will handle multiple types of metals, others will not.
     - Sodium chloride contains sodium chloride salt, which melts to form an oxygen-excluding crust over the metal. A thermoplastic additive such as nylon is added to allow the salt to more readily form a cohesive crust over the burning metal. It is useful on most alkali metals, including sodium and potassium, and other metals including magnesium, titanium, aluminum, and zirconium.

- Copper-based dry powder was developed for hard-to-control lithium and lithium-alloy fires. The powder smothers and acts as a heat sink to dissipate heat, but also forms a copper-lithium alloy on the surface, which is noncombustible and cuts off the oxygen supply. It will cling to a vertical surface. It is used for lithium only.
- Graphite-based powder contains dry graphite that smothers burning metals. The first type developed, designed for magnesium, works on other metals as well. Unlike sodium chloride powder extinguishers, the graphite powder fire extinguishers can be used on very hot burning metal fires such as lithium, but unlike copper powder extinguishers, will not stick to and extinguish flowing or vertical lithium fires. Like copper extinguishers, the graphite powder acts as a heat sink as well as smothering the metal fire.
- Sodium carbonate–based powder is used where stainless steel piping and equipment could be damaged by sodium chloride–based agents to control sodium, potassium, and sodium–potassium alloy fires. It has limited use on other metals. It smothers the metal fire and forms a crust.

	Fire Type			
Extinguishing Agent	**Ordinary Solid Materials**	**Flammable Liquids**	**Electrical Equipment**	**Combustible Metals**
	Water Foam • Removes heat • Removes air and heat	Foam CO_2 • Removes air	CO_2 • Removes air	Special Agents • Usually removes air
	Dry chemical • Breaks chain reaction	Dry chemical halon • Breaks chain reaction	Dry chemical halon • Breaks chain reaction	

Figure 28 Types of Portable Fire Extinguishers

- **Dry chemical** is a powder-based agent that extinguishes by separating the four parts of the fire tetrahedron. It prevents the chemical reactions involving heat, fuel, and oxygen (combustion), thus extinguishing the fire. During combustion, the fuel breaks down into free radicals, which are highly reactive fragments of molecules that react with oxygen. The substances in dry chemical extinguishers can stop this process.
  - Monoammonium phosphate, also known as *tri-class*, *multipurpose*, or *ABC* dry chemical, is used on Class A, B, and C fires. It receives its Class A rating from the agent's ability to melt and flow to smother the fire.
  - Sodium bicarbonate, *regular* or *ordinary*, is used on Class B and C fires. In the heat of a fire, it releases a cloud of carbon dioxide that smothers the fire. That is, the gas drives oxygen away from the fire, thus stopping the chemical reaction. This agent is not generally effective on Class A fires because the agent is expended and the cloud of gas dissipates quickly, and if the fuel is still sufficiently hot, the fire starts up again.
  - Potassium bicarbonate (the principal constituent of Purple-K) is used on Class B and C fires. About twice as effective on Class B fires as sodium bicarbonate, it is the preferred dry chemical agent of the oil and gas industry. It is the only dry chemical agent certified for use in aircraft rescue and firefighting (ARFF) by the NFPA. It is colored violet to distinguish it.
  - Potassium bicarbonate and urea complex is used on Class B and C fires. It is more effective than all other powders due to its ability to decrepitate (where the powder breaks up into smaller particles) in the flame zone, creating a larger surface area for free radical inhibition.
  - MET-L-KYL/PYROKYL is a specialty variation of sodium bicarbonate for fighting pyrophoric (ignites on contact with air) liquid fires. In addition to sodium bicarbonate, it also contains silica gel particles. The sodium bicarbonate interrupts the chain reaction of the fuel and the silica soaks up any unburned fuel, preventing contact with air. It is effective on other Class B fuels, as well.

- **Foams** are applied to fuel fires as either an aspirated (mixed and expanded with air in a branch pipe) or nonaspirated form to create a frothy blanket or seal over the fuel, preventing oxygen reaching it. Unlike powder, foam can be used to progressively extinguish fires without flashback.
  - An aqueous film-forming foam (AFFF), used on Class A and B fires and for vapor suppression, is the most common type of portable foam extinguisher. Alcohol-resistant aqueous film-forming foams (AR-AFFF) are used on fuel fires containing alcohol; they form a membrane between the fuel and the foam, preventing the alcohol from breaking down the foam blanket.
  - Film-forming fluoroprotein (FFFP) contains naturally occurring proteins from animal by-products and synthetic film-forming agents to create a foam blanket that is more heat resistant than the strictly synthetic AFFF foams. FFFP works well on alcohol-based liquids and is used widely in motorsports.
  - Compressed air foam system (CAFS) extinguishers differ from standard stored-pressure premix foam extinguishers in that they operate at a higher pressure of 140 psi, aerate the foam with an attached compressed gas cylinder instead of an air-aspirating nozzle, and use a drier foam solution with a higher concentrate-to-water ratio. They are generally used to extend a water supply in wildland operations. The are used on Class A fires and with very dry foam on Class B fires for vapor suppression.
  - Arctic Fire is a liquid fire-extinguishing agent that emulsifies and cools heated materials more quickly than water or ordinary foam. It is used extensively in the steel industry. It is effective on Class A, B, and D fires.
- **Wet chemical** (potassium acetate, potassium carbonate, or potassium citrate) extinguishes the fire by forming an air-excluding soapy foam blanket over the burning oil through the chemical process of saponification (an alkali reacting with a fat to form a soap) and by the water content cooling the oil below its ignition temperature. It is generally used on Class A and K fires.
- **Water-type extinguishers** cool burning materials and are very effective against fires in furniture, fabrics, etc. (including deep-seated fires), but they can be safely used only in the absence of electricity. NFPA 10 is the Standard for Portable Fire Extinguishers.

7. Answer: **B**. The term BLEVE is the acronym for a Boiling Liquid Expanding Vapor Explosion, which is a major container rupture due to a form of pressure release explosion. This can be caused from external heating such as an adjacent container fire. For this reason, the fire attack scenario of a tank fire would include hose streams directed on adjacent containers, as well as on the burning tank.

8. Answer: **C**

   Fume – Solid particles generated by condensation from the gaseous state, generally after volatilization from a melted substance (e.g., welding), and often accompanied by a chemical reaction such as oxidation. Gases and vapors are not fumes.

   Mist – An aerosol consisting of liquid particles generated by condensation of a substance from the gaseous to the liquid state

   Gas – A substance that is in the gaseous state at room temperature and pressure

   Smoke – A visible suspension of carbon or other particles in air, typically emitted from a burning substance.

9. Answer: **C**. Static electricity is best described as a condition of high voltage with low current. A static electrical charge may be either positive (+) or negative (−) and is manifested when some force has separated the positive electrons from the negative protons of an atom. Typical forces include flowing, mixing, pouring, pumping, filtering, or agitating materials where there is forceful separation of two like or unlike materials. Examples of static generation are common with operations involving the movement of liquid hydrocarbons, gases contaminated with particles (e.g., metal scale and rust), liquid particles (e.g., paint spray, steam), and dust or fibers (e.g., drive belts, conveyors). The static electric charging rate is increased greatly by increasing the speed of separation (e.g., flow rate and turbulence), low-conductivity materials (e.g., hydrocarbon liquids), and surface area of the interface (e.g., pipe or hose length, and micropore filters). Protection from the effects of static electricity include identification

Domain 4: Fire Prevention and Protection   123

of potential static buildup areas; measures to reduce the rate of static electricity generation; and provisions to dissipate accumulated static electricity charges. Control measures include bonding and grounding, inerting, and humidity control. The lower the humidity, the higher the potential for static electricity buildup.

10. Answer: **B**. GFCIs are designed to interrupt the circuit when leakage current (amps) occurs between a conductor and the shield. The definition of a ground fault circuit interrupter (GFCI) is located in Article 100 of the NEC and is as follows: "A device intended for the protection of personnel that functions to de-energize a circuit or portion thereof within an established period of time when a current to ground exceeds the values established for a Class A device." A Class A GFCI trips when the current to ground has a value in the range of 4 milliamps to 6 milliamps, and references UL 943, the Standard for Safety for Ground Fault Circuit Interrupters. OSHA 1910.399 defines a ground fault circuit interrupter, or GFCI, as "a device whose function is to interrupt the electric circuit to load when a fault current to ground exceeds some predetermined value, that is less than that required to operate the overcurrent protective device of the supply circuit." A voltmeter is a tool used to detect current leakage. NFPA 70 (2001)

11. Answer: **D**. A **panic bar** (also known as a **crash bar**, **exit device**, **panic device**, or a **push bar**) is a type of door handle that permits opening the door quickly during emergency conditions. The mechanism consists of a spring-loaded metal bar fixed horizontally to the inside of an outward-opening door. When the lever is either pushed or depressed, it activates a mechanism which unlatches the door, allowing occupants to quickly exit the building.

12. Answer: **C**. According to *The NFPA Fire Protection Handbook*, for combustion to occur four components are necessary: oxygen (oxidizing agent); fuel (substrate); heat (ignition); and a self-sustained chemical reaction (also referred to as the chain reaction). These components can be graphically described as the "fire tetrahedron." Each component of the tetrahedron must be in place for combustion to occur. Remove any one of the four components and combustion will not occur. If ignition has already occurred, the fire is extinguished when one of the components is removed from the reaction.

13. Answer: **A**. The U.S. Department of Defense defines CBRNE as chemical, biological, radiological, nuclear, and (high-yield) explosive.

14. Answer: **B**. As described in *Counter Terrorism for Emergency Responders*, 2nd edition, a chemical explosion, like fire, requires oxidizer, fuel, ignition, and a chemical reaction, but more importantly, it requires confinement of the oxidizer and fuel. Without confinement, the materials will not explode; they will merely burn with great intensity.

15. Answer: **D**. Class II, Division 2 locations are those in which combustible dust is not normally present but might be, due to abnormal or periodic operations. During those times, sufficient dust may be present in the air to produce explosive or ignitable mixtures. A Class II, Division 2 location is an area normally free of dust, but due to some incident, dust may be introduced. Mechanical breakdown of a valve or a break in a pipe are examples of conditions that would require an area to be classified as Division 2.

The NEC Class II hazard classification includes combustible dusts (**Table 12**). Refer NFPA 70 Article 500.

Table 12 NEC Class II Hazard Classification

CLASS	DIVISION 1	DIVISION 2
I Gases, Vapors, and Liquids (ART501)	Normally explosive and hazardous	Not normally present in an explosive concentration (but may accidentally exist)
II Dusts (ART502)	Ignitable quantities of dust normally are or may be in suspension, or conductive dust may be present	Dust not normally suspended in an ignitable concentration (but may accidentally exist) Dust layers are present
III Fibers and Flyings (ART503)	Textiles, woodworking, etc. (easily ignitable but not likely to be explosive)	Stored or handled in storage (exclusive of manufacturing)

Article 500 of the National Electrical Code (NEC), NFPA 70, 2017 edition, National Fire protection Association

Domain 5: Emergency Response Management (ERM)

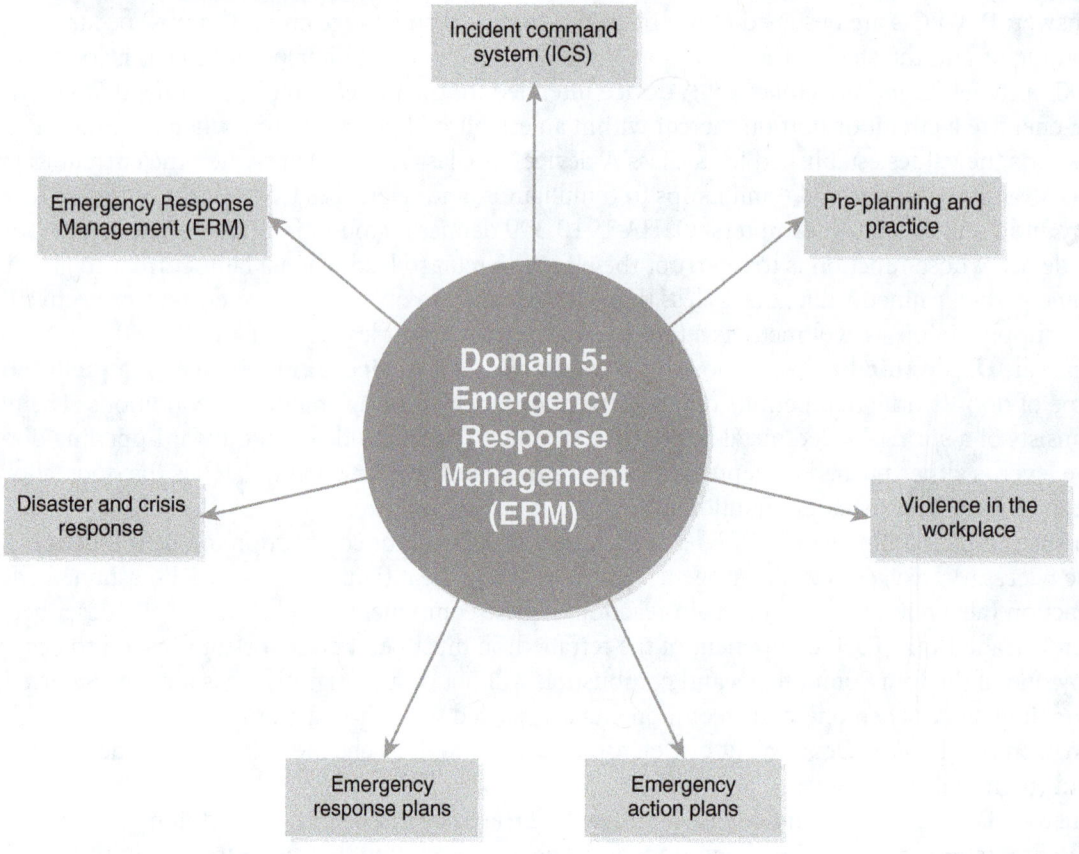

Modified from ASP® Exam Blueprint (ASP10), November 10, 2019

Domain 5 Quiz 1 Questions

1. Which of the following, according to the National Safety Council, is not included in good accident investigation procedures?
    A. Identify basic causal factors.
    B. Determine who is to blame for the accident.
    C. Identify deficiencies in the management system.
    D. Suggest corrective action alternatives for the management system.

2. All the following are recognized methods of smoke management by NFPA except:
    A. airflow.
    B. buoyancy.
    C. compartmentalization.
    D. dispersion.

3. If a small mobile crane with rubber tires has struck a power line and the line is apparently dead, lying across the crane boom, what is the best course of action for the crane operator?

   A. Jump from the crane and run away.
   B. Stay in the crane until the emergency crew arrives.
   C. Have an oiler knock the power line from the boom with a wood pole.
   D. Swing the boom back and forth until the line breaks or falls off.

4. Which of the following is not considered a phase of emergency management?

   A. Response
   B. Recovery
   C. Mitigation
   D. Litigation

5. Under ICS, the Command Staff positions include:

   A. Safety Officer, Public Information Officer, and Liaison Officer.
   B. Liaison Officer, Operations Section Chief, and Finance and Administration Section Chief.
   C. Public Information Officer, Chief Executive Officer, and Safety Officer.
   D. Logistics Section Chief, Safety Officer, and the Contracting Officer.

6. The Incident Command System (ICS) recognizes that field response is where response personnel carry out tactical decisions and activities in direct response to an incident, under the command of:

   A. the federal government.
   B. an appropriate authority.
   C. the local government.
   D. private contractors.

7. The primary consideration when preparing for a potential disaster is:

   A. selecting the emergency committee.
   B. identifying a person to be the on-scene commander.
   C. doing advance emergency planning.
   D. having a list of necessary state and federal directives.

8. Which visual correctly identifies a DOT oxidizer placard?

   A. Background yellow, information black
   B. Lower half black, upper half white
   C. Lower part white, upper triangle yellow
   D. Background red, information white/black

9. Cleaning up a flammable or combustible material spill requires following all guidelines below except:

   A. immediately notify OSHA of the spill.
   B. isolate the spill site from nonrequired personnel.
   C. block off the spill area to prevent access.
   D. remove electric hazards, incompatible chemicals or wastes, physical hazards, and sources of ignition.

10. What are the colors on a corrosive placard?

    A. Red, yellow
    B. Red, white
    C. Black, white
    D. Yellow, black

126 ASP Exam Study Workbook

11. **What does the number "3" indicate on the Hazardous Material Label?**
    A. Flammable material
    B. Adhesive material
    C. Hazard class
    D. Third label in the series

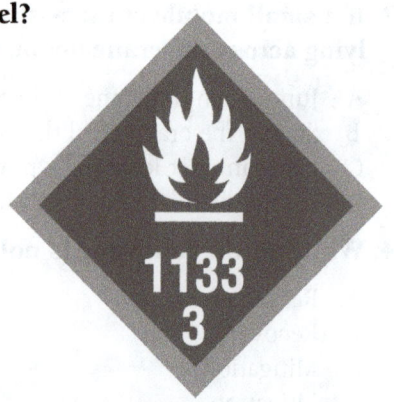

Figure 29 Hazardous Material Label
Courtesy of American Lablemark Corp.

12. **An emergency in which planning efforts are more focused on mitigation and recovery than on prevention is a:**
    A. natural disaster.
    B. chemical disaster.
    C. fire disaster.
    D. explosion disaster.

13. **In the theory of fire, understanding the fire tetrahedron is important for understanding how to extinguish a fire. The four elements that must be present for a fire to occur are a fuel, heat, an oxidizing agent (usually oxygen), and a chemical chain reaction. One method used to reduce the possibility of a fire hazard is use of an inerting gas to reduce the oxidizing agent concentration. The most important property of this gas is:**
    A. heat capacity.
    B. molecular weight.
    C. vapor pressure.
    D. content of hydrogen.

14. **A local fire department has responded to a blaze on the surface of a combustible liquid in a laboratory setting. If firefighters apply AFFF, what hazard is associated with this approach?**
    A. The foam will not work at 100°C or higher.
    B. The high temperature will increase foam solubility and slow down its ability to smother the fire.
    C. Foam is not a recommended extinguisher for a combustible liquid fire.
    D. Foam will form an emulsion of steam, air, and fuel that may cause frothing of the burning liquid.

15. **A rate-of-rise detector responds to which condition?**
    A. Smoke particulate in the air
    B. Water pressure in fire-suppression piping
    C. Indoor humidity
    D. Heat

16. **What is the purpose of a jockey pump?**
    A. To pump water through a sprinkler system to extinguish a fire
    B. To maintain system pressure when the sprinkler system is not in use
    C. To open the sprinkler heads to the proper size based on the rate of rise
    D. To deliver water through the pipes so that the system can continue to put out the fire

Domain 5: Emergency Response Management (ERM)   127

17. A flood destroys a company's operational ability. After emergency management issues are addressed, the business implements several plans for recovery of critical files and information that had been stored off site, establishes a temporary facility from which operations can be conducted, and informs customers of the circumstances and how customers will be served. These plans are examples of a comprehensive loss control activity called:

   A. emergency management/emergency response.
   B. situational awareness.
   C. disaster recovery/business continuity planning.
   D. business impact analysis.

18. Pre-emergency management planning is the best way to minimize potential loss from natural or technological disasters and accidents. The primary responsibilities of emergency planning must exclude:

   A. establishing continuity of operations for the customers' sake.
   B. providing for the safety of employees and public.
   C. protecting property and environment.
   D. establishing methods to restore operations to a new normal as soon as possible.

19. Many different agencies might be responsible for controlling and cleaning up complex hazardous materials incidents. Which of the following is the critical first step in responding to a chemical release when multiple agencies are involved?

   A. Approve the Incident Action Plan.
   B. Establish the Incident Command System.
   C. Approve resource requests.
   D. Order demobilization.

20. The National Incident Management System (NIMS) is the responsibility of the:

   A. Department of State (DOS).
   B. Department of Health and Human Services (DHHS).
   C. Department of Defense (DOD).
   D. Department of Homeland Security (DHS).

21. You are checking on a confined space but do not see the attendant. You look into the space and see two people who appear to be unconscious. What is the first action you take?

   A. Immediately call for assistance.
   B. Immediately approach the victims and try to render first aid.
   C. Immediately call out to them both to see if they are okay.
   D. Immediately check the atmosphere to see if it is safe to enter.

22. Which training level applies to employees who are likely to witness or discover a hazardous substance release and who need to be trained to initiate an emergency response sequence by notifying the proper authorities of the release?

   A. Awareness level
   B. Operations level
   C. Hazardous materials technicians
   D. Specialist employees

23. The Clean Air Act (CAA) places responsibility for the prevention of accidental chemical releases on both OSHA and EPA. OSHA has implemented the Process Safety Management (PSM) Rule. Which of the following represents the EPA's related program for threshold quantities of extremely hazardous substances?

    A. Risk Mitigation Process (RMP) Rule.
    B. Response Management Protocols (RMP) Rule.
    C. Response Mitigation Program (RMP) Rule.
    D. Risk Management Program (RMP) Rule.

24. The public resists change for all the following reasons except:

    A. fear of the unknown.
    B. false confidence.
    C. loss of face.
    D. lack of purpose.

25. The most important spokesperson characteristics for effective risk communication to the public are:

    A. expertise and authoritative presence.
    B. appearance and empathy.
    C. authoritative presence and credibility.
    D. credibility and technical competency.

Domain 5 Quiz 1 Answers

1. Answer: **B**. According to the NSC, good accident investigation procedures:
   - Provide information needed to determine injury rates, identify trends or problem areas, permit comparisons, and satisfy workers' compensation requirements.
   - Identify, without placing blame, the basic causal factors that contributed directly or indirectly to each accident
   - Identify deficiencies in the management system
   - Suggest corrective action alternatives for a given accident
   - Suggest corrective action alternatives for the management system
   - Recognize that (in reconstruction of a vehicle accident) the most important element is to consider the possibility of multiple causes

2. Answer: **D**. Smoke management refers to methods employed to modify smoke movement for the benefit of evacuating occupants or firefighters, or to reduce property losses and damage. Airflow, buoyancy, compartmentation, dilution, and pressurization are mechanisms of smoke management that are utilized individually or in combination to reduce harmful effects of a fire. Dispersion is related to the distribution of water from a fire sprinkler head or of the agent from a fire extinguisher.

3. Answer: **B**. Each power line contact situation poses different problems. However, the generally accepted guidance is for the crane operator to stay in the cab until power company emergency crews arrive. Often power lines are equipped with fault-clearing re-closers, which will reapply power to a faulted line after a few minutes. The re-closer can cycle three or four times before the line is really disconnected and then it is still unsafe because of cross-feed situations. Departing the cab should only be considered if a fire or other situation requires it. Jumping from the cab with feet together is the only safe departure method. Those involved must avoid contact with the energized crane and earth and step potential must be kept at a minimum.

4. Answer: **D**. The coordinated response to and recovery from an emergency event is the mainstay of emergency management. **Preparedness** is planning how to respond in case an emergency or disaster occurs and working to increase the resources that are available to respond effectively. **Response** involves the effective and efficient application of assets and activities to resolve the immediate impacts of an event. In the case of a planned event, response activities include the application of sufficient resources to ensure that the event occurs without undue or unexpected undesirable outcomes. **Recovery** activities occur until

all community systems return to normal or nearly normal conditions. This includes both short-term and long-term recovery actions. **Mitigation** refers to those actions and activities taken to reduce or eliminate the chance of occurrence or the effects of a disaster.

5. Answer: **A**. ICS is organized into three components: Incident Command, Command Staff, and General Staff positions. Incident Command can be comprised either of a single Incident Commander or a Unified Command. An example an ICS organizational chart is shown below.

   The Command Staff (CS) members perform incident-wide tasks and report directly to the IC. The three most common CS positions include:

   Safety Officer – Responsible for the safe operations of all tasks performed on site. The Safety Officer has the essential authority to terminate any operations deemed to be unsafe, and even to override the authority of the IC to do so.

   Public Information Officer – The PIO is responsible for passing information regarding the incident to the public and to the media. Traditionally, the PIO was responsible for press releases and public warning statements issued through the media. In recent years, with the huge increase in use of social media, the PIO position has expanded greatly.

   Liaison Officer – This position is responsible for interacting and coordinating with other response entities not represented in the incident to provide their input on legal issues and resource availability.

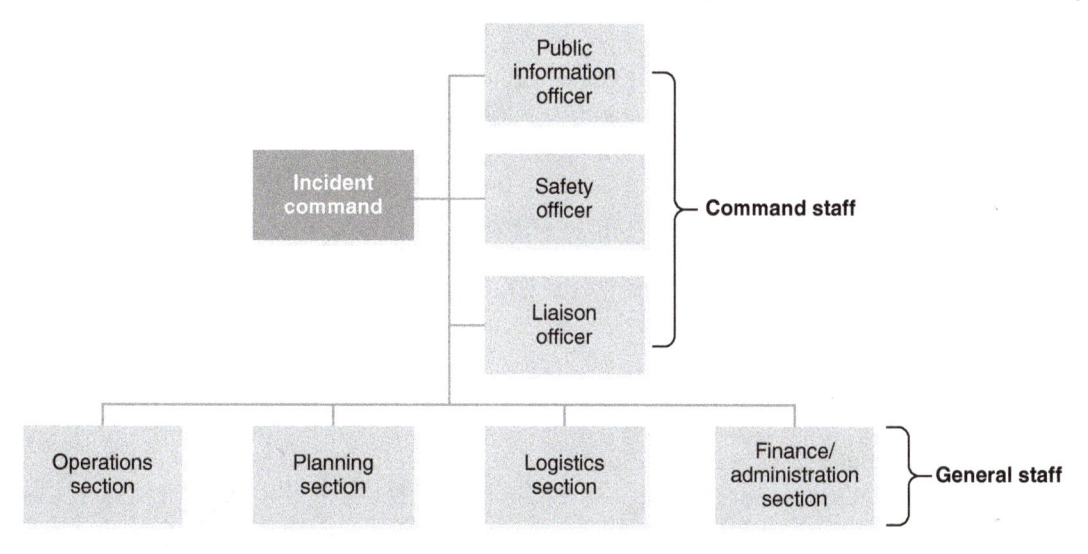

   Figure 30 ICS Organizational Chart Example
   fema.gov

6. Answer: **B**. ICS recognizes that field response is where response personnel, under the command of an appropriate authority, carry out tactical decisions and activities in direct response to an incident. ICS has 14 management characteristics that make it useful when responding to a hazardous materials emergency (DHS, 2008):

   Use of Common Terminology – Common terminology allows all responders unambiguous information flow. Common terminology applies to organizational functions of the ICS, resource descriptions (such as resource typing), and common names for incident facilities.

   Modular Organization – The ICS structure is driven by the nature of the incident. While a full-blown ICS (involving perhaps thousands of responders at the largest scale) can be managed, the modular organization allows for management of the smallest incident as well by staffing only those ICS elements necessary to accomplish the tasks at hand.

   Management by Objectives – ICS identifies incident objectives through a planning process. All activities are performed in support of one or more of those objectives. Once all of the incident objectives are accomplished, the incident is over. Staffing of the incident is increased or decreased in response to the incident objectives. While not specified under ICS, it is always valuable to develop **SMART objectives—objectives that are Specific, Measurable, Achievable, Realistic, and Time-constrained**—as part of any incident action plan.

- **Incident Action Planning** – ICS calls for centralized incident action planning and only one action plan for the entire response. This ensures that all response activities are focused on the same objectives, improving the effectiveness and efficiency of the response.
- **Manageable Span of Control** – Every supervisor has a manageable number of directly reporting staff. ICS calls for a span of control of from 3 to 7, with 5 being optimum.
- **Predesignated Incident Facilities and Locations** – Incident facilities, such as the Command Post and the Staging Area, are defined. All responders know what takes place at each facility.
- **Comprehensive Resource Management** – One entity is responsible for tracking the status and location of all resources. This ensures that all resources are accounted for and put to optimum use. No resource individual or group has the authority to free-lance or perform a mission they are not assigned.
- **Integrated Communications** – All methods of communication (radios, written reports, etc.) are coordinated to provide common situational awareness and interaction. A common communications plan and processes—including communications discipline—are integrated for the entire incident.
- **Establishment and Transfer of Command** – Every incident has a clearly identified commander appointed by the agency or entity with jurisdiction. If the Incident Commander changes, this transfer of command is clear and transparent to everyone.
- **Chain of Command and Unity of Command** – The chain of command establishes the line of authority and decision-making at an incident. Unity of command ensures that everyone present has one (and only one) supervisor. These principles eliminate multiple conflicting directives.
- **Unified Command** – In our federal system no one entity has all of the authority necessary to bring an incident to a successful conclusion. Unified command allows those entities with some portion of the authority to pool their resources and work together without losing any entity's authority, responsibility, or accountability. Typically, the Unified Command will consist of one representative from each level of government (federal, state, local, and responsible party, for instance) or geographic entity (adjacent counties impacted by the incident) to perform the duties of the Incident Commander, such as determining incident objectives and priorities.
- **Accountability** – Keeping track of all personnel and resources at an incident is critical to ensuring presence, health and safety, and responsibility.
- **Dispatch and Deployment** – Resources respond to the incident and are deployed only as directed by Incident Command. This reduces the occurrence of self-dispatch of resources and freelancing at the incident scene.
- **Information and Intelligence Management** – ICS provides a mechanism for collecting, analyzing, and disseminating incident-related information and intelligence.

These 14 elements make ICS a flexible yet powerful tool for managing hazardous materials incidents.

7. Answer: **C**. According to the NSC, "advanced emergency management planning is the best way to minimize potential loss from natural or human-caused disasters or accidents."
8. Answer: **A**.
Answer B is the color for a **corrosive** sign or placard.
Answer C is the color for a **radioactive** sign or placard.
Answer D is the color for a **combustible** sign or placard.

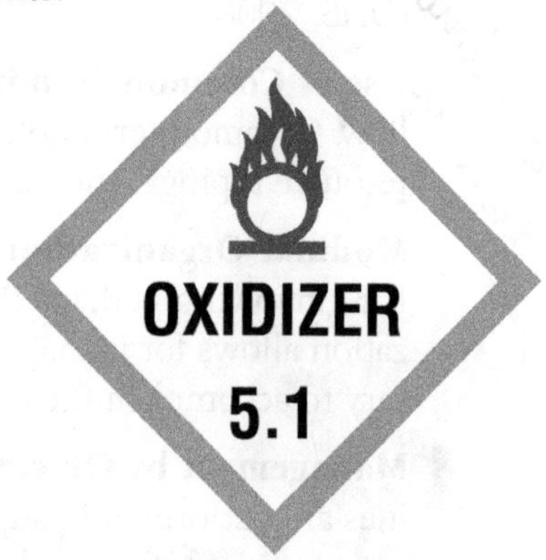

Figure 31 DOT oxidizer placard

9. Answer: **A**. Supervisors are not required to notify OSHA for a minor spill. However, the supervisor must isolate the area for cleanup and arrange for removal of all hazards, including ignition sources, especially if the spill is flammable.
10. Answer: **C**. DOT hazard class 8 is for corrosives and is black and white.

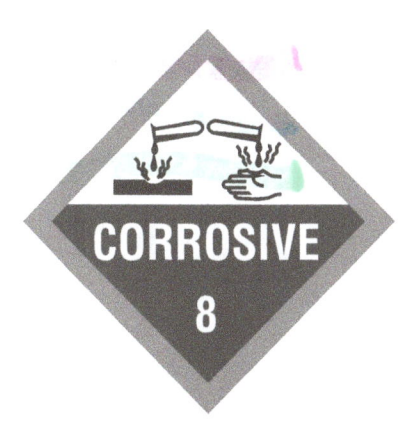

Figure 32 Corrosive Placard

Class 1	Explosives[1]
Division 1.1	Explosives with a mass explosion hazard. A mass explosion is one that affects almost the entire load instantaneously.
Division 1.2	Explosives with a projection hazard but not a mass explosion hazard
Division 1.3	Explosives with a fire hazard and either a minor blast hazard or a minor projection hazard or both, but not a mass explosion hazard
Division 1.4	Explosives with a minor explosion hazard. The explosive effects are largely confined to the package and no projection of fragments of appreciable size or range is to be expected.
Division 1.5	Very insensitive explosives. This division is comprised of substances that have a mass explosion hazard but are so insensitive that there is very little probability of initiation.
Division 1.6	Extremely insensitive articles that do not have a mass explosion hazard
Class 2	**Gases**
Division 2.1	Flammable gases
Division 2.2	Nonflammable, nonpoisonous compressed gases
Division 2.3	Poisonous gases
Class 3	**Flammable and Combustible Liquids**
Class 4	**Flammable Solids**
Division 4.1	Flammable solids
Division 4.2	Spontaneously combustible materials
Division 4.3	Materials that are dangerous when wet
Class 5	**Oxidizers**
Division 5.1	Oxidizers
Division 5.2	Organic peroxides

132 ASP Exam Study Workbook

Class 6	Poisonous Materials
Division 6.1	Poisonous materials
Division 6.2	Infectious substances
Class 7	Radioactive Materials
Class 8	Corrosive Materials
Class 9	Miscellaneous Hazardous Materials

[1] Review the *Emergency Response Guidebook*, http://phmsa.dot.gov/.

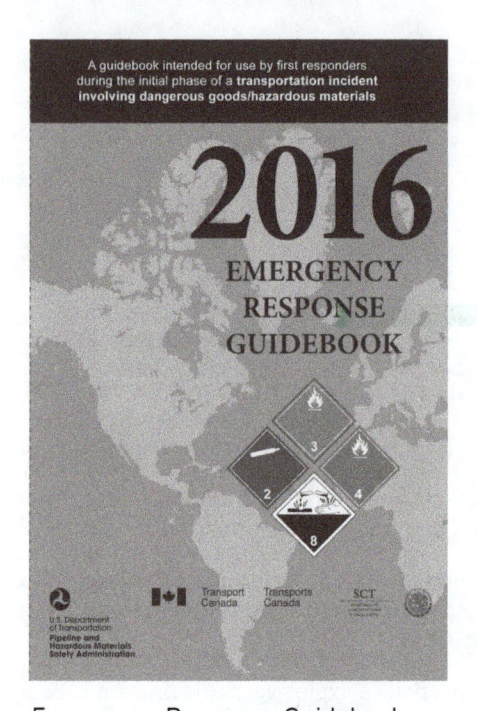

Emergency Response Guidebook
United States Department of Transportation, PHMSA, Emergency Response Guidebook,
Retrieved from http://phmsa.dot.gov/

11. Answer: **C**. The flame symbol on the top indicates a flammable material, the number 1133 is the UN number, and the "3" indicates the hazard class. Examples of UN numbers: 1033 is for dimethyl ether (Class 2); 1133 is for adhesives (Class 3); and 1333 is for cerium (Class 4).

12. Answer: **A**. Generally, preventing natural disasters is beyond the control of mankind. Emergency preparedness efforts should be focused on mitigation, loss reduction, and business continuity instead of prevention.

13. Answer: **A**. According to the *Fire Protection Handbook*, the most important property is the heat capacity of a gas.

14. Answer: **D**. According to the *Fire Protection Handbook*, if the temperature of the liquid itself is above the boiling point of water used to create the foam, a frothy and voluminous emulsion of steam, air, and burning fuel may occur upon application of the foam to the surface of the fire.

15. Answer: **D**. There are three types of heat detectors candidates should be familiar with for the examination. They are listed below with their general characteristics:

    Fixed-Temperature: Designed to alarm when the temperature of the operating element reaches a specified point. These units are susceptible to "thermal lag."

    Rate Compensation: Designed to alarm when the temperature of surrounding air reaches a predetermined level, regardless of rate of temperature rise. Element configuration compensates for thermal lag.

Rate-of-Rise: Designed to alarm when the rate of temperature increase exceeds a predetermined value (usually 12°F to 15°F per minute). An example of use would be on a petroleum-based hydraulic pump to prevent explosions.

16. Answer: **B**. A jockey pump, or a pressure-maintenance pump, is a small apparatus that works together with a fire pump as part of a fire-protection sprinkler system. It is designed to keep the pressure in the system elevated to a specific level when the system is not in use, so that the fire pump doesn't have to run all the time and the system doesn't go off randomly. It can also help prevent the system from damage when a fire happens and water rushes into the pipes. These devices consist of a three-part assembly. In many places, there are governmental guidelines and recommendations for installing these devices to make sure they work properly. To understand how a jockey pump works, it's important to understand how a fire sprinkler system works. Sprinkler systems consist of pipes with pressurized water in them and heads that are designed to open when they reach a certain temperature. When the heads open, the water pressure in the pipes drops, since water is flowing out of them. When this happens, a large device called a fire pump starts to send more water through the pipes so that the system can continue to put out the fire. The purpose of the jockey pump is to keep the water pressure in the pipes within a specific range when there's not a fire, so that the sprinklers won't go off randomly. Because pipes leak, over time the water pressure inside them automatically goes down. The jockey pump senses this, and then fills them back up to normal pressure. If a fire happens and the pressure drops dramatically, the jockey pump won't be able to keep up, and the pressure drop will trigger the large fire pump to start sending water. Secondarily, this pump prevents sprinkler systems from being damaged when the fire pump begins sending water. If a system does not have a jockey pump keeping it pressurized, it may have relatively low pressure. When the fire pump starts sending highly pressurized water through the pipes, the sudden change in pressure can damage or destroy the system.

17. Answer: **C**. According to *Risk Analysis and the Security Survey*, 3rd edition, business continuity planning is a key part of a loss-control program. Such plans should include recovering corporate information, setting up operations, and financing temporary operations until a new facility can be commissioned. Depending upon the risk of a natural disaster, some companies purchase business interruption insurance to help finance operations.

18. Answer: **A**. According to the National Safety Council, advance emergency management planning should include the following items and they should be ranked as they are sequenced.
    a. Provide for the safety of employees and public.
    b. Protect property and the environment.
    c. Establish methods to restore operations to normal as soon as possible.

    When developing emergency management plans, sometimes the fundamental purpose is lost, which is to protect life, property, and the environment. Though command and communication responsibilities are important and must be part of the planning process, fundamental strategies must be developed to protect people, property, and the environment, and then tactics can be applied.

    When developing a risk management plan, one must anticipate what will go wrong and make timely attempts to overcome identified loss scenarios. The risk management process consists of the following steps:
    - Identify loss scenarios.
    - Develop alternatives to control them.
    - Implement best solution(s).
    - Manage and control risk(s).

19. Answer: **B**. According the NFPA *Hazardous Materials/WMD Response Handbook* (2008), all the answers are tasks for the Incident Commander. A vital step during pre-incident planning is to identify these agencies. The first thing to establish is the Incident Command System and designate who is in charge. The National Incident Management System, FEMA, 2017, establishes the following functions as the Incident Commander's (IC's) primary responsibilities:
    - Have clear authority and know agency policy.
    - Ensure incident safety.

134   ASP Exam Study Workbook

- Establish the incident command post (ICP).
- Set priorities, and determine incident objectives and strategies.
- Establish an incident command system (ICS).
- Approve an incident response plan (IAP).
- Coordinate command and general staff activities.
- Approve resource requests and use of volunteers and auxiliary personnel.
- Order demobilization as needed.
- Ensure after-action review.

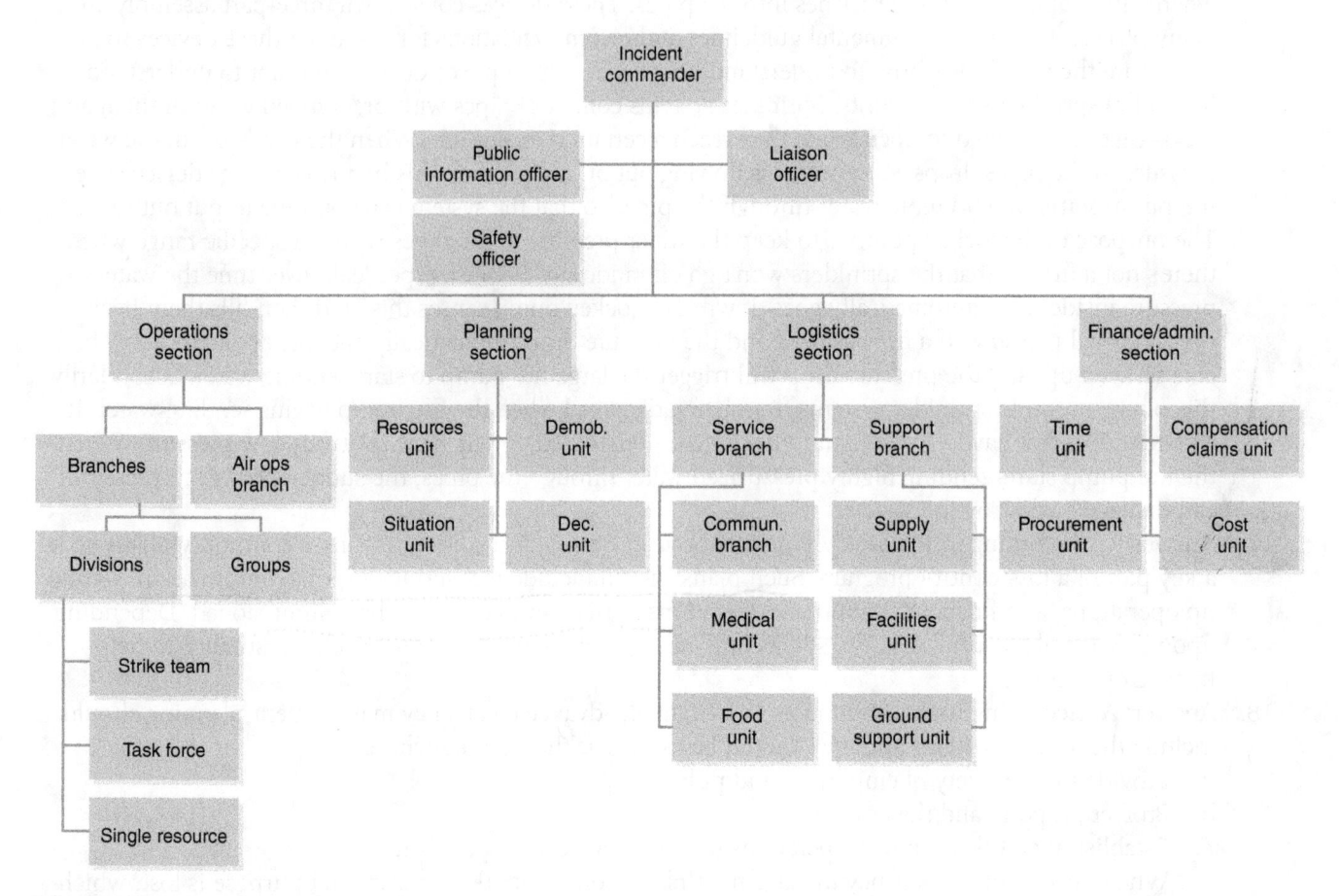

Figure 33 ICS Organizational Chart Example 2
fema.gov

20. Answer: **D**. The **National Incident Management System (NIMS)** is the responsibility of the Department of Homeland Security (DHS). It provides a consistent template for managing incidents in a companion document to the National Response Framework and provides standard command and management structures that apply to response activities. This system provides a consistent, nationwide template to enable federal, state, tribal, and local governments, the private sector, and nongovernmental organizations (NGOs) to work together to prepare for, prevent, respond to, recover from, and mitigate the effects of incidents, regardless of cause, size, location, or complexity. This consistency provides the foundation for utilization of the NIMS for all incidents, ranging from daily occurrences to incidents requiring a coordinated federal response.

21. Answer: **A**. The first action taken any time there is an indication that someone is unconscious in a confined space is to summon assistance. From there, the actions may vary based on the company's policy and procedures; however, you never want to enter the space without proper training or preparation and it is not recommended to take any action that could delay a proper rescue (by calling out to them or testing the atmosphere before sounding the alarm).

22. Answer: **A**. The OSHA 1910.120 standard defines several levels of training for hazardous materials emergency responders. These include:
    - **Awareness Level** – First responders at the awareness level are individuals who are likely to witness or discover a hazardous substance release and who have been trained to initiate an emergency response sequence by notifying the proper authorities of the release. They would take no further action beyond notifying the authorities of the release.
    - **Operations Level** – First responders at the operations level are individuals who respond to releases or potential releases of hazardous substances as part of the initial response to the site for protecting nearby persons, property, or the environment from the effects of the release. They are trained to respond in a defensive fashion without trying to stop the release. Their function is to contain the release from a safe distance, keep it from spreading, and prevent exposures.
    - **Hazardous Materials Technician** – Hazardous materials technicians are individuals who respond to releases or potential releases for the purpose of stopping the release. They assume a more aggressive role than a first responder at the operations level, in that they will approach the point of release to plug, patch, or otherwise stop the release of a hazardous substance.
    - **Hazardous Materials Specialist** – Hazardous materials specialists are individuals who respond with and provide support to hazardous materials technicians. Their duties parallel those of the hazardous materials technician; however, their duties require a more directed or specific knowledge of the various substances they may be called upon to contain. The hazardous materials specialist would also act as the site liaison with federal, state, local, and other government authorities regarding site activities.
    - **On-Scene Incident Commander** – Incident commanders assume control of the incident scene beyond the first responder awareness level.
    - **Skilled Support Personnel** – Personnel, not necessarily an employer's own employees, who are skilled in the operation of certain equipment, such as mechanized earth moving or digging equipment, or crane and hoisting equipment, and who are needed temporarily to perform immediate emergency support work that cannot reasonably be performed in a timely fashion by an employer's own employees, and who will be or may be exposed to the hazards at an emergency response scene.
    - **Specialist Employees** – Employees who, in the course of their regular job duties, work with and are trained in the hazards of specific hazardous substances, and who will be called upon to provide technical advice or assistance at a hazardous substance release incident to the individual in charge.

    Each of these classes of employees must receive the appropriate level of training for the tasks they are to perform. The standard prescribes a minimum duration of training and many organizations require longer training courses. Similar standards and guidance are provided from other sources, such as the National Fire Protection Association (NFPA) 472.

23. Answer: **D**. OSHA has responsibility for the protection of workers, the public, and the environment from accidental chemical releases under the Process Safety Management (PSM) standard. The EPA has responsibility for protection of the public and the environment from accidental chemical releases, and promulgated the Risk Management Program (RMP). The RMP ensures that the public will be properly informed about chemical risks in their communities, and that federal, state, and local regulators will have more effective tools to assist with lowering chemical accident risk. The PSM and RMP programs regulate toxic, reactive, and flammable substances, many of which are listed in both rules. As a result, if an employer were required to implement the PSM standard for a covered process, that same process may also be subject to RMP rules. Both the PSM and RMP are important elements of an integrated approach to chemical safety. Though there are similarities between the two chemical safety regulations, the two have significant differences: OSHA requires no reporting of a facility's Process Safety Management (PSM) program, but EPA does require a facility to submit its Risk Management Plan (online using "e-Submit" software). Also, EPA's "off-site consequence analysis" (OCA) is required for each "covered process" in order to determine the facility's "Worst-Case Release Scenario" and its "Alternative Release Scenario." But the obvious differences stop there, and unfortunately there are several other significant requirements that can cause serious compliance issues for facilities that must comply with the RMP rules. To determine if a process is covered by either standard, one must determine the quantity in the process and compare that

to the **threshold quantities** prescribed by the standard to determine if the process is covered by one or both standards. In some cases, the process may be covered by RMP and not OSHA, or vice versa. For instance, a facility that uses one-ton chlorine cylinders would be covered by OSHA's PSM but would *not* be covered by EPA's RMP rule. This is because OSHA's threshold for chlorine is 1500 pounds and EPA's threshold is 2500 pounds. The other difference in the "threshold determination" is that OSHA lumped ALL FLAMMABLE LIQUIDS (FP < 100°F) together and set their threshold at 10,000 pounds. EPA treats flammable liquids differently, in that the SPECIFIC FLAMMABLE LIQUID must be listed by CAS number to be considered an "Extremely Hazardous Substance" (EHS).

24. Answer: **B**. Some of the common reasons that people resist change are:
    - Fear of the unknown
    - Disrupted habits
    - Loss of confidence
    - Loss of control
    - Poor timing
    - Work overload
    - Loss of face
    - Lack of purpose

25. Answer: **A**. Spokespersons allow the public to put a face to the act of responding to, investigating, and resolving a crisis. How a spokesperson handles public and media inquiries, in addition to what he or she says, helps establish credibility for an organization. It also contributes to the public's transition from the crisis stage to the resolution and recovery stages. An organization should carefully choose the personnel who will represent it.

    The selection should be based on two factors:
    - The individual's familiarity with the subject matter
    - His or her ability to talk about it clearly and with confidence

Risk communication (RC) is a complex, multidisciplinary, multidimensional, and evolving process of increasing importance in protecting the public's health. Public health officials use RC to give citizens necessary and appropriate information and to involve them in making decisions that affect them, such as where to build waste disposal facilities. The National Research Council (NRC) defines risk communication as "an interactive process of exchange of information and opinion among individuals, groups, and institutions." The definition includes "discussion about risk types and levels and about methods for managing risks." NIOSH (1998) Specifically, this process is defined by levels of involvement in decisions, actions, or policies aimed at managing or controlling health or environmental risks. There are seven cardinal rules for the practice of risk communication, as first expressed by the U.S. Environmental Protection Agency:
- Accept and involve the public as a legitimate partner.
- Plan carefully and evaluate your efforts.
- Listen to the public's specific concerns.
- Be honest, frank, and open.
- Coordinate and collaborate with other credible sources.
- Meet the needs of the media.
- Speak clearly and with compassion.

Communicating with the Public: 10 Questions To Ask
- Why are we communicating?
- Who is our audience?
- What do our audiences want to know?
- What do we want to get across?
- How will we communicate?
- How will we listen?
- How will we respond?
- Who will carry out the plans? When?
- What problems or barriers have we planned for?
- Have we succeeded?

Factors Influencing Risk Perception

Risk perceptions more likely to be accepted	Risk perceptions less likely to be accepted
Voluntary	Imposed
Under an individual's control	Controlled by others
Have clear benefits	Have little or no benefit
Fairly distributed	Unfairly distributed
Natural	Manmade
Statistical	Catastrophic
Generated by a trusted source	Generated by an untrusted source
Familiar	Exotic
Affect adults	Affect children

According to FEMA, the person who delivers the messages plays a critical role in both risk and crisis communications. Communications experts have identified six traits of successful risk communicators:

- Communicator's speaking ability
- Reputation among audience members (trustworthiness and credibility)
- Subject matter knowledge
- Image of authority
- Obvious lack of vested interest
- Ability to connect, sympathize, or empathize with the audience

During a crisis or emergency, the messenger(s) puts a human face on disaster response and this person(s) is critical to building confidence among the public that people will be helped, and their community will recover. Public Information Officers (PIOs) regularly deliver information and messages to the media and the public. However, the primary face of the disaster response should be an elected or appointed official (i.e., mayor, governor, county administrator, city manager) or the director of the emergency management agency, or both.

These individuals bring a measure of authority to their role as a messenger, and in the case of the emergency management director, as the person who oversees response and recovery operations. The public wants to hear from an authority figure, and the media wants to know that the person they are talking to is the one making the decisions. Emergency management agencies should also designate appropriate senior managers who will be made available to both the traditional and new media to provide specific information on their activities and perspective. This is helpful in even the smallest disaster; persons with expertise in specific facets of the response can be very effective in delivering disaster response information and messages. Any official who serves as a communicator during and after a crisis should receive media training before the crisis. Ultimately, communicators will seek to create actual messages that transmit certain knowledge, whether factual (awareness) or action based (operational).

Six principles of effective crisis and risk communication are:

1. Be First: Crises are time-sensitive. Communicating information quickly is almost always important. For members of the public, the first source of information often becomes the preferred source.
2. Be Right: Accuracy establishes credibility. Information can include what is known, what is not known, and what is being done to fill in the gaps.
3. Be Credible: Honesty and truthfulness should not be compromised during crises.
4. Express Empathy: Crises create harm, and the suffering should be acknowledged in words. Addressing what people are feeling, and the challenges they face, builds trust and rapport.
5. Promote Action: Giving people meaningful things to do calms anxiety, helps restore order, and promotes a restored sense of control.
6. Show Respect: Respectful communication is particularly important when people feel vulnerable. Respectful communication promotes cooperation and rapport. Centers for Disease Control and Prevention (2014)

Domain 6: Industrial Hygiene and Occupational Health

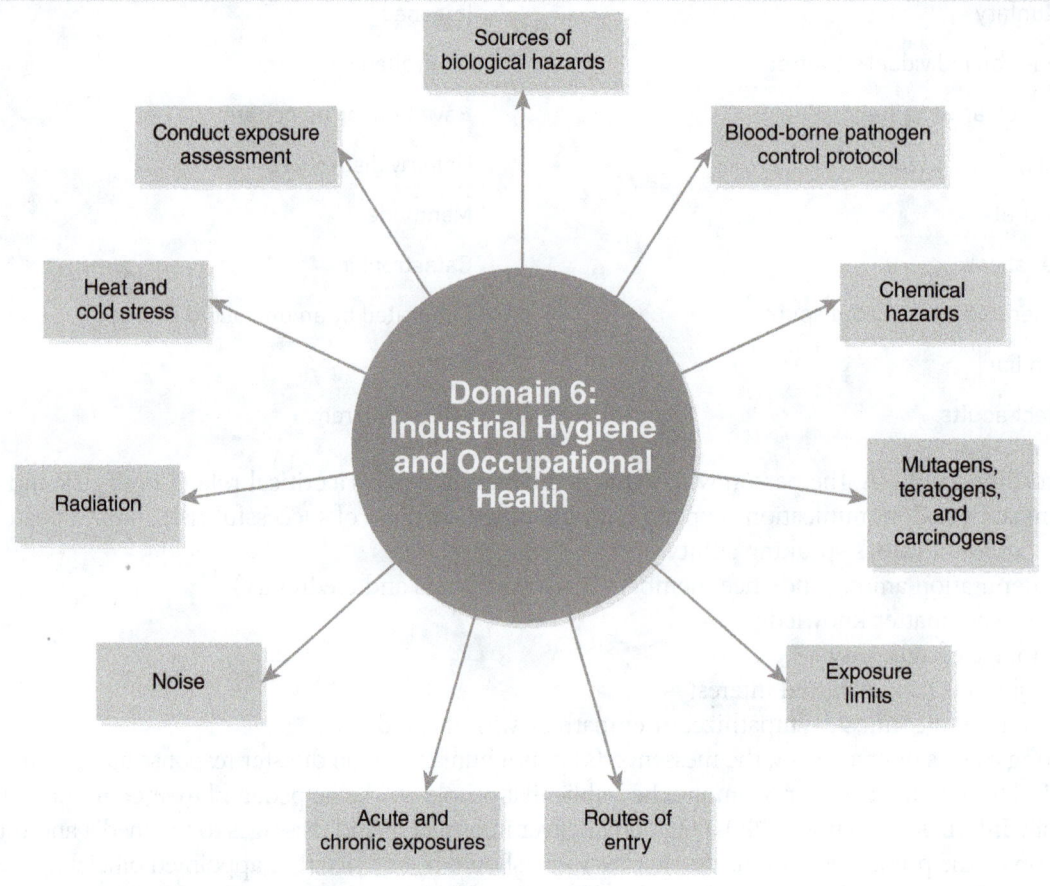

Modified from ASP® Exam Blueprint (ASP10), November 10, 2019

Domain 6 Quiz 1 Questions

1. Due to a portion of a company's workforce being exposed to chromium (VI), employee testing has begun. Where should test results be filed?

    A. On the safety manager's computer
    B. In the safety manager's file cabinet
    C. In employees' personnel files
    D. In employees' medical records

2. When skin is exposed to solvents, workers may experience inflammation (dermatitis) because of:

    A. scraping of dermal layers.
    B. defatting of the skin.
    C. deep cuts.
    D. chemical injection.

3. A disease of the inner ear that can cause vertigo, tinnitus, and hearing loss is called:

    A. rhinosinusitis.
    B. Barrett's esophagus.
    C. byssinosis.
    D. Ménière's disease.

4. "Metal fume fever" is primarily caused by inhalation of:

   A. zinc oxide fumes.
   B. hexavalent chrome fumes.
   C. fuming silver nitrate.
   D. silicon oxide fumes.

5. If a plant worker is diagnosed with *mesothelioma*, his/her supervisor should suspect which agent as a likely cause?

   A. Carbon monoxide
   B. Nitrous oxide
   C. Toluene
   D. Chrysotile

6. Gamma globulin proteins found in blood and used by the immune system to identify and neutralize foreign objects, such as bacteria and viruses, are called:

   A. antibodies.
   B. white blood cells.
   C. pathogens.
   D. chromosomes.

7. Which medical conditions include cotton worker's lung, cotton bract disease, mill fever, and brown lung?

   A. Osteoporosis
   B. Byssinosis
   C. Pneumoconiosis
   D. Occupational bronchitis

8. A toxic agent or substance that inhibits, damages, or destroys the cells and/or tissues of the kidneys is called a:

   A. nephrotoxin.
   B. neurotoxin.
   C. hemotoxin.
   D. hepatoxin.

9. The term synonymous with oncogenesis is:

   A. homeostasis.
   B. carcinogenesis.
   C. myogenesis.
   D. glycogenesis.

10. Inhalation of iron oxide causes a pneumoconiosis called:

    A. anthracosis.
    B. siderosis.
    C. silicosis.
    D. silicosiderosis.

11. Neutron radiation's effect on the human body is best described as:

    A. neutrons causing secondary release of protons.
    B. neutrons changing the structure of body atoms.
    C. neutron radiation ionizing water in the body.
    D. neutron radiation causing release of secondary radiation in the body.

12. Aging causes a vascular and neural degeneration of the inner ear, resulting in a decrease in hearing ability called:

    A. sensorineural.
    B. sociocusis.
    C. presbycusis.
    D. tinnitus.

13. Which responsibility is not assigned to the National Institute for Occupational Safety and Health (NIOSH)?

    A. Research and identification of occupational safety/health hazards
    B. Recommending changes to safety/health regulations
    C. Training of safety/health personnel
    D. Enforcement of occupational safety/public health standards within the regulated community

14. Which is the most correct statement concerning the affliction of frostbite?

    A. Frostbite causes uncontrolled shivering.
    B. Frostbitten skin is soft, puffy, and darker than normal.
    C. The first symptoms of frostbite are "pins and needles" sensations, followed by numbness.
    D. Frostbite is characterized by irregular heartbeat and respiration.

15. Which disease is characterized by white fingers and numbness?

    A. Siderosis
    B. Raynaud's syndrome
    C. Lead poisoning
    D. Tetanus

16. Which pair of common vectors has the capability of transmitting causative agents, resulting in an infection in humans?

    A. Mosquito and beetle
    B. Tick and beetle
    C. Beetle and bird
    D. Mosquito and tick

17. Which illness would you associate with a framing carpenter?

    A. De Quervain syndrome
    B. Epicondylitis
    C. Carpal tunnel syndrome
    D. Raynaud's syndrome

18. Liver-damaging substances such as carbon tetrachloride, chloroform, tannic acid, and trichloroethylene are called:

    A. nephrotoxins.
    B. hematoxins.
    C. hepatotoxins.
    D. lacrimators.

19. A mercury exposure during a spill would have the greatest impact on:

    A. the central nervous system.
    B. the gastrointestinal system.
    C. the circulatory system.
    D. the integumentary system.

20. **How does alcohol ingestion increase the likeliness of hypothermia?**
    A. Alcohol is a vasoconstrictor.
    B. Alcohol is a vasodilator.
    C. Alcohol restricts blood flow to the extremities.
    D. Alcohol causes an endothermic reaction in the liver.

Domain 6 Quiz 1 Answers

1. Answer: **D**. According to 1910, employee exposure records are part of medical records. 1910.1020(c)(5): "Employee exposure record" means a record containing any of the following kinds of information: 1910.1020(c)(5)(i): Environmental (workplace) monitoring or measuring of a toxic substance or harmful physical agent, including personal, area, grab, wipe, or other form of sampling, as well as related collection and analytical methodologies, calculations, and other background data relevant to interpretation of the results obtained; 1910.1020(c)(5)(ii): Biological monitoring results which directly assess the absorption of a toxic substance or harmful physical agent by body systems (e.g., the level of a chemical in the blood, urine, breath, hair, fingernails, etc.) but not including results which assess the biological effect of a substance or agent or which assess an employee's use of alcohol or drugs.
2. Answer: **B**. Direct contact of solvents with the skin can cause irritation, defatting of the skin, and dermatitis. Some solvents, especially less polar (lipophilic) solvents, can penetrate the skin, so dermal exposure to solvents can be an additional route of exposure. Experiments have demonstrated that solvent vapors can also be absorbed through the skin. Occupational dermatitis can be caused by chemical, mechanical, physical, and biological agents and plant poisons. Chemical agents are the predominant causes of dermatitis in manufacturing industries. Cutting oils and similar substances are significant because the oil dermatitis they cause is probably of greater interest to industrial concerns than is any other type of dermatitis (*Fundamentals of Industrial Hygiene*, 6th edition).
3. Answer: **D**. Ménière's disease is a disorder of the inner ear that causes severe dizziness (vertigo), ringing in the ears (tinnitus), hearing loss, and a feeling of fullness or congestion in the ear. Ménière's disease usually affects only one ear.
4. Answer: **A**. Metal fume fever (MFF) is an acute affliction that produces flu-like symptoms (fever and chills). Recovery is normally complete within one to two days. Daily exposure will cause immunity; however, any disruption such as a weekend off will result in reoccurrence of symptoms, usually with greater severity. The cause of MFF is almost always inhalation of high concentrations of zinc oxide fumes. But there are instances arising from exposure to cadmium, magnesium oxide, and copper oxides.
5. Answer: **D**. Some people exposed to asbestos in industrial environments have developed a cancer called *mesothelioma*. Mesothelioma affects mesothelial tissue used by the body for linings or sacs. These linings/sacs are found in the body's pulmonary and abdominal cavities. Persons known to develop these types of cancers include insulation workers who inhale gross amounts of asbestos, especially *chrysotile*.
6. Answer: **A**. Antibodies are plasma proteins capable of combining chemically with specific antigens that introduced their formation. An antibody is any of the body globulins that combine specifically with antigens to neutralize toxins, agglutinate bacteria or cells, and precipitate soluble antigens.
7. Answer: **B. Byssinosis,** also called "brown lung disease" or "Monday fever," is an occupational lung disease caused by exposure to cotton dust in inadequately ventilated working environments. Byssinosis commonly occurs in workers who are employed in the yarn and fabric manufacture industries. It is not believed that cotton dust directly causes the disease, and some believe that the causative agents are endotoxins from cell walls of gram-negative bacteria growing on cotton. Although bacterial endotoxin is a likely cause, the absence of similar symptoms in workers in other industries exposed to endotoxins makes this theory uncertain.
8. Answer: **A**. Nephrotoxins target kidneys, neurotoxins target nerve cells, hemotoxins target red blood cells, and hepatoxins target the liver.
9. Answer: **B. Carcinogenesis** or **oncogenesis** is literally the creation of cancer. It is a process by which normal cells are transformed into cancer cells. It is characterized by a progression of changes at the

cellular and genetic levels that ultimately reprogram a cell to undergo uncontrolled cell division, thus forming a malignant mass.

10. Answer: **B**. **Anthracosis** is a pneumoconiosis caused by exposure to coal dust (Black Lung).

    Siderosis is a lung disease caused by inhalation of iron oxide or other metallic particles.

    Silicosis is a pneumoconiosis caused by inhalation of stone dust, sand, or flint containing silica.

    Silicosiderosis is a pneumoconiosis in which inhaled dust is that of silica and iron.

11. Answer: **D**. Most of the damage in the human body from exposure to neutron radiation is due to the secondary release of gamma, beta, or alpha radiation within the body. This secondary radiation causes tissue damage. Determining the dose within the human body is difficult and depends on the amount of neutrons absorbed and energy distribution.

12. Answer: **C**. **Presbycusis** is hearing loss due to the normal process of aging. **Sociocusis** refers to hearing loss due to nonoccupational noise sources, such as household noise, TV, radio, traffic, etc. *Tinnitus* is ringing in the ears. **Sensorineural** hearing loss is loss of hearing due to occupational exposure.

13. Answer: **D**. The National Institute for Occupational Safety and Health (NIOSH) is administratively located within the Centers for Disease Control (CDC), which reports to the Department of Health and Human Services (HHS). NIOSH was originally founded within the Department of Health, Education, and Welfare that is now HHS, under the provisions of the OSH Act (1970).

    It has prime responsibility for research on occupational health and safety hazards and criteria development in dealing with toxic materials. NIOSH has the responsibility to identify hazards and recommend regulation changes. It performs testing and certification of workers' personal protective equipment, mainly respirators. NIOSH has a very active training grant program that supports university training throughout the country and conducts excellent courses at regional centers.

    NIOSH also does workplace investigations under 42 CFR Part 85, largely to conduct epidemiological methods research and studies. It does not, however, provide enforcement actions. Each year it publishes a list of toxic substances by generic family or other useful groupings.

14. Answer: **C**. The symptoms of frostbite are a "pins and needles" sensation followed by numbness. Frostbitten skin is hard, pale, and cold, and has *no feeling*. When the skin is thawed, it becomes red and very painful. Severe cases may blister and become gangrenous, resulting in hard frozen skin, sometimes all the way to bone. Answer selections A, B, and D are all symptoms of hypothermia.

15. Answer: **B**. A combination of cold and vibration often causes Raynaud's phenomenon, or traumatic vasospastic disease. This is a condition, usually of the fingers and hands, characterized by pallor caused by a greatly diminished blood supply resulting from spasm of the blood vessel walls. In addition to white fingers, the victim may also experience numbness of the affected area. The disease is most prevalent among those who work with vibrating machinery in the cold. Typical occupations are chain saw operators, jackhammer operators, tamping tool operators, etc.

16. Answer: **D**. Vector-borne infection results when a causative agent is transmitted to a host mechanically or biologically by a living vector (such as a mosquito or tick) through a bite, directly through the skin in rare cases, or by mechanical means. Biological transmission involves propagation, multiplication, cyclic development, or a combination of these in the host before the arthropod can transmit the infective form of the agent. Infected ticks and mosquitoes have transmitted Rocky Mountain spotted fever, malaria, and yellow fever to investigators in the laboratory and in the field and are a potential hazard for other outdoor workers (*Fundamentals of Industrial Hygiene*, 6th edition).

17. Answer: **B**.
    - Carpal tunnel syndrome—inflammation of the tendons in the wrist that affects the median nerve
    - De Quervain syndrome—swelling of the tendon sheath of the thumb
    - Epicondylitis—carpenter's elbow
    - Raynaud's syndrome—constriction of the blood vessels in the hand; usually due to vibrations
    - Tendinitis—swelling of a tendon

- Tenosynovitis—swelling of the sheath surrounding a tendon
- Trigger finger—a particular type of tenosynovitis in which the tendon becomes nearly locked, which pulls the finger toward the palm with a jerky movement

18. Answer: **C**. Substances capable of damaging the liver are called **hepatotoxins.** The liver is the main processing organ for toxins. It may convert toxins into nontoxic forms; however, the liver may generate a more toxic by-product, which can cause cellular and tissue damage. Examples of hepatotoxins are carbon tetrachloride, chloroform, tannic acid, and trichloroethylene. Examples of chemicals that cause cirrhosis (a fibrotic disease that results in liver dysfunction and jaundice) are carbon tetrachloride, alcohol, and aflotoxin. Other effects can range from tumors to enlargement of the liver and fat accumulation.

    The main function of the kidneys is to filter the blood and eliminate wastes. Because waste gets concentrated in the process, toxins can be at much higher levels in the kidneys. Toxins that damage this organ are known as **nephrotoxins**. Most heavy metals fall into this category, including mercury, arsenic, and lithium. Many halogenated (i.e., chlorinated) organic compounds are also nephrotoxins, such as tetrachloroethylene, carbon tetrachloride, and chloroform. Other chemicals that damage the kidneys include carbon disulfide, methanol, toluene, and ethylene glycol.

    Substances capable of producing blood disorders are called **hematoxins**. Chemicals that affect the bone marrow, which is the source of most of the components of blood, are arsenic, bromine, methyl chloride, and benzene. Chemicals that affect platelets, which are cell fragments that help in the process of blood clotting, are aspirin, benzene, and tetrachloroethane. Chemicals that affect white blood cells, which help the body defend against infection, are naphthalene and tetrachloroethane.

    Lacrimators are chemicals that can cause instant tearing at low concentrations. Examples are tear gas and MACE. Other chemicals can cause cataracts, optic nerve damage, and retinal damage by circulating through the bloodstream and reaching the eye. Examples of these are naphthalene, methanol, and thallium.

19. Answer: **A**. Mercury is a neurotoxin; health being affected by an exposure to mercury depends on many factors:
    - The form of mercury (for example, methylmercury or elemental (metallic) mercury)
    - The amount of mercury in the exposure
    - The age of the person exposed (a fetus is the most vulnerable)
    - How long the exposure lasts
    - How the person is exposed (through breathing, eating, skin contact, etc.)
    - The health of the person exposed

    Exposures to metallic mercury most often occur when metallic mercury is spilled, or when products that contain metallic mercury break, so that mercury is exposed to the air. Metallic mercury mainly causes health effects when inhaled as a vapor, where it can be absorbed through the lungs. Symptoms of prolonged and/or acute exposures include:
    - Tremors
    - Emotional changes (such as mood swings, irritability, nervousness, excessive shyness)
    - Insomnia
    - Neuromuscular changes (such as weakness, muscle atrophy, twitching)
    - Headaches
    - Disturbances in sensations
    - Changes in nerve responses
    - Poor performance on tests of mental function

    Higher exposures may also cause kidney effects, respiratory failure, and death.

20. Answer: **B**. Alcohol is a vasodilator, meaning that it causes blood vessels to dilate. Alcohol may make your body feel warm inside, but the vasodilation it causes results in more rapid heat loss from the surface of the skin. The body's natural shivering response is diminished in people who've been drinking alcohol. In addition, the use of alcohol or recreational drugs can affect a person's judgment about the need to get inside or wear warm clothes in cold weather conditions. If a person is intoxicated and passes out in cold weather, he or she is likely to develop hypothermia.

Domain 6 Quiz 2 Questions

1. What effect in the lung tissue is caused by asbestos and silica dust?
   A. Cystosis
   B. Fibrosis
   C. Necrosis
   D. Scoliosis

2. One occupational illness not caused by a virus is:
   A. HIV/AIDS.
   B. tuberculosis.
   C. hepatitis B.
   D. West Nile.

3. The human body is:
   A. more capable of coping with heat loss than heat gain.
   B. less capable of coping with heat loss than heat gain.
   C. equally capable of coping with heat loss or heat gain.
   D. unaffected by environments with potential of heat loss or gain.

4. Which device does not electronically store data?
   A. Data logger
   B. Colorimetric tube
   C. Portacount® equipment
   D. Holter monitor

5. For protection against chlorinated solvents in jobs requiring dexterity and sensitivity, which type of chemical-resistant gloves is preferred?
   A. Butyl
   B. Neoprene
   C. Nitrile
   D. Polyvinyl alcohol (PVA)

6. An output power up to 500 mW, sufficient to cause eye injury, is produced by Class ____ lasers.
   A. 1
   B. 2
   C. 3
   D. 4

7. The most difficult material(s) to remove during decontamination is/are:
   A. those chemically permeated into PPE material.
   B. dried solid materials caked onto PPE.
   C. liquid material spread into crevices and pleats of PPE.
   D. sludges splattered onto PPE.

8. Chemicals or substances that cause damage or death to a developing fetus, but cannot be passed on to further generations, are called:
   A. irritants.
   B. sensitizers.
   C. mutagens.
   D. teratogens.

9. Which of the following is not a protection method used for external radiation exposure?

   A. Time
   B. Distance
   C. Dose exposure
   D. Shielding

10. A plant manager goes from a quiet office to the plant floor, where loud noises are present. What type of occupational noise exposure does the plant manager encounter?

    A. Intermittent
    B. Continuous
    C. Impact
    D. Peak

11. If an industrial hygienist is conducting a sound-level survey at a plant, the sound-level meter should be set to which scale/weight to assess the noise hazard?

    A. A-weighted
    B. B-weighted
    C. C-weighted
    D. D-weighted

12. Dermatitis would be a major concern with the permeability of neoprene gloves if selected for protection for which of the following?

    A. Motor oil
    B. Propane
    C. Carbon tetrachloride
    D. Hexane

13. A work operation is being conducted in a large three-story underground vault. The operation consists of stick welding steel pipe on the third floor, with local exhaust ventilation and continuous air monitoring. A crew of two laborers is assigned to support the welders by transporting the large sections of steel pipe from the first floor, where they are off-loaded by a mobile crane. The temperature in the vault is about 90°F, with a humidity of 85%. After about two hours of operation, one of the laborers is overcome and must be removed from the area. His symptoms include a pale, pasty-white complexion, nausea, headache, rapid pulse, and low blood pressure. Which of the following best describes the condition that most likely caused this illness?

    A. Heat exhaustion
    B. Carbon dioxide poisoning
    C. Carbon monoxide poisoning
    D. Metal fume fever

14. What is the general purpose of a globe thermometer?

    A. It is a device used to measure radiant heat.
    B. It is a device used to measure relative humidity.
    C. It collects data on the absolute moisture content of the air and water vapor pressure.
    D. It measures surface temperature.

15. Which of the following is not a common type of heat transfer?

    A. Radiation
    B. Condensation
    C. Convection
    D. Conduction

16. A specific eye, mouth, other mucous membrane, nonintact skin, or parenteral contact with blood or other potentially infectious materials that results from the performance of an employee's duties is called a/an:

   A. pathogenic incident.
   B. contamination incident.
   C. exposure incident.
   D. universal precaution.

17. One substance, having very low or no significant toxicity, enhances the toxicity of another substance (e.g., 0 + 5 = 15); the result is a more severe injury than that which the toxic substance would have produced by itself. This is termed the:

   A. additive effect.
   B. synergistic effect.
   C. potentiating effect.
   D. antagonistic effect.

18. In which of the following conditions would the use of dilution ventilation be most appropriate?

   A. The source of contamination is constant and highly toxic.
   B. The source of contamination is a heavy particulate.
   C. Workers are in close contact with the source of contamination.
   D. The source of contamination is constant and nontoxic.

19. An office environment is experiencing increased sick building syndrome complaints from employees. The HVAC system is found to be operating and well maintained. What could be a physical cause for concern?

   A. Poor maintenance of air filtration
   B. Poor air quality or distribution
   C. Carpal tunnel syndrome
   D. Job stress due to personal factors

20. Three employees at a call center report headache and fatigue, and are concerned with indoor air quality. The results of indoor air quality sampling do not indicate any airborne hazards. The only change in the call center environment is a 30% increase in staff to handle the large call volume. What is a likely psychological cause of the symptoms?

   A. Air quality
   B. HVAC system problems
   C. Job stress
   D. Ventilation

Domain 6 Quiz 2 Answers

1. Answer: **B**. Fibrosis is a condition in which the lung becomes scarred and inflexible, making the lung unable to expand and contract.
2. Answer: **B**. Answers A, C, and D are caused by a virus, whereas tuberculosis is caused by bacteria.
3. Answer: **B**. The human body is designed to work optimally at a temperature of 98.6°F ± 1.8°F. The human body is less capable of coping with heat loss than with heat gain. Exposure to cold temperatures (air temperatures less than 61°F) can reduce manual dexterity. While adaptive mechanisms (e.g., sweating and acclimation) are crucial during heat stress exposures, the physiological adaptations to cold stress have less dramatic effects. The first physiological response to cold stress is to conserve body heat by reducing blood circulation through the skin, effectively making the skin an insulating layer. The second physiological response is boosting the body's metabolism through shivering, a sign of significant cold stress.
4. Answer: **B**. A *data logger* is an electronic instrument used to take measurements from sensors and store those measurements for future use. Some common measurements include temperature, pressure, current,

velocity, strain, displacement, and other physical phenomena. A ***colorimetric tube*** (Dreager-tubes®) provides a color change to indicate concentration levels of specific contaminants. It is used to perform quick, on-the-spot measurement of specific toxic and combustible substances at relatively low cost. It does not electronically store data. A ***PortaCount***® is a device used to measure quantitative respirator fit testing. A ***Holter monitor*** is a portable device for continuously monitoring various electrical activity of the cardiovascular system for at least 24 hours.

5. Answer: **C**.

   Chemical-Resistant Gloves
   - ***Butyl***: High-resistance protection from gas or water vapors. Also, resistant to common acids and alcohols.
   - ***Hot-Mill or Aluminized***: Reflective and insulating protection, for welding, furnace, and foundry work.
   - ***Latex***: Protection from most aqueous solutions of acids, alkalis, salts, and ketones. Latex gloves resist abrasions during grinding, sandblasting, and polishing. These general-purpose, pliable, and comfortable gloves are used for common industrial applications, food processing, maintenance, construction, and lab work.
   - ***Natural Rubber***: Liquid-proof protection against acids, caustics, and dye stuffs.
   - ***Neoprene***: Protection against hydraulic fluids, gasoline, alcohols, organic acids, and alkalis. Neoprene gloves offer good pliability and finger dexterity, high density, tensile strength, and high tear resistance.
   - ***Neoprene Latex***: Protection against detergents, salts, acids, and caustic solutions.
   - ***Nitrile/Natural Rubber***: Protection from chlorinated solvents. Nitrile/rubber gloves are intended for jobs requiring dexterity and sensitivity. The blend resists abrasions, cuts, tears, and punctures.
   - ***N-DEX***: These nitrile gloves provide splash and spill protection against a wide variety of chemicals, although they are not intended for extended immersion activities. Available in low-power and powder-free options.
   - ***Polyvinyl Alcohol (PVA)***: Resistance to strong solvents such as chlorinated and aromatic solvents. This material is water soluble (polyvinyl alcohol) and cannot be used in water or water-based solutions.
   - ***Polyvinyl Chloride (PVC)***: Resistance to abrasives such as materials coated or immersed in grease, oil, acids, or caustics. Available lined or unlined, depending on dexterity requirements.
   - ***Silver Shield***: Protection against a wide range of solvents, acids, and bases. These lightweight laminate gloves are flexible, but not form fitting, which affects user dexterity.
   - ***Vinyl***: Resistance to a variety of irritants.
   - ***Viton***: Resistance to PCBs, chlorinated and aromatic solvents, gas, and water vapors. These gloves can be used in water-based solutions.

6. Answer: **C**. A **laser** is a device that emits light through a process of optical amplification based on the stimulated emission of electromagnetic radiation. The term "laser" originated as an acronym for "light amplification by stimulated emission of radiation." This fits the definition of a Class 3B laser. Laser eyewear must be selected with the specific laser wavelength in mind.

   The International Electrotechnical Commission (IEC) publishes standards on laser safety. The IEC also sets out five classes of laser: 1, 2, 3A, 3B, and 4. This classification gives the user an indication of the degree of laser hazard.

   Class 1 lasers have an output power that is below the level at which eye injury can occur.

   Class 2 lasers emit visible light and are limited to a maximum output power of 1 milliwatt (mW). A person receiving an eye exposure from a Class 2 laser will be protected from injury by their natural blink reflex, an involuntary response that causes the person to blink and turn their head, thereby avoiding eye exposure.

   Class 3A lasers may have a maximum output power of 5 mW. This limit restricts the power entering a fully dilated human eye (taken as a 7 mm aperture) to 1 mW. Thus, accidental exposure to a Class 3A laser should be no more hazardous than exposure to a Class 2 laser. However, Class 3A laser pointers are hazardous when viewed with an optical aid such as binoculars and are therefore unsuitable for the general consumer.

Class 3B lasers have an output power up to 500 mW, sufficient to cause eye injury. The extent and severity of any eye injury will depend upon several factors, including the laser power entering the eye and the exposure duration.

Class 1, Class 2, Class 3A, and Class 3B lasers do not have sufficient power to cause a skin injury.

Class 4 lasers have an output power greater than 500 mW; are capable of causing injury to both the eye and skin; and will be a fire hazard if sufficiently high-output powers are used. ANSI Z136.1 (2007)

7. Answer: **A**. Chemicals permeated into PPE material are the most difficult to remove. Most PPE manufacturers recommend disposal of permeated PPE.

8. Answer: **D**. **Irritants** are chemicals that will irritate various tissues, causing redness, rashes, swelling, coughing, or even hemorrhaging. Chlorine and ammonia are two examples of irritants.

    Another name for **sensitizers** is allergens. These chemicals cause an allergic type of reaction due to sensitivity from prior exposure. An acute response may be swelling of the breathing tubes, which causes breathing difficulty. Sensitizers can cause chronic lung disease. Some common examples are epoxies, aromatic amines, formaldehyde, nickel metal, and maleic anhydride.

    Mutagens cause alterations in the genes of an exposed person. The result may be malfunction of a specific organ or tissue, depending upon the type of cell in which the mutation took place. Gene damage can be passed on to children if the mutation occurred in either parent's sperm or egg. Examples of mutagens are ethylene oxide, benzene, and hydrazine.

    Teratogens cause damage or death to a developing fetus. This damage cannot be passed on to further generations, as it does not affect the genetic code. Examples of teratogens are thalidomide, dioxins, lead, and cadmium.

9. Answer: **C**. For external radiation exposure hazards, the basic protection measures are associated with time, distance, and shielding (**Table 13**). Shielding is a barrier that protects workers from harmful radiation released by radioactive materials. Lead bricks, dense concrete, water, and earth are examples of materials used for shielding (*Fundamentals of Industrial Hygiene*, 6th edition). Use of the ALARA concept as a guideline originated in the atomic energy field and stands for "as low as reasonably achievable." According to the Nuclear Regulatory Commission, ALARA means making every reasonable effort to maintain exposures to ionizing radiation (**Table 14**) as far below the dose limits as practical.

Table 13 Basic Protection Measures for External Radiation Exposure

TYPE	EFFECTS	SHIELDING
Alpha	Short range: < 4" in air Chemically similar to calcium (can collect in kidneys, bones, liver, lungs, and spleen) Eyes are an internal exposure	Skin, paper, thin film of water
Beta	Secondary release of gamma radiation Higher energies can cause skin burns	Light metals (like aluminum)
Neutron	Secondary release of gamma radiation	Carbon or high hydrogen content (like water)
Gamma and X-ray	Most penetrating Electromagnetic radiation: Gamma (natural) and X-ray (manmade)	Heavy metals (like lead)

Table 14 Exposure Limits for Ionizing Radiation

Exposure	Limit	Source
Whole body; head and trunk; active blood-forming organs, 1.25 rem per calendar quarter lens of eyes; gonads	1.25 rem per calendar quarter	OSHA, NRC
Hands and forearms; feet and ankles	8.75 rem per calendar quarter 18.75 rem per calendar quarter	NRC OSHA
Skin of whole body	0.5 rem per calendar quarter 7.5 rem per calendar quarter	NRC OSHA
Individuals younger than 18 years of age	1/10 of above limits	OSHA, NRC
Drinking water: Radium (226 Ra and 228 Ra) and gross alpha particle	5 pCi/l	EPA
Drinking water: gross alpha particle activity (excluding radon and uranium)	15 pCi/l	EPA
Drinking water: beta particles and photons from artificial sources to total body or any internal organ	4 mrem/yr	EPA
Air quality, exposure of the public Whole body Critical organ	25 mrem/yr 75 mrem/yr	EPA
Average person	500 mrem/yr, 2 mrem/hr; 100 mrem/7 days	NRC
Nuclear industry worker	5 (*N*–18) rem/yr, 3 rem/quarter	NRC

10. Answer: **A**. There are three general classes into which occupational noise exposures can be grouped: continuous noise, intermittent noise, and impact-type noise.

    Continuous noise is normally defined as broadband noise of approximately constant level and spectrum to which an employee is exposed for a period of 8 hours per day, 40 hours per week. A large number of industrial operations fit into this class of noise exposure. Most damage-risk criteria are written for this type of noise exposure because it is the easiest to define in terms of amplitude, frequency content, and duration.

    Exposure to intermittent noise can be defined as exposure to a given broadband sound-pressure level several times during a normal working day. The inspector or facility supervisor who periodically makes trips from a relatively quiet office into noisy production areas may be subject to this type of noise.

    With steady noises, it is sufficient to record the A-weighted sound level attained by the noise. With noises that are not steady, such as impulsive noises, impact noises, and the like, the temporal character of the noise requires additional specification. Both the short-term and long-term variations of the noise must be described. Non-steady noise exposure measurements are most easily made using dosimeters.

    Impact-type noise is a sharp burst of sound, and sophisticated instrumentation is necessary to determine the peak levels for this type of noise. Noise types other than steady ones are commonly encountered. In general, sounds repeated more than once per second can be considered as steady. Impulsive or impact noise, such as that made by hammer blows or explosions, is generally less than one-half second in duration and does not repeat more often than once per second. Employees should not be exposed to impulsive or impact noise that exceeds a peak sound pressure level of 140 dB.

11. Answer: **A**. The A-weighted sound level measurement is important in the assessment of overall noise hazard because it represents human hearing. It is thought to provide a rating of industrial broadband noises that indicates the injurious effects such noise has on human hearing.

    The A-weighted sound level has been adopted as the measurement for assessing noise exposure by the American Conference of Governmental Industrial Hygienists (ACGIH). The A-weighted sound level as the preferred unit of measurement was also adopted by the US Department of Labor as part of its Occupational Safety and Health Standards. The A-weighted sound level has also been shown to provide reasonably good assessments of speech interference and community disturbance conditions and has been adopted by the U.S. Environmental Protection Agency (EPA) for these purposes.

12. Answer: **C**. A common mistake is to recommend "rubber" or neoprene gloves for use as a hand protection against a solvent, regardless of the kind of solvent in use. Many solvents can quickly penetrate latex rubber or neoprene gloves and come in contact with the skin. Neoprene is good for protection against most common oils, aliphatic hydrocarbons, and certain other solvents, but is not satisfactory against aromatic hydrocarbons, halogenated hydrocarbons, ketones, and many other solvents. Some solvents, such as benzene, carbon tetrachloride, and methyl alcohol, can be absorbed in amounts great enough to cause injury to organs other than the skin.

13. Answer: **A**. Several workplace conditions could cause these symptoms. However, the symptoms listed are the classic signs of heat exhaustion. Inhalation of large amounts of carbon dioxide causes increased heart rate and rapid pulse, but increased blood pressure. Carbon monoxide poisoning would result in the same symptoms except for the lack of cyanosis (blue lips and skin). Metal fume fever is characterized by flu-like symptoms.

14. Answer: **A**. An ordinary dry bulb thermometer alone will not measure radiant heat. A **black globe thermometer** is a hollow copper sphere painted on the outside with a matte black finish to measure the radiant energy from direct sunlight or other sources (e.g., machinery and hot structures near the workplace).

15. Answer: **B**. Three common types of heat transfer are radiation, convection, and conduction. Radiation: Solid bodies of different temperatures have a net heat flow from the hotter surface to the cooler surface by electromagnetic radiation (primarily infrared radiation). The rate of heat transfer by radiation depends on the average temperature of the surrounding solid surfaces, skin temperature, and clothing. Convection: The exchange of heat between the skin and the surrounding air is referred to as convection. The direction of heat flow depends on the temperature difference between the skin and air. The rate of convective heat exchange depends on the magnitude of the temperature difference, the amount of air motion, and clothing. Conduction: When two solid bodies are in contact, heat will flow from the warmer body to the cooler body. The rate of heat transfer depends on the difference in temperatures between the skin and the solid surface, the thermal conductivity of the solid body that the person contacts, and clothing that may separate the person from the solid surface. Radiant heat is a form of electromagnetic energy similar to light, but of longer wavelength. Radiant heat (from such sources as red-hot metal, open flames, and the sun) has no appreciable heating effect on the air it passes through, but its energy is absorbed by any object it strikes, thus heating the person, wall, machine, or whatever object it falls on. Protection requires placing opaque shields or screens between the person and the radiating surface.

16. Answer: **C**. *OSHA 1910.1030(b) Bloodborne Pathogen Standard* defines **exposure incident** as a specific eye, mouth, other mucous membrane, nonintact skin, or parenteral contact with blood or other potentially infectious materials that results from the performance of an employee's duties.

17. Answer: **C**. People are never exposed to only one chemical at a time. We are always exposed to mixtures of chemicals, whether we are in the workplace, at home, or in the ambient outdoor environment. Most chemicals do not cause a similar degree of injury in all the tissues or organs they encounter. Major adverse effects usually occur in the **target organs**. For example, benzene usually affects the bone marrow, *n*-hexane affects the peripheral nervous system, and paraquat affects the lungs. The majority of the available toxicological data comes from controlled studies where test subjects have been exposed to only a single substance. There are few data from studies in which test subjects have been exposed to two or more substances simultaneously.

Based on the available data and other observations, toxicologists have identified five ways in which chemicals may interact with each other in the body to produce responses. These interactions are:
- **Independent effect**: Substances exert their own toxicity independently of each other.
- **Additive effect**: The combined effect of exposure to two chemicals that have both the same mechanism of action and target organ, is equal to the sum of the effects of exposure to each chemical when given alone (e.g., 3 + 5 = 8). In the absence of any data to the contrary, chemicals are assumed to interact in an additive manner (example: two different organophosphate insecticides and inhibition of acetylcholinesterase at neuromuscular junctions).

- **Synergistic effect**: The combined effect of exposure to two chemicals is much greater than the sum of the effects of each substance when given alone (e.g., 3 + 5 = 30); each substance magnifies the toxicity of the other.
- **Potentiating effect**: One substance, having very low or no significant toxicity, enhances the toxicity of another (e.g., 0 + 5 = 15); the result is a more severe injury than that which the toxic substance would have produced by itself.
- **Antagonistic effect**: An exposure where two chemicals together interfere with each other's toxic actions (e.g., 4 + 6 = 8), or one chemical interferes with the toxic action of the other chemical, such as in antidotal therapy (e.g., 0 + 4 = 2).

18. Answer **D**. Dilution ventilation is the preferred solution when relatively nontoxic emissions are produced, when the source is mainly gases or vapors (not primarily heavy particulates), and when employees do not work in the immediate vicinity or direct path of the emission source. The old adage "no pollution through more dilution" is often very appropriate; however, when toxic, heavy, direct path, time inconsistent, or large sources of emissions are encountered, the solution is point source removal through local exhaust ventilation. Local exhaust ventilation and dust collection systems shall be designed, constructed, installed, and maintained in accordance with good practices such as those found in the American National Standard – Fundamentals Governing the Design and Operation of Local Exhaust Systems, ANSI Z9.2-1979.

19. Answer: **B**. In approximately 500 indoor air quality investigations in the last decade, the National Institute for Occupational Safety and Health (NIOSH) found that the primary sources of indoor air quality problems are:

Inadequate ventilation	52%
Contamination from inside building	16%
Contamination from outside building	10%
Microbial contamination	5%
Contamination from building fabric	4%
Unknown sources	13%

20. Answer: **C**. In a recent NIOSH document, Stress Management in Work Settings, occupational stress is discussed in terms of assessment methods, stress management, and programs and training necessary to reduce occupational stress. The synergistic effect of multiple stressors appears to indicate that building-related problems may be more than an air quality problem. The combined effect of these multiple stressors may interact with employees and could result in acute adverse emotional or physical reactions. In the short term, these reactions may lead to decreased productivity, absenteeism, and high turnover rates, and if prolonged may lead to a variety of illnesses including hypertension, coronary heart disease, ulcers, alcoholism and mental illness. These office-related health problems can be evaluated by a consultant through employee interviews and analysis of job demands.

    Often employee complaints result from items such as cigarette smoke, odors, low-level contaminants, poor air circulation, thermal gradients, humidity, job pressures, lighting, work-station design, or noise. (OSHA TED 1-0.15A)

    The following potential problems may need to be addressed:

    Physical hazards including noise from nearby sources such as air conditioning systems and printers, inadequate lighting, stress from the operation of video display terminals (VDT's), vibration sources, extremes of heat, cold and humidity, drafts, and poor air circulation.

    Ergonomic problems such as carpal tunnel syndrome or inflammatory disorders of the tendons and joints of keyboard operator's due to tasks requiring repetitive motions. Proper design of fixed work stations where employees are required to perform repetitive tasks includes proper lighting to prevent glare, maintaining temperature and humidity in a comfortable range with minimum temperature variations, maximum flexibility in work station design including adjustable chair, keyboard, and screen height, and a work-rest regimen that allows breaks to reduce psychological distress.

152 ASP Exam Study Workbook

Reduction of job stress by: (a) adequate flow of information from management to employees; (b) explanation of any changes introduced into the workplace including new chemicals, ventilation, production modification, and work schedules; (c) maximizing employee participation in planning and implementing changes; (d) stress reduction techniques including exercise, biofeedback, and assertiveness training; and (e) training workers to understand chemicals they may be working with and their health effects, dose/response relationships, and results of environmental evaluation.

Domain 6 Quiz 3 Questions

1. Toxicologists have learned that many chemicals act together in certain ways on biological systems. When exposure to two different toxic chemicals produces a more severe effect than simply doubling the dose of either one alone, such as isopropyl alcohol and chloroform, this reaction is called:
    A. the additive effect.
    B. the synergistic effect.
    C. potentiation.
    D. antagonism.

2. When a person is doing drugs to relax or escape from a situation, this type of drug use is called:
    A. experimental.
    B. recreational.
    C. compulsory.
    D. addiction.

3. What are the three parts of a wellness program?
    A. Lifestyle change for the better, health programs, counseling programs
    B. Violence prevention, medical assurance, counseling programs
    C. Counseling programs, violence prevention programs, substance abuse program
    D. Health programs, medical insurance, and lifestyle change programs

4. The shortest wavelength is:
    A. ultraviolet.
    B. visible.
    C. infrared.
    D. microwave.

5. The part of the eye that turns light waves into a signal that is transmitted to the brain by the optic nerve is called the:
    A. cornea.
    B. lens.
    C. retina.
    D. pupil.

6. Toxic materials enter the body through which major routes?
    A. Inhalation, skin absorption, ingestion, injection
    B. Inhalation, capillary absorption, intravenous
    C. Inhalation, respiration, breathing, capillary absorption
    D. Inhalation, skin absorption, intravenous, eye absorption

7. The PPE that provides the greatest level of skin and respiratory protection is:
    A. Level A.
    B. Level B.
    C. Level C.
    D. Level D.

8. Which authority publishes TLVs?

    A. ACGIH
    B. OSHA
    C. MSHA
    D. NIOSH

9. In a poorly ventilated office space, the best way to check air quality is to measure:

    A. carbon dioxide (CO_2) levels.
    B. carbon monoxide (CO) levels.
    C. oxygen (O_2) levels.
    D. the *Stachybotrys* mold spore count.

10. What is Legionnaires' disease?

    A. Virus-induced influenza
    B. Bacteria-induced pneumonia
    C. Fungi-induced histoplasmosis
    D. Chrome-induced dermatitis

11. The National Institutes of Health (NIH) publishes biosafety guidelines commonly used for containment of biohazardous agents in workplaces (Biosafety in Microbiological and Biomedical Laboratories). How many biosafety levels (BSL) are there?

    A. 2
    B. 3
    C. 4
    D. 5

12. Which is the best method to prevent infection from escaping a surface in a lab?

    A. Use of disposable personal protective equipment (PPE)
    B. Decontamination procedures for PPE
    C. An industrial hygiene program
    D. Containment

13. Professionals dedicated to the science that studies harmful, or toxic, properties of substances are:

    A. industrial hygienists.
    B. industrial toxicologists.
    C. health physicists.
    D. medical pathologists.

14. In the lungs, oxygen is absorbed into the bloodstream by passing through the membrane of the _____ in the lungs.

    A. pleural cavity
    B. bronchioles
    C. alveoli
    D. trachea

15. A full-facepiece-supplied air respirator in positive pressure mode has a protection factor of:

    A. 1000 APF.
    B. 100 APF.
    C. 10 APF.
    D. 10,000 APF.

16. Using the chart below, determine the maximum use concentration (MUC) for a half-mask respirator with dust/mist filters for aluminum metal dust. The TLV for aluminum metal dust is 10 mg/m^3.

TYPE OF RESPIRATOR	Respirator Assigned Protection Factors		
	Qualitative	Quantitative	IDLH
Particulate filter, vapor or gas, quarter or half mask. Includes combination filters.	10	Per-individual max of 100	NO
Particulate filter, vapor or gas, full face piece. Includes combination filters.	100	Per-individual max of 100	NO
Powered particulate filter, vapor or gas, full face piece, any respiratory inlet covering.	No test required due to positive pressure. Max protection is 3000 with high-efficiency filter.		NO

A. 10 mg/m^3
B. 1 mg/m^3
C. 100 mg/m^3
D. 10,000 mg/m^3

Domain 6 Quiz 3 Answers

1. Answer: **B**

    Additive Effect (2 + 2 = 4) Some toxic chemicals add their effects together in producing a biological effect. In this case the effect is the same as being exposed to double the dose of either chemical alone. Example: acetaminophen and ibuprofen.

    Synergistic Effect (2 + 2 = 6) Synergism is the exposure to two different toxic chemicals that produce a more severe effect than simply doubling the dose of either one alone. An example is isopropyl alcohol and chloroform. The alcohol ties up enzymes that would normally break down chloroform.

    Potentiation (0 + 2 = 10) In some cases a chemical without any known toxic effect may act together with a known toxic substance to make the toxic substance even more potent and thus more dangerous. Ethanol (ethyl alcohol) and chloroform together affect the liver in just such a manner.

    Antagonism (4 + 6 = 8) The interaction of two toxic chemicals may be such that the effect produced is actually less than would be expected. Phenobarbital and benzopyrene together is an example. The phenobarbital increases the enzyme activity that detoxifies benzopyrene.

2. Answer: **B**. Recreational drugs are used for enjoyment, escape, or leisure purposes, rather than for medical reasons. Users may feel drugs help them forget their worries or problems. When they first use a drug, people may perceive what seem to be positive effects; they also may believe that they can control their use. However, drugs can quickly take over a person's life. Over time, if drug use continues, other pleasurable activities become less pleasurable, and taking the drug becomes necessary for the user just to feel "normal." Users may then compulsively seek and take drugs even though it causes tremendous problems for themselves and their loved ones. Some people may start to feel the need to take higher or more frequent doses, even in the early stages of their drug use. These are the telltale signs of an addiction. Addiction is defined as a chronic, relapsing brain disease that is characterized by compulsive drug seeking and use, despite harmful consequences. It is considered a brain disease because drugs change the brain—they change its structure and how it works. These brain changes can be long-lasting and can lead to the harmful behaviors seen in people who abuse drugs.

3. Answer: **A**. Ultimately a wellness program involves **lifestyle change for the better**. A wellness program allows an employer or plan to offer premium discounts, cash rewards, gym memberships, and other incentives to participate. Some examples of wellness programs include programs to assist smoking cessation, diabetes management programs, weight-loss programs, and preventive health screenings. Many employee assistance programs offer counseling and substance abuse programs.

4. Answer: **A**. The **visible spectrum** (sometimes called the optical spectrum) is the portion of the electromagnetic spectrum that is visible to (can be detected by) the human eye. Electromagnetic radiation in this range of wavelengths is called **visible light** or simply light. A typical human eye will respond to wavelengths in air from about 380 to 750 nm (some references use 400 to 780 nm). Infrared (IR) radiation and microwave radiation are electromagnetic radiation types with wavelengths longer than that of visible light, and ultraviolet (UV) light is electromagnetic radiation with a wavelength shorter than that of visible light.
5. Answer: **C**. When light enters the **eye**, it first passes through the **cornea**; the cornea's main function is to refract, or bend, light. The **lens** focuses light rays onto the light-sensitive **retina**, where it is changed into a signal that is transmitted to the brain by the **optic nerve**. The signal is received and interpreted by the brain as a visual image. The **pupil** is the opening of the iris. The pupil may appear to open (dilate) and close (constrict), but it is really the iris that is the prime mover; the pupil is merely the absence of iris. The pupil determines how much light is let into the eye.
6. Answer: **A**. The most common ways for toxic materials to enter the body is through inhalation, eye and skin absorption, ingestion, and injection. Inhalation is the major route for industrial contaminants. Inhalation is significant not only because it is the most common path but because of the rapidity with which a toxic material can be absorbed in the lungs, or nasal passages, passed to the bloodstream, and reach the brain. Skin absorption is generally recognized to be the next most frequent route of entry, followed by ingestion. Puncture wounds are the least frequent. Exposure depends on the environment. For example, the most common route of entry in the off-duty (home) environment is ingestion.
7. Answer: **A**. Before a technician responds to a hazardous material incident, he/she must be familiar with the types and levels of protective clothing available. The Occupational Safety and Health Administration has developed a classification scheme for the various levels (**Table 15**) of chemical protective clothing (29CFR 1910.120, Appendix B). The levels are defined as follows: Level A: protection that should be worn when the highest level of respiratory, skin, eye, and mucous membrane protection is needed (for example, SCBA and a gas-tight, totally encapsulating chemical suit). Level B: protection that should be selected when the highest level of respiratory protection is needed with a lesser level of skin and eye protection (for example, SCBA plus an encapsulated suit with an exhaust port or a hooded suit, gloves, and boots). Level B protection is the minimum level recommended on initial site entries until the hazards have been further identified and defined by monitoring, sampling, and other reliable methods of analysis. Level C: protection that should be selected when the type of airborne substance is known, concentration is measured, criteria for using air-purifying respirators are met, and skin and eye exposures are unlikely. Periodic monitoring of the air must be performed. Level D: primarily, a work uniform. It should not be worn on any hazardous materials site.

Table 15 Modified Chart of EPA/OSHA Levels of Protection

Level	Skin	Respiratory	When
A	Fully encapsulating, chemical-resistant suit, inner gloves, chemical-resistant safety boots	Pressure-demand, full-facepiece SCBA or pressure-demand supplied-air respirator with escape SCBA	Highest level of protection indicated by high concentration of atmospheric vapors, gases, or particulates, or when splash hazard exists
B	Chemical-resistant clothing (overalls and long-sleeved jacket; hooded, one- or two-piece chemical splash suit; disposable chemical-resistant one-piece suit), inner and outer gloves, chemical-resistant safety boots, hard hat	Pressure-demand, full-facepiece SCBA or pressure-demand supplied-air respirator with escape SCBA	High level of respiratory protection required, but less skin protection. IDLH, less than 19.5% oxygen.

(Continues)

Table 15 Modified Chart of EPA/OSHA Levels of Protection (*Continued*)

Level	Skin	Respiratory	When
C	Chemical-resistant clothing (overalls and long-sleeved jacket; hooded, one- or two-piece chemical splash suit; disposable chemical-resistant one-piece suit), inner and outer gloves, chemical-resistant safety boots, hard hat	Full-facepiece, air-purifying, canister-equipped respirator	The contaminants, splashes, or direct contact will not affect exposed flesh. Canister will remove contaminant.
D	Overalls, safety boots, safety glasses or chemical splash goggles, hard hat	No respiratory protection and minimal skin protection	The atmosphere contains no known hazard. Splashes, immersion, or inhalation improbable.

When the use of PPE cannot be avoided, the program should include these elements:
- Selection based on the hazards that are present
- Use and limitations on use
- Work duration while using
- Maintenance and storage requirements
- Decontamination and disposal procedures
- Training and fitting requirements
- Donning and doffing procedures
- Inspection procedures
- Temperature limitations

8. Answer: **A**. The American Conference of Governmental Industrial Hygienists (ACGIH) publishes the Threshold Limit Values (TLVs) in wide use in industry. OSHA publishes the Permissible Exposure Limits (PELs). NIOSH publishes the RELs.

Threshold Limit Values (TLVs)
- Established by the American Conference of Governmental Industrial Hygienists (ACGIH)
- Represent *recommended* exposure limits
- Include different types of limits:
  - **TLV - Time-Weighted Average (TLV-TWA)**
  - **TLV - Short-Term Exposure Limit (TLV-STEL)**
  - **TLV - Ceiling Limit (TLV-C)**
  - **Skin notation**
- **Short-term exposure limit (STEL):**
  - Indicates the maximum concentration workers can be exposed to for a short time period (**usually 15 minutes**)
  - Indicates the concentration to which it is believed workers can be exposed continuously for a short period of time
  - Represents a 15-minute exposure for no more than 4 times a day with at least 60 minutes between each exposure
  - Must not cause irritation, chronic tissue damage, or **narcosis** that increases the possibility of accidental injury, impairment of self-rescue, or reduced work efficiency
  - Does not exceed the daily TLV-TWA
- **Skin notation:**
  - Indicates that dermal exposure may contribute significantly to overall exposure

*List of PELs: 29 CFR Part 1910, Subpart Z, and 1926

TLV - Ceiling (TLV-C)
- Should *not* be exceeded during any part of the working exposure
- Differs from the TWA:
  - The TWA permits **excursions** above the TLV, provided they are compensated for by equivalent excursions below the TWA.
  - The **ceiling limit** places a definite boundary that concentrations *must not* be permitted to exceed.
- **PELs**   OSHA Permissible Exposure Limits are time-weighted average (TWA) concentrations that must not be exceeded during any 8-hour work shift of a 40-hour workweek.
- **IDLHs**   NIOSH definition Immediately Dangerous to Life or Health concentrations represent the maximum concentration from which, in the event of a respirator failure, one could escape within 30 minutes without a respirator and without experiencing any escape-impairing (e.g., severe eye irritation) or irreversible health effects.

9. Answer: **A**. To check for indoor air quality, use a direct reading instrument to detect carbon dioxide (CO_2) levels. Carbon monoxide is another common contaminant usually found in work environments with combustion engines and poor air exchange. *Stachybotrys chartarum* is a species of mold, also called black mold or toxic black mold, that causes health problems impacting the respiratory system.

10. Answer: **B**. Legionnaires' disease is a form of bacterial pneumonia. It is spread chiefly by bacteria-laden water droplets coming through air conditioning and similar systems. The Centers for Disease Control and Prevention (CDC) first identified *Legionella pneumophila* in 1977 as the cause of an outbreak of pneumonia that caused 34 deaths at a 1976 American Legion Convention in Philadelphia. *L. pneumophila* had undoubtedly caused previous pneumonia outbreaks, but the organism's slow growth and special growth requirements prevented earlier discovery. The species of *Legionella* that have been associated with cases of Legionnaires' disease are called Legionnaires' disease bacteria (LDB).

11. Answer: **C**. There are 4 biosafety levels:

    BSL-1: Agents not known to consistently cause disease in healthy adults

    BSL-2: Agents associated with human disease; hazard is from percutaneous injury, ingestion, mucous membrane exposure

    BSL-3: Indigenous or exotic agents with potential for aerosol transmission; disease may have serious or lethal consequences

    BSL-4: Dangerous/exotic agents that pose a high risk of life-threatening disease; aerosol-transmitted lab infections; or related agents with unknown risk of transmission BMBL (2009)

12. Answer: **D**. Containment is the mechanism for ensuring that workers, the immediate work environment, and the community, including those outside the immediate workplace, are protected or shielded from exposure during workplace activities involving infectious or biological agents. As stated in the fifth edition of BMBL (2009), "the term 'containment' is used in describing safe methods, facilities and equipment for managing infectious materials in the laboratory environment where they are being handled or maintained." Varying configurations of these components are used depending on the hazard category of the work. The CDC and NIH have designated four default configurations of work practices, safety equipment, and facility design as biosafety levels (BSLs) for work involving infectious agents or activities in which experimentally or naturally infected vertebrate animals are manipulated. The combination must be specifically appropriate for the operations performed, the documented or suspected routes of transmission of the agent, and the laboratory function or activity. The use of increasingly stringent procedures and more complex laboratory facilities permits higher risk activities to be carried out safely. Specific mitigation measures should be selected based on the identified risks. As a simple example, minimizing sharps would be a good practice for handling an agent that causes disease through percutaneous exposure. Depending on the sophistication of the mitigation measures, containment can be expensive to operate and maintain and/or procedurally burdensome, so optimizing the control measures for the identified risks ideally provides the best return on investment to improve safety.

13. Answer: **B**. According to the *Fundamentals of Industrial Hygiene*, an **industrial toxicologist** is one who studies the harmful, or toxic, properties of substances and determines dose thresholds.

An **industrial hygienist** is one devoted to the art and science of anticipation, recognition, evaluation, and control of those environmental factors in the workplace that may cause sickness or impaired health and well-being.

A **health physicist** studies the field of science concerned with radiation physics and radiation biology, with the goal of providing technical information and proper techniques regarding safe use of ionizing radiation.

Pathologists are physicians who diagnose and characterize disease in living patients by examining biopsies or bodily fluid. Pathologists may also conduct autopsies to investigate causes of death.

14. Answer: **C**. An **alveolus** (plural: **alveoli**) is an anatomical structure that has the form of a hollow cavity. Found in the lung parenchyma, the pulmonary alveoli are the terminal ends of the respiratory tree, which outcrop from either alveolar sacs or alveolar ducts, which are both sites of gas exchange with the blood as well. The alveolar membrane is the gas-exchange surface. Carbon dioxide–rich blood is pumped from the rest of the body into the alveolar blood vessels where, through diffusion, it releases its carbon dioxide and absorbs oxygen.

The **pleural cavity** is the thin fluid-filled space between the two pulmonary pleurae (visceral and parietal) of each lung. The outer pleura (parietal pleura) is attached to the chest wall. The inner pleura (visceral pleura) covers the lungs and adjoining structures, including blood vessels, bronchi, and nerves.

The **bronchioles** or **bronchioli** are the passageways by which air passes through the nose or mouth to the alveoli (air sacs) of the lungs, in which branches no longer contain cartilage or glands in their submucosa. They are branches of the bronchi, and are part of the conducting zone of the respiratory system. The bronchioles divide further into smaller **terminal** bronchioles, which are still in the conducting zone, and these then divide into the even smaller **respiratory** bronchioles, which mark the beginning of the respiratory region.

The **trachea**, colloquially called the **windpipe**, is a cartilaginous tube that connects the pharynx and larynx to the lungs, allowing the passage of air.

15. Answer: **A**. Assigned Protection Factor (APF) means the workplace level of respiratory protection that a respirator or class of respirators is expected to provide to employees when the employer implements a continuing, effective respiratory protection program as specified by this section.

Assigned Protection Factors

Type of Respirator	Quarter mask	Half mask	Full facepiece	Helmet/Hood	Loose-fitting facepiece
1. Air-Purifying Respirator	5	10	50	—	—
2. Powered Air-Purifying Respirator (PAPR)	—	50	1000	25/1000	25
Supplied-Air Respirator (SAR) or Airline Respirator • Demand mode • Continuous flow mode • Pressure-demand or other positive-pressure mode	— — —	10 50 50	50 1000 1000	— 25/1000 — —	— 25 — —
Self-Contained Breathing Apparatus (SCBA) • Demand mode • Pressure-demand or other positive-pressure mode (e.g., open/closed circuit)	— —	10 —	50 10,000	50 10,000	— —

OSHA 3352-02 2009 Assigned Protection Factors for the Revised Respiratory Protection Standard.

OSHA 3352-02 2009, Assigned Protection Factors for the Revised Respiratory Protection Standard, Retrieved from https://www.osha.gov/Publications/3352-APF-respirators.pdf

16. Answer: **C**. The MUC for respirators is calculated by multiplying the APF for the respirator by the PEL. The MUC is the upper limit at which the class of respirator is expected to provide protection. The Protection Factor for a half-mask respirator from the chart is 10.

$$\begin{aligned} MUC &= TLV \times APF \\ &= 10 \text{ mg/m}^3 \times 10 \\ &= 100 \text{ mg/m}^3 \end{aligned}$$

End-of-service-life indicator (ESLI) means a system that warns the respirator user of the approach of the end of adequate respiratory protection—for example, that the sorbent is approaching saturation or is no longer effective.

Domain 7: Environmental Management

Domain 7: Environmental Management components:
- Water
- Air
- Land and conservation
- Waste elimination, reduction, minimization
- Hierarchy of conservation
- Environmental management systems
- Waste removal, treatment, and disposal
- Sustainability
- Environmental hazards awareness
- Hazardous waste characteristics

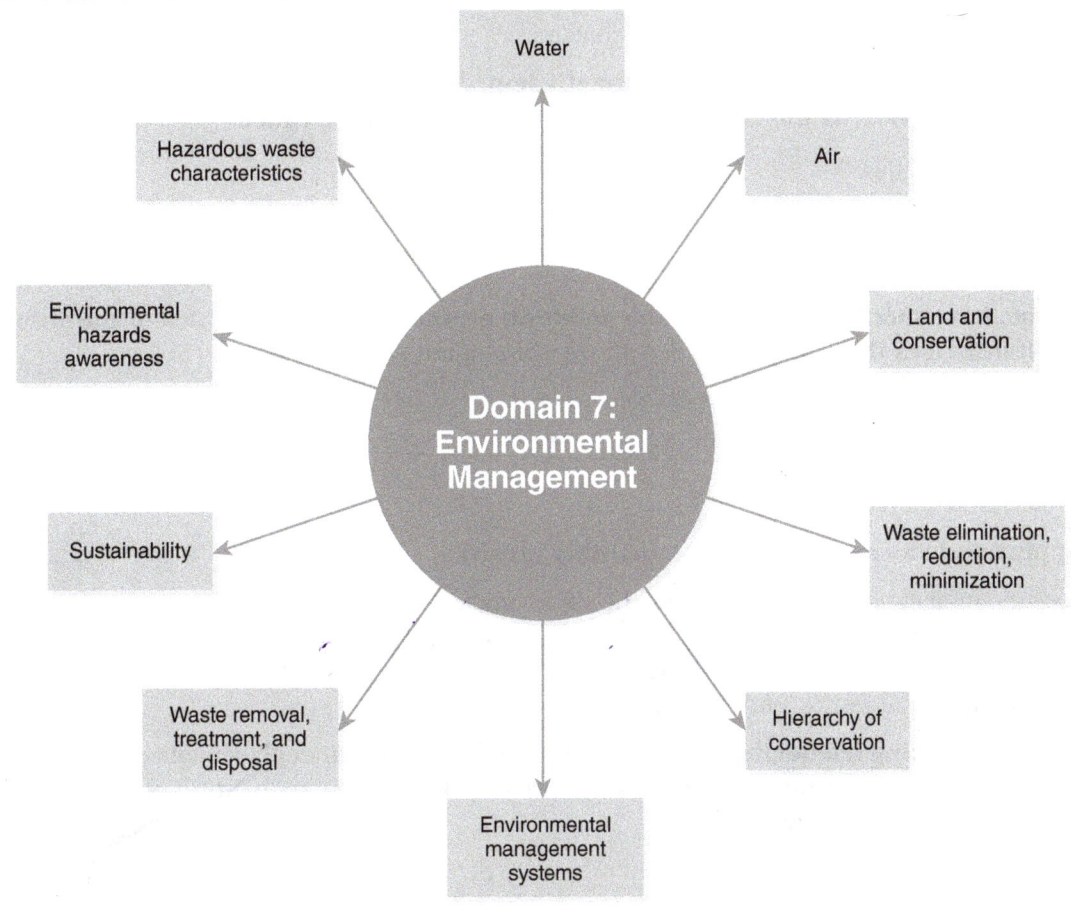

Modified from ASP® Exam Blueprint (ASP10), November 10, 2019

Domain 7 Quiz 1 Questions

1. The most common natural cause of wildfires is from which type of lightning?
   A. Cloud-to-cloud
   B. Dry lightning
   C. Rocket lightning
   D. Ribbon lightning

2. Transporting hazardous materials requires a commercial motor vehicle to display placards in which of the following locations?
   A. Front, rear, and both sides of vehicle
   B. Front, rear, and both sides of hazmat container
   C. Front, rear, top, and both sides of vehicle
   D. Front, rear, top, and both sides of hazmat container

3. Highly efficient filtration devices that minimally impede the flow of gases and easily remove fine particulate matter such as dust and smoke from the airstream are called:
   A. electrostatic precipitators.
   B. wet scrubbers.
   C. bag houses.
   D. stack scrubbers.

4. Many terms have specific meanings in the pollution prevention context. Which of the following terms best describes the storage and distillation of a spent solvent?
   A. Disposal
   B. Preconsumer recycled content
   C. Closed-loop recycling
   D. Postconsumer recycled content

5. Overlapping systems required for sustainability involve:
   A. resources, human needs, and preserving the environment.
   B. people, the environment, and profits.
   C. partnerships, collaboration, and outreach.
   D. conservation, social justice, and consequences.

6. Renovation (including remodeling or redecorating) of buildings or replacement of utility systems increases the potential for disturbing ACM. Before conducting any renovation or remodeling work, the building owner should first:
   A. review asbestos inspection and assessment records to determine where ACM may be located.
   B. visually reinspect the area.
   C. evaluate the likelihood that ACM will be disturbed.
   D. conduct sampling.

7. Hazardous waste profiles from several chemical processes yield nonpotable water, lithium metal, acetone, and halogenated hydrocarbons. What is the greatest concern for a waste site worker segregating waste streams into 55-gallon drums?
   A. Mixing lithium metal and nonpotable water
   B. Mixing lithium metal and acetone
   C. Mixing spent acetone and nonpotable water
   D. Mixing halogenated hydrocarbons and acetone

8. Any activity that decreases or prevents the creation of a waste or decreases the toxicity of the waste stream without treatment is called:
   A. waste minimization.
   B. source reduction.
   C. oxidation reduction.
   D. waste reduction.

9. The RQ listed on shipping papers of hazardous materials refers to:
   A. Requested Quality.
   B. Reserve Quantity.
   C. Reportable Quantity.
   D. Regulated Quantity.

10. Following a defined set of procedures, sometimes called a protocol, is advised when making an environmental audit. Which of the following is not considered one of the three basic parts of an environmental protocol?
    A. Previsit activities
    B. Visit activities
    C. Determination of liability
    D. Postvisit activities

11. What is a useful indicator for determining the adequacy of water treatment and the integrity of the distribution system?
    A. Viscosity
    B. Turbidity
    C. Total coliforms
    D. Clarity

12. If sewage is present in a body of water, what are the potential effects on the body of water?
    A. Depletes oxygen
    B. Introduces oxygen
    C. Increases water temperature
    D. Decreases water temperature

13. Which of the following electrical devices would most likely contain polychlorinated biphenyls (PCBs)?
    A. Transformers, capacitors, fluorescent light ballasts
    B. Fuses, wiring, and meters
    C. Circuit breakers, panel boards, and Unistrut
    D. Meters, relays, and switches

14. What UN agency impacts international hazardous waste transportation overseas?
    A. IATA
    B. IMO
    C. IAIA
    D. UNCE

15. Who is ultimately responsible for hazardous waste from start to finish?
    A. Shipper of the manifested hazardous waste
    B. Chemical manufacturer of the hazardous waste constituents
    C. Large- and small-quantity generators of the hazardous waste
    D. Hazardous waste treatment and storage and disposal facility

16. Required placards for shipping hazardous material are required by whom?
   A. Driver
   B. Carrier
   C. Shipper
   D. Manufacturer

17. A large generator is least likely subject to hazardous waste regulations when the waste is:
   A. determined by the generator as a hazardous waste and properly stored.
   B. listed by authorities as exhibiting a hazardous waste profile by characteristic.
   C. untreated solid waste that is segregated and disposed of in a remote, permitted landfill.
   D. a mixture of an acutely hazardous waste effectively diluted by a nonhazardous waste stream.

18. The use of source reduction and/or environmentally sound recycling methods prior to treating or disposing of hazardous wastes is called:
   A. waste minimization.
   B. e-cycling.
   C. hazard determination.
   D. footprint reduction.

19. An environmental Life Cycle Assessment (LCA) is best described as:
   A. stable procedure with few changes over time.
   B. generally simple and low cost for small firms.
   C. a systematic set of procedures for evaluating the environmental impacts of a product, service, or system.
   D. a government requirement to develop enforcement-based environmental regulations.

20. Which cause is frequently associated with hazardous material releases from underground storage tanks?
   A. Tampering
   B. Corrosion
   C. Soil subsidence
   D. Thermal shock

21. The certification process for new building construction and renovations that includes a rating system designed to guide and distinguish high-performance buildings that have less impact on the environment and are healthier to work within is called:
   A. GREEN.
   B. ALARA.
   C. LEED®.
   D. ASHARE.

22. Environmental management guidelines are generally composed of a series of interlinking and supporting components that include:
   A. a set of principles, tools to achieve environmental objectives, management programs, and a management framework.
   B. a set of regulatory standards, tools to achieve environmental objectives, management programs, and a management framework.
   C. a set of principles, tools to achieve environmental objectives, and management programs.
   D. a set of regulatory standards, tools to achieve environmental objectives, and a management framework.

23. **Considering the waste hierarchy of controls, which is the least desirable?**
    A. Source reduction/elimination
    B. Recovery/reuse/recycle
    C. Waste exchange/energy recovery
    D. Treatment/destruction/disposal

24. **Which is the gas with the most impact on the greenhouse effect?**
    A. Methane
    B. Carbon monoxide
    C. Carbon dioxide
    D. Sulfur dioxide

25. **Generally, system life cycle phases include:**
    A. concept, development, operation, and disposal.
    B. initiation, development, design, and evaluation.
    C. analysis, design, production, and disposal.
    D. concept, sustainment, reliability, and disposal.

Domain 7 Quiz 1 Answers

1. Answer: **B**. In the United Sates, **dry lightning** is a term for lightning that occurs with no precipitation at the surface. This type of lightning is the most common natural cause of wildfires. Cloud-to-cloud lightning discharges may occur between areas of cloud having different potentials without contacting the ground. These are most common between the anvil and lower reaches of a given thunderstorm. This lightning can sometimes be observed at great distances at night as so-called "heat lightning." In such instances, the observer may see only a flash of light without thunder. The "heat" portion of the term is a folk association between locally experienced warmth and the distant lightning flashes. Cloud-to-ground lightning is a great lightning discharge between a cumulonimbus cloud and the ground initiated by the downward-moving leader stroke. This is the second most common type of lightning and poses the greatest threat to life and property of all known types. Some references define a lightning bolt as a visual manifestation of the **equalization** of a large electrical difference between clouds or clouds and the ground.

2. Answer: **A**. According to 49 CFR 172.504, placards should be attached while loading and before driving the vehicle. The placards must appear on both sides and ends of the vehicle. Each placard must be easily seen from the direction it faces.
    Placards must be placed so the words or numbers are level and read from left to right, and must be at least three inches from other markings.

3. Answer: **A**. An **electrostatic precipitator (ESP)**, or electrostatic air cleaner, is a particulate collection device that removes particles from a flowing gas (such as air) using the force of an induced electrostatic charge. Electrostatic precipitators are highly efficient filtration devices that minimally impede the flow of gases through the device, and can easily remove fine particulate matter such as dust and smoke from the airstream. In contrast to wet scrubbers, which apply energy directly to the flowing fluid medium, an ESP applies energy only to the particulate matter being collected and therefore is very efficient in its consumption of energy (in the form of electricity).

4. Answer: **C**. *Closed-loop recycling* is a system in which a process waste is conveyed through closed systems to tank storage and then recycled in tanks before returning the reprocessed material to the production system. An example could be the storage and distillation of a spent solvent. *Disposal* means either the destruction of a waste (for example, incineration, energy recovery, or chemical reaction) or putting it in the ground (for example, landfilling or land application). *Preconsumer recycled content* is the fraction of feedstock used in manufacturing a material that is derived from wastes captured during or just after

the manufacturing process. An example is repulping scrap paper shaved from the ends of a paper roll to produce the next batch. *Postconsumer recycled content* means the fraction of feedstock used in manufacturing a material that is derived from materials that have been used by the public, discarded, and collected for reprocessing.

5. Answer: **B**. Although there are various definitions of sustainability, the general concept involves overlapping systems impacting people, the environment, and profits. The current paradigm in environmental management is based on concepts of sustainable development. Sustainable development has four interlocking dimensions: economic, human, environmental, and technological.

   With greater public expectations for corporate environmental stewardship and increased demand for green (environmentally friendly) products and services, corporate leaders began taking a fresh look at their environmental management programs. Many have found that undertaking a serious pollution prevention effort is a successful business response because it reduces their regulatory burden, increases public confidence, reduces long-term risk, and nearly always cuts costs. Pollution prevention is also being furthered as a natural outcome of Environmental Management Systems (EMS), a business-oriented approach that has emerged and rapidly gained acceptance.

   Sustainable development has been defined by the United Nations World Commission on Environment and Development as meeting the needs of the world's current population without making it impossible for the world's future citizens to meet their needs. The global nature of this definition often makes implementation challenging within business organizations. According to Krieger (2000), this definition can mean anything to anyone and provides little concrete guidance. Therefore, more precise definitions of sustainable development have been attempted but even these provide minimal direction:

   - *Physical definition:* Use of renewable natural resources in a manner that does not eliminate or degrade them (i.e., diminish renewability for future generations), while maintaining adequate resources such as soil, groundwater, and biomass.
   - *Economic definitions:* Maximizing the net benefits of economic development, subject to maintaining the services and quality of natural resources. "Our economic systems should be managed so that we live off the dividend of our resources, maintaining and improving the asset base."
   - *Social definition:* Development that improves health care, education, and social well-being and involves local peoples in decisions that impact their lives. Gary R. Krieger (2000)

   Businesses that are ready to make sustainable development operational begin by transforming principles, behaviors, and practices involved in their basic internal workings. Those base principles and behaviors have to do with transparency in business objectives and practices; governance practices, including business environmental ethics; social responsibility programs, including community, workforce, and other involved stakeholders' environmental health; and safety processes based on continuous improvement. Sustainable development, like EMS, requires the development of indicators (leading or lagging), and metrics by which to measure and verify improvements in the categories mentioned. These measures go together with the concept of the triple bottom line, under which stakeholders evaluate companies not only on financial performance, but also on environmental and social performance. As an extension of this, many businesses now include environmental and social performance in their annual reporting to shareholders. Environmental aspects that readily lend themselves to the development of metrics include consideration of residuals (e.g., air emissions, waste water, and solid and hazardous waste); energy and material inputs and outputs associated with a process; and the life cycle environmental costs of the product or service produced.

6. Answer: **A**. Before conducting any renovation or remodeling work, the building owner should have the APM review asbestos inspection and assessment records to determine where ACM may be located, visually reinspect the area, and evaluate the likelihood that ACM will be disturbed. Any suspect or assumed ACM that could be disturbed during the renovation work should either be sampled and analyzed to determine whether it contains asbestos, or the work should be carried out as if the materials did contain asbestos. The APM should also ensure that no new ACM is introduced into the building as part of the renovation work.

7. Answer: **A**. The consequences of mixing incompatible chemicals together are potentially severe from a health and safety perspective. From a disposal perspective, mixing of wastes can be costly. Mixed wastes can result in the need for sequential treatment using different technologies at different facilities. It is

unlikely that random mixing of different waste materials together will reduce the toxicity of the mixture. Lithium metal is water reactive and should not be mixed. It is therefore of greatest concern in this scenario.

8. Answer: **B**. *Source reduction* means any activity that decreases or prevents the creation of a waste or decreases the toxicity of the waste stream without treatment. It can also mean an activity (other than treatment or ordinary recycling) that prevents a contaminant from entering any waste stream (including fugitive emissions) or being otherwise released into the environment. It is the preferred management strategy. *Waste minimization* means the reduction, to the extent feasible, of hazardous waste that is generated or subsequently treated, stored, or disposed. It includes any source reduction or recycling activity that results in reduction of the total volume or the toxicity of hazardous waste generated, so long as the reduction is consistent with the goal of minimizing present or future threats to human health and the environment. *Pollution prevention (P2)* means source reduction. In addition, the terms *pollution prevention* and *waste minimization* are often used interchangeably. *Waste reduction* means any activity that decreases the amount of waste materials that require waste management efforts. *Waste stream* means the continuing production of abandoned materials that are collected and managed for the purpose of disposal or recycling (U.S. Environmental Protection Agency [EPA]). Unlike most areas of environmental management, pollution prevention is driven more by business interests than by existing laws and regulations.

9. Answer: **C**. RQ is a regulatory acronym representing Reportable Quantity, and is associated with hazardous substances. USEPA's List of Hazardous Substances and Reportable Quantities is found in 40 CFR Part 302.

10. Answer: **C**. According to the NSC Environmental Management Accident Prevention Manual, the Environmental Audit Protocol consists of three parts, the previsit at which contact is established, the preparation of a questionnaire, and establishment of reporting relationships.

    During the visit phase, trainers conduct the entrance briefing, tour the facility, record, interview, review records, inspect, record findings, and conduct an exit briefing.

    During the postactivity, trainers follow up to resolve outstanding issues and provide audit reports. Determining liability is **not** part of audit protocol.

    The purpose of an audit is to measure and verify actual performance against established objectives for the purpose of process improvement. Comprehensive audits are conducted by multidisciplinary teams that are knowledgeable of the work processes and independent of line management.

11. Answer: **C**. Total coliforms are a group of related bacteria that are not harmful to humans. A variety of bacteria, parasites, and viruses, known as pathogens, can potentially cause health problems if humans ingest them. EPA considers total coliforms a useful indicator of other pathogens for drinking water. Total coliforms are used to determine the adequacy of water treatment and the integrity of the distribution system.

    Coliform bacteria counts are an indicator of the disease potential of a wastewater stream. Although coliform bacteria are not necessarily pathogens and are naturally present in feces or warm-blooded animals, the presence of a large number of coliforms is an indication that other disease-carrying bacteria can be present (*Accident Prevention Manual for Business and Industry: Environmental Management*, 2nd edition and epa.gov).

12. Answer: **A**. Biological oxygen demand (BOD) is a measure of the potential impact of wastewater organic matter on a stream or river. High levels of organics deplete the oxygen within a water body. As the oxygen is consumed by biological activity, the ability of a body of water to support healthy populations of fish is diminished. High BOD concentrations also lead to the rapid growth of algae, which, in turn, lowers oxygen levels even further (*Accident Prevention Manual for Business and Industry: Environmental Management*, 2nd edition).

13. Answer: **A**. Polychlorinated biphenyls (PCBs) are found in certain electrical devices such as transformers, capacitors, fluorescent light ballasts, etc., as well as in heat-transfer enclosures and investment casting waxes in foundries. In 1978, the EPA under TSCA banned the use of PCBs in light ballasts, transformers, and capacitors; however, it is still possible to find equipment containing PCBs.

14. Answer: **B. IMO – The International Maritime Organization (IMO)** is the United Nations' specialized agency with responsibility for the safety and security of shipping and the prevention of marine pollution

by ships. The International Maritime Dangerous Goods Code (IMDGC) relates to the safe carriage of dangerous goods by sea.

The **United Nations Environment Programme (UNEP)** is an agency of the United Nations and coordinates its environmental activities, assisting developing countries in implementing environmentally sound policies and practices.

IAIA – The International Association for Impact Assessment (IAIA) is an international association of professionals involved with impact assessment, including both social impact assessment and environmental impact assessment.

IATA – The International Air Transport Association (IATA) is a trade association representing airlines. IATA works closely with local governments and the International Civil Aviation Organization (ICAO), a specialized agency of the United Nations, in the development of regulations. The IATA Dangerous Goods Regulations (DGR) manual is the global reference for shipping dangerous goods by air and is the only standard recognized by airlines.

15. Answer: **C**. In keeping with the cradle-to-grave concept, waste continues to be the property of the generator. Any discrepancies in waste shipment must be reported to EPA. The current hazardous waste manifest system is a set of forms, reports, and procedures designed to seamlessly track hazardous waste from the time it leaves the generator facility where it was produced until it reaches the off-site waste management facility that will store, treat, or dispose of the hazardous waste. The system allows the waste generator to verify that its waste has been properly delivered, and that no waste has been lost or unaccounted for in the process. The current Hazardous Waste Manifest is a joint undertaking by EPA and the Department of Transportation (DOT). EPA is responsible for regulating hazardous waste under a federal statute known as the Resource Conservation and Recovery Act (RCRA). This Act requires that all hazardous waste shipped off-site be tracked from **"cradle-to-grave"** using a manifest that provides information about the generator of the waste, the facility that will receive the waste, a description and quantity of the waste (including the number and type of containers), and how the waste will be routed to the receiving facility. Because hazardous waste is also regulated by the DOT under its hazardous materials laws, the manifest (**Table 16**) was developed to meet both EPA's requirements for a manifest and DOT's requirements for "shipping papers."

    Conditionally Exempt Small Quantity Generator (CESQG)
    - Generated
        - Less than 100 kg/mo of any hazardous waste
        - Less than 1 kg/mo of P-listed (acutely hazardous) waste
        - Less than 100 kg/mo of cleanup waste
    - Accumulated
        - Less than 1000 kg of any hazardous waste
        - Less than 1 kg of P-listed (acutely hazardous) waste
        - Less than 100 kg of cleanup waste

    Small Quantity Generator (SQG)
    - Generated
        - 100 and 1000 kg per month of hazardous waste
        - No more than 1 kg of acutely hazardous waste
    - Have limitations on accumulation as follows:
        - Accumulation time without permit is less than or equal to 180 days
        - Accumulation quantity is limited to 6000 kg
        - Accumulation is allowed in tanks or containers only

Large Quantity Generator (LQG)
- Is subject to full Subtitle C regulation
- Generates more than SQG and CESQG
    - More than 1000 kg/mo of any hazardous waste
    - More than 1 kg/mo of acutely hazardous waste
- Accumulates more than SQG and CESQG
    - More than 6000 kg of hazardous waste
    - More than 1 kg of acutely hazardous waste
    - More than 100 kg of contaminated soil, waste, or debris

Table 16 Table of Hazardous Waste Regulations

Agency	Purpose	Basic Requirements	Extent of Coverage
RCRA	40 CFR 260 to 271. Regulate hazardous-waste generators and transporters; manage treatment, storage, and disposal facilities (TSDFs) and cradle to grave regulations.	Permits, technical standards, and ground water monitoring; corrective action for releases; transportation manifest forms; and UST standards.	Hazardous wastes as defined by EPA; TSDFs; generators of more than 100 kg of hazardous wastes a month.
CERCLA	40 CFR 300.61 to 300.71. Locate, assess, and clean potential hazardous waste sites and emergency spills; grant EPS authority to initiate investigations, testing, and monitoring of disposal sites; implement site remediation.	Place a site on the National Priority List because the site poses a threat to human health and the environment.	Removal and response actions; establish strict liability resulting from hazardous wastes; finance response actions through a hazardous-substance response trust fund; notification requirements for hazardous-waste spills and releases; Title III of SARA Community Right-to-Know provisions.
CWA	40 CFR 121 to 135, and 403. Protect U.S. waters (surface and groundwater) from direct, indirect, and hazardous point-source pollution discharges.	Establish water-quality standards; set discharge limits.	Restrict pollutant discharges into water; impose monitoring requirements.
CAA	40 CFR 69. Protect and enhance U.S. air quality; maintain National Ambient Air Quality Standards (NAAQS); establish National Emissions Standards for Hazardous Air Pollutants (NESHAP).	Prevent air-quality deterioration; set NAAWS and emission standards.	Hazardous air pollutants and VOCs; NAAQS for NO, CO, sulfur dioxide, lead, ozone and particulate matter.
DOT	49 CFR 172, 173, 178, 179. Establish standards for the safe transport of hazardous wastes through package and container requirements; establish a labeling system applicable to hazardous-waste transportation; document transport to ensure proper treatment and disposal; notification of roadside spills.	Requirements for registration, labeling, vehicle and driver safety; "manifest" documents for shipments of hazardous wastes.	Transportation of hazardous wastes.

(Continues)

Table 16 Table of Hazardous Waste Regulations (*Continued*)

Agency	Purpose	Basic Requirements	Extent of Coverage
OSHA	29 CFR Ensure safe and healthy employment conditions; address the proper management of hazardous materials in the workplace by setting standards designed to prevent injury and illness.	Address exposure limits, labeling, protective equipment, control procedures, monitoring, and measuring employee exposure, medical exams, and access to records.	Applicable to facilities with 10 or more workers; OSHA regulations addressing hazardous wastes including health standards, cancer policy, Hazard Communication Standard, and Hazardous waste Operation and Emergency Response rules.
TSCA	Screen new chemicals; test new chemicals identified as potential hazards; regulate toxic substance disposal.	Notification of substantial risk by chemical manufacturers who become aware of a chemical threat.	Chemicals that are hazardous, toxic, corrosive, flammable, irritants, or oxidizers.

16. Answer: **C**. To transport products by truck, railroad, ship, or airplane, the shipper must:
    - determine the product's proper shipping name, hazard class, identification number, correct packaging, correct placard, and correct tables and markings.
    - package materials, label and mark the packages, prepare shipping paper, and supply the placards.
    - certify on shipping paper that there is proper compliance with shipment rules.

17. Answer: **C**. A waste will be subject to the hazardous waste regulations if it meets any of the following conditions: **Characteristic Waste.** Waste exhibiting any of the four characteristics of a hazardous waste: ignitibility, corrosivity, reactivity, or toxicity. **Listed Hazardous Waste.** Wastes specifically listed in Subpart D of the regulations: Nonspecific Source (F-Listed); Specific Source (K-Listed); Acute Hazardous Waste (P-Listed); Toxic Hazardous Waste (U-Listed). **Mixtures.** The waste is a mixture of a listed hazardous waste and a nonhazardous waste. **Declared to be Hazardous**. The waste has been declared to be hazardous by the generator. The Resource Conservation and Recovery Act (RCRA) extended protection to the environmental medium of land. As the name suggests, the law set forth an intent to promote conservation of resources through reduced reliance on landfilling. **This law covers both solid waste and hazardous waste. All hazardous waste is considered solid waste by definition, but not all solid waste is considered hazardous waste.**

18. Answer: **A**. Waste minimization refers to the use of source reduction and/or environmentally sound recycling methods prior to treating or disposing of hazardous wastes. Waste minimization includes source reduction practices that reduce or eliminate waste generation at the source and environmentally sound recycling practices where source reduction is not economically practical. Waste minimization does not include waste treatment (i.e., any process designed to change the physical, chemical, or biological character or composition of a hazardous waste or waste disposal). For example, compacting, neutralizing, diluting, and incineration are not waste minimization practices. EPA's preferred hierarchical approach to solid waste disposal includes source reduction as the first solution, followed by recycling, then incineration, then disposal in landfills. Source reduction includes any practice that reduces the quantity and/or toxicity of pollutants entering a waste stream prior to recycling, treatment, or disposal. Examples include equipment or technology modifications, reformulation or redesign of products, substitution of less toxic raw materials, improvements in work practices, maintenance, worker training, and better inventory control. Recycling includes the use, reuse, and/or reclamation of waste residuals (that may be designated as hazardous waste) or materials in a hazardous waste. A material is "used or reused" if it is used as an ingredient in an industrial process to make a product or if it is used as an effective substitute for a commercial product. A material is "reclaimed" if it is processed to recover a usable product, or if it is regenerated.

19. Answer: **C**. As a means of relieving government of costly enforcement of environmental regulations, some countries are establishing product-oriented incentives that are intended to yield environmental benefits. The basis for evaluating such incentives is the province of Life Cycle Assessment (LCA). ISO 14040, the Life Cycle Assessment Guideline, defines LCA as a systematic set of procedures

for compiling and examining the inputs and outputs of materials and energy and the associated environmental impacts directly attributable to the functioning of a product or service system throughout its life cycle.

20. Answer: **B**. According to EPA studies, the releases from underground storage tanks (USTs) are typically associated with these problems: (1) piping failure, (2) corrosion, (3) spills and overfilling.
21. Answer: **C**. Designed primarily for new construction of office buildings, the **Leadership in Energy and Environmental Design (LEED)** certification process has been applied to many other commercial building types. LEED certification is a performance-oriented rating system where building projects earn points for satisfying criteria designed to address specific environmental impacts inherent in the design, construction, operations, and management of a building. The LEED certification system is organized into six environmental categories: Sustainable Sites, Water Efficiency, Energy and Atmosphere, Materials and Resources, Indoor Environmental Quality, and Innovation and Design.
22. Answer: **A**. Environmental management guidelines are generally composed of a series of interlinking and supporting components:
    - A set of *principles* to help understand environmental management;
    - A series of *tools* that can be used to achieve environmental objectives;
    - A series of *management programs* traditionally used to solve environmental issues; and
    - A *management framework* to integrate environmental issues into the core business processes and decision making.

    Some tools have been specifically developed as environmental management guidelines (ISO 14001, for example), and some have been adopted from other management practices.
23. Answer: **D**. EPA developed the nonhazardous materials and waste management hierarchy in recognition that no single waste management approach is suitable for managing all materials and waste streams in all circumstances. The hierarchy ranks the various management strategies from most to least environmentally preferred.

    According to EPA, the hierarchy places emphasis on reducing, reusing, and recycling as key to sustainable materials management. Source reduction, also known as waste prevention, means reducing waste at the source, and is the most environmentally preferred strategy. It can take many different forms, including reusing or donating items, buying in bulk, reducing packaging, redesigning products, and reducing toxicity. Source reduction also is important in manufacturing. Lightweighting of packaging, reuse, and remanufacturing are all becoming more popular business trends. Purchasing products

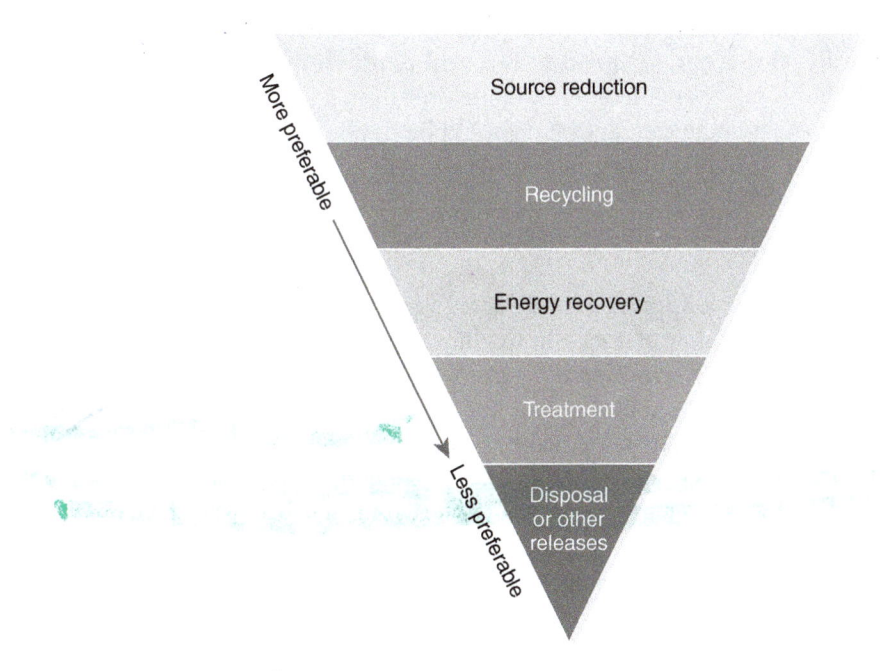

Figure 34 Hazardous Waste Management Hierarchy

that incorporate these features supports source reduction. Recycling is a series of activities that includes collecting used, reused, or unused items that would otherwise be considered waste; sorting and processing the recyclable products into raw materials; and remanufacturing the recycled raw materials into new products. Consumers provide the last link in recycling by purchasing products made from recycled content. Recycling also can include composting of food scraps, yard trimmings, and other organic materials. Energy recovery from waste is the conversion of nonrecyclable waste materials into useable heat, electricity, or fuel through a variety of processes, including combustion, gasification, pyrolization, anaerobic digestion, and landfill gas (LFG) recovery. This process is often called waste to energy (WTE). Converting nonrecyclable waste materials into electricity and heat generates a renewable energy source and reduces carbon emissions by offsetting the need for energy from fossil sources and reduces methane generation from landfills. After energy is recovered, approximately ten percent of the volume remains as ash, which is generally sent to a landfill. Prior to disposal, treatment can help reduce the volume and toxicity of waste. Treatments can be physical (e.g., shredding), chemical (e.g., incineration), and biological (e.g., anaerobic digestion). Landfills are the most common form of waste disposal and are an important component of an integrated waste management system. Modern landfills are well-engineered facilities located, designed, operated, and monitored to ensure compliance with state and federal regulations. Landfills that accept municipal solid waste are primarily regulated by state, tribal, and local governments. EPA, however, established national standards that these landfills must meet in order to stay open. The federal landfill regulations eliminated the open dumps (disposal facilities that do not meet federal and state criteria) of the past. Today's landfills must meet stringent design, operation, and closure requirements. Methane gas, a by-product of decomposing waste, can be collected and used as fuel to generate electricity. After a landfill is capped, the land may be used for recreation sites such as parks, golf courses, and ski slopes.

24. Answer: **C**. The term *greenhouse gas* generally describes gases that are highly transparent to incoming solar radiation but are relatively opaque to long-wave radiation, similar (for descriptive purpose) to glass in a greenhouse. Atmospheric gases differ greatly in their absorptive properties. The most important atmospheric constituent of the greenhouse effect is water vapor (H_2O). Water vapor, together with CO_2 and clouds, creates about 90% of the total effect. The remaining 10% of the greenhouse effect is due to the presence of trace amounts of ozone (O_3), methane (CH_4), and nitrous oxide (N_2O) (Krieger, 2000). So, although methane is more impactful than carbon dioxide—it has a "global warming potential" of 21 compared to carbon dioxide's potential of only 1, according to the EPA's "Greenhouse Gas Overview"[1]—carbon dioxide is the *most* impactful because of the quantity of carbon dioxide.[2]

25. Answer: **A**. According to Haight (2012), there are four major phases of development in a system life cycle: (1) **concept**, (2) **system development**, (3) **production and deployment**, and (4) **sustainment and disposal**. Each phase includes safety engineering tasks that result in a formal decision about proceeding to the next phase. A system-safety management plan should be developed during the concept phase in order to design safety into the system and maintain it throughout the system's life. Incorporating system safety early in development increases the probability that hazards can be addressed more economically and with greater efficiency. A formal decision earmarks the acceptance of risks to that point of development or operation.

    System safety is a comprehensive approach for integrating safety as part of the design—and implementing requirements throughout other phases—in the life cycle of a system, product, process, or facility. The primary function of system safety is to identify and control hazards in each phase of the life cycle, from concept through decommissioning and disposal. In system development, anticipating potential hazards and conditions is a key aspect of safety engineering work. It is a challenge to anticipate the hazards of a system before it is developed; however, safety engineering activities designed into each phase promote a systematic process of anticipating and identifying hazards as the system is developed. According to Brauer (1990), "System safety is . . . the systematic, forward-looking identification and control of hazards . . . ." Safety engineers assess the existing and potential conditions that could affect a system.

---

[1] https://www.epa.gov/enviro/greenhouse-gas-overview
[2] https://www.epa.gov/ghgemissions/overview-greenhouse-gases

Domain 8: Training, Education, and Communication

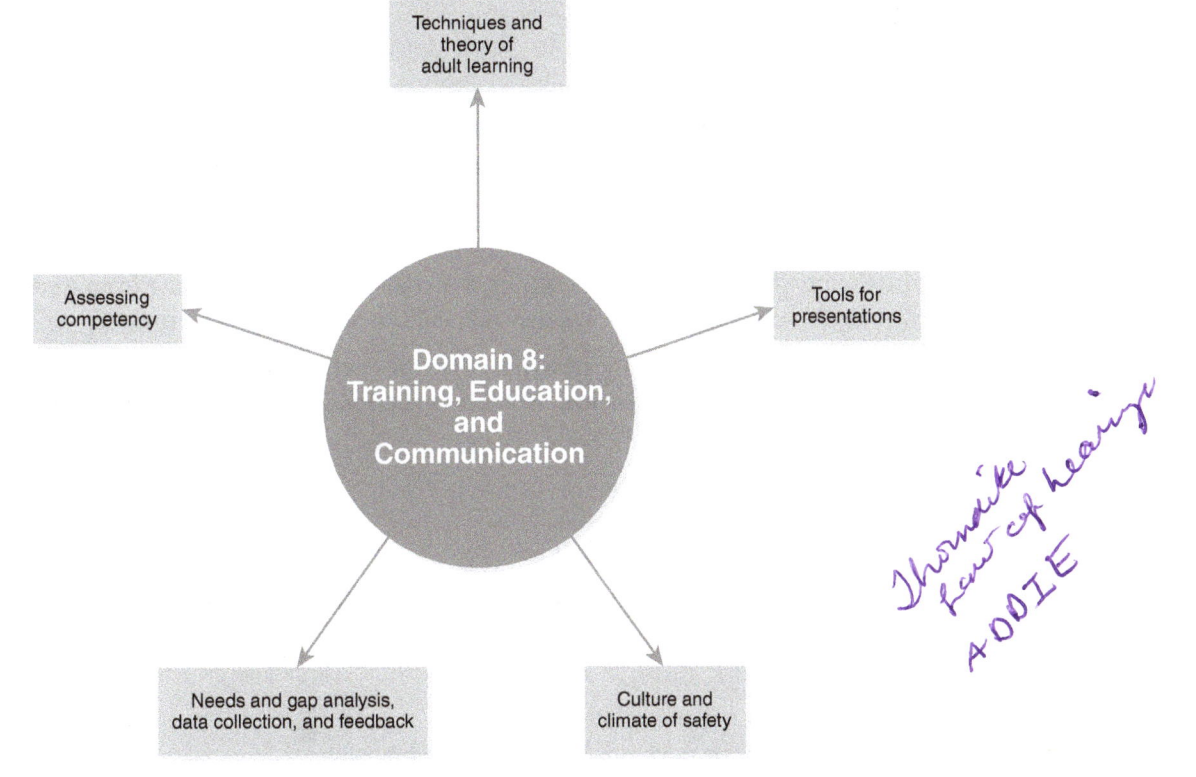

Modified from ASP® Exam Blueprint (ASP10), November 10, 2019

Domain 8 Quiz 1 Questions

1. The least important measurement of a safety training program effectiveness is:
   A. Behavior – What behaviors were changed because of the training?
   B. Knowledge – What skills were learned and demonstrated?
   C. Reaction – How well did students like the training?
   D. Interaction – How did students interact and exchange ideas in class?

2. Selecting the media to be used for presenting instructional content:
   A. requires only a knowledge of specific course objectives.
   B. should be done only after a planning process that includes content analysis, audience analysis, and other steps.
   C. partly determines what content can be included and should precede content analysis.
   D. is the first step in instructional design.

3. Which of the following represent the best training methods for retention?
   A. Experience, visual pictures
   B. Words, auditory
   C. Multimedia presentation, auditory
   D. Demonstrations, words

4. Learner reaction to instruction is greatly impacted by facilitator behaviors. Which learner performance outcome is least likely to occur?
   A. Observers learn by watching and imitating others; they tend to behave as they have seen others behave.
   B. Observers will imitate a model who is passionate about his/her topic.
   C. Observers will imitate a model when they see the model being rewarded for his/her actions.
   D. Observers will imitate a model when they see the model being punished for his/her actions.

5. Which training method allows for the least amount of student-instructor interaction?
   A. Lecture
   B. Role-playing
   C. Case study
   D. Facilitated discussion

6. Adult learning theory has established universal assumptions of adult learner needs. Which statement is least likely considered when designing hazard awareness training?
   A. Adults have experience and need to control their learning.
   B. Adults need to know why learning information is relevant.
   C. Adults need to be provided with written training materials to acquire meaning from learning content.
   D. Adults need to know how to apply knowledge and skill for successful performance.

7. Following employees' introduction to a new process, an evaluation sheet is administered to obtain employee feedback on the training session. Which is the least appropriate question?
   A. Was the course content accurate?
   B. Did the instructor display enthusiasm?
   C. Did the instructor maintain your interest?
   D. Was the presentation organized/easy to follow?

8. Tests and evaluation development for a training program should not utilize which guideline?
   A. Test items must be reliable.
   B. Evaluations are norm-referenced.
   C. Each test item must have criterion-related validity.
   D. The evaluation tool should be developed before training begins.

9. Which of the following is not a shortfall of one-way communication?
   A. Information will be transmitted correctly.
   B. Information flows in only one direction.
   C. Lack of feedback will occur.
   D. The receiver may not comprehend the message.

10. Which of the following is not an advantage to building and maintaining group cohesiveness?
    A. The group develops a "we" concept.
    B. Each member feels that they are part of the group.
    C. It acts as a bonding agent.
    D. It starts with and maintains a standardized structure.

11. What is the most effective type of workplace communication?
    A. Face-to-face group lecture
    B. Face-to-face group two-way communication
    C. Face-to-face individual two-way communication
    D. Written individual two-way communication

12. In behavioral science, Abraham Maslow's human needs theory is often cited, identifying a need as a deficiency a person feels a compulsion to satisfy. Central to this theory is the progressive principle, arranging needs in a hierarchy; only after a lower-level need is satisfied can the next higher level become active. Which of the following needs are at the lowest level in Maslow's hierarchy?
    A. Individual needs
    B. Group needs
    C. Rational needs
    D. Developmental needs

13. Define *communication*.
    A. Sharing information and/or ideas with others and being understood
    B. Sharing information and/or ideas with others and gaining approval
    C. Sharing opinions and/or ideas with others and being understood
    D. Sharing opinions and/or ideas with others and gaining approval

14. A primary desirable attribute of a safety training instructor is that he/she:
    A. always uses PowerPoint® presentations.
    B. covers course content and adds many personal-experience stories.
    C. enhances the presentation with many scientific and technical terms.
    D. covers the quantity of material outlined by the course objectives.

15. To effectively work with people, a crucial human characteristic that must be understood is that:
    A. the behavior of one person is not the same as another person's.
    B. the physical characteristics of one person are not the same as another person's.
    C. everyone is average.
    D. all human behaviors fit a standard pattern.

16. Which statement is most accurate about using the conference method as a communication technique?
    A. Individual understanding of the content is not important after a conference method session.
    B. The conference method is inappropriate for small-group problem-solving sessions.
    C. The success of the conference method is largely dependent upon the skills of the facilitator.
    D. The success of the conference method depends entirely on the amount of material covered.

17. Safety trainers often attempt to change the way an audience views their procedures or actions. A primary way to help facilitate change is by:
    A. allowing everyone to express their point of view.
    B. following the lesson plan without interruptions.
    C. allowing a limited number of questions at the end of the presentation.
    D. pointing out how change will affect the workplace.

18. A common safety training technique used when facilitating work team learning is the case study. Which is most correct about the use of a case study as a learning strategy?
    A. Case studies must always involve fictitious situations or incidents so that no one group or individual will feel threatened.
    B. Case studies should be written and distributed as handouts to be most effective, because most trade employees have short attention spans.
    C. Case studies are good problem-solving tools and can be used effectively with brainstorming activities and group discussions.
    D. Case studies involving real situations should only be used if they can be presented by the actual employees/responders involved in the situation or incident.

19. Successful communications include:
    A. sender and message.
    B. sender and receiver.
    C. message and receiver.
    D. sender, message, and receiver.

20. Often group methods are used to increase the effectiveness of training and active student participation. What is the best use of the *role-playing* technique?
    A. In human relations training
    B. For job instruction training in a one-on-one situation
    C. To illustrate the complexities of a step-by-step detailed industrial task
    D. For in-depth technical subjects

Domain 8 Quiz 1 Answers

1. **Answer: C.** Reaction is least valuable at the end of training, since students do not know the actual use of skills or knowledge gained until they put them into action. That is why most training experts recommend a second critique after six months to obtain a valid student reaction.
2. **Answer: B.** The target audience is the group of learners. A good training needs analysis provides the trainer with intelligence about target audience demographics. Relevant details include:
   - Educational background
   - Level of experience with the training topic
   - Job duties and responsibilities
   - Risk factors
   - History of training
   - Length of employment
   - Organizational climate
   - Attitudes toward training
   - Mastery of prerequisite skills/knowledge/abilities
   - Medical requirements

   The more a trainer knows about the target audience, the more appropriate the training will be. To avoid delivering a workshop that is too elementary or too advanced for a particular audience, the trainer can make adjustments in the instructional strategies. These adjustments can vary between peer groups or individuals; the purpose is that they can accomplish the learning objective.

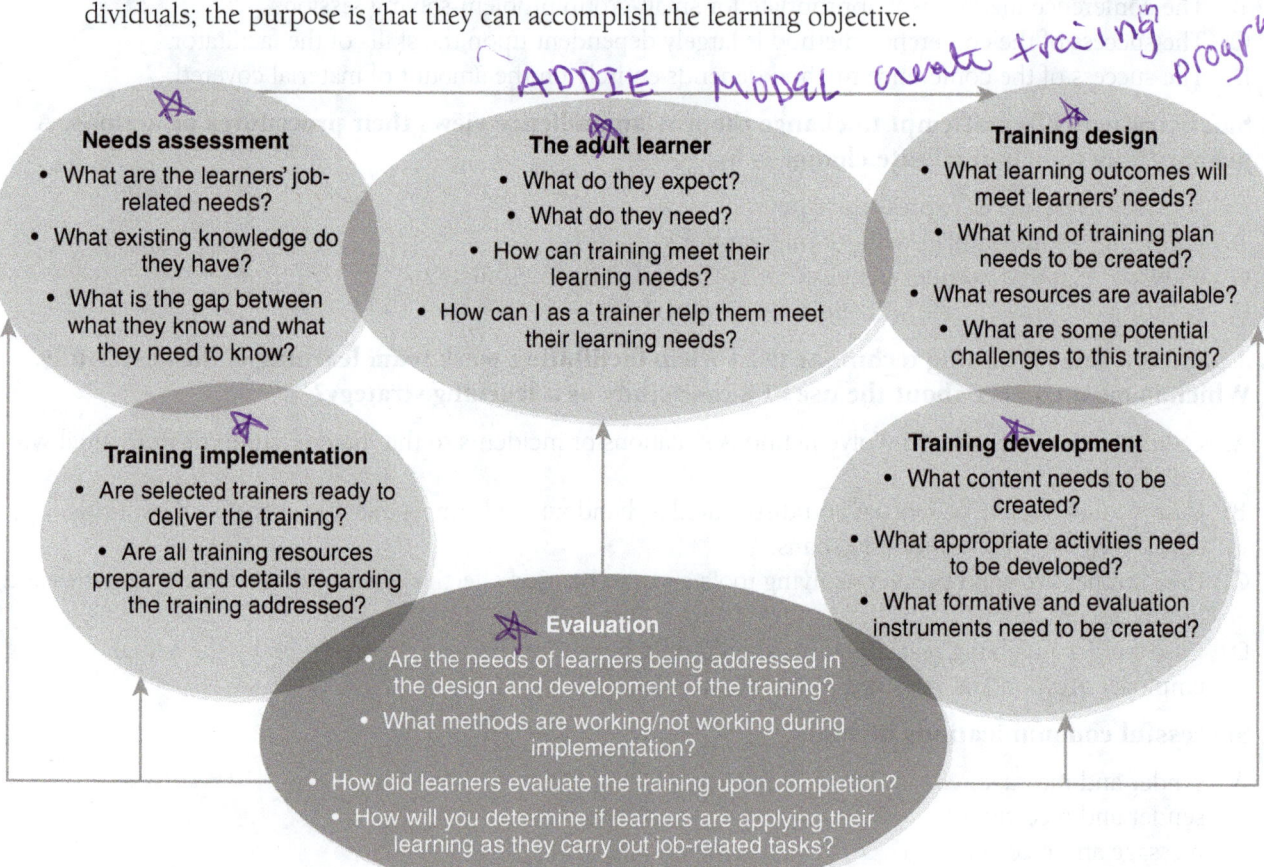

Needs assessment
- What are the learners' job-related needs?
- What existing knowledge do they have?
- What is the gap between what they know and what they need to know?

The adult learner
- What do they expect?
- What do they need?
- How can training meet their learning needs?
- How can I as a trainer help them meet their learning needs?

Training design
- What learning outcomes will meet learners' needs?
- What kind of training plan needs to be created?
- What resources are available?
- What are some potential challenges to this training?

Training implementation
- Are selected trainers ready to deliver the training?
- Are all training resources prepared and details regarding the training addressed?

Training development
- What content needs to be created?
- What appropriate activities need to be developed?
- What formative and evaluation instruments need to be created?

Evaluation
- Are the needs of learners being addressed in the design and development of the training?
- What methods are working/not working during implementation?
- How did learners evaluate the training upon completion?
- How will you determine if learners are applying their learning as they carry out job-related tasks?

Figure 35 Creating a Training Program Using the ADDIE Model

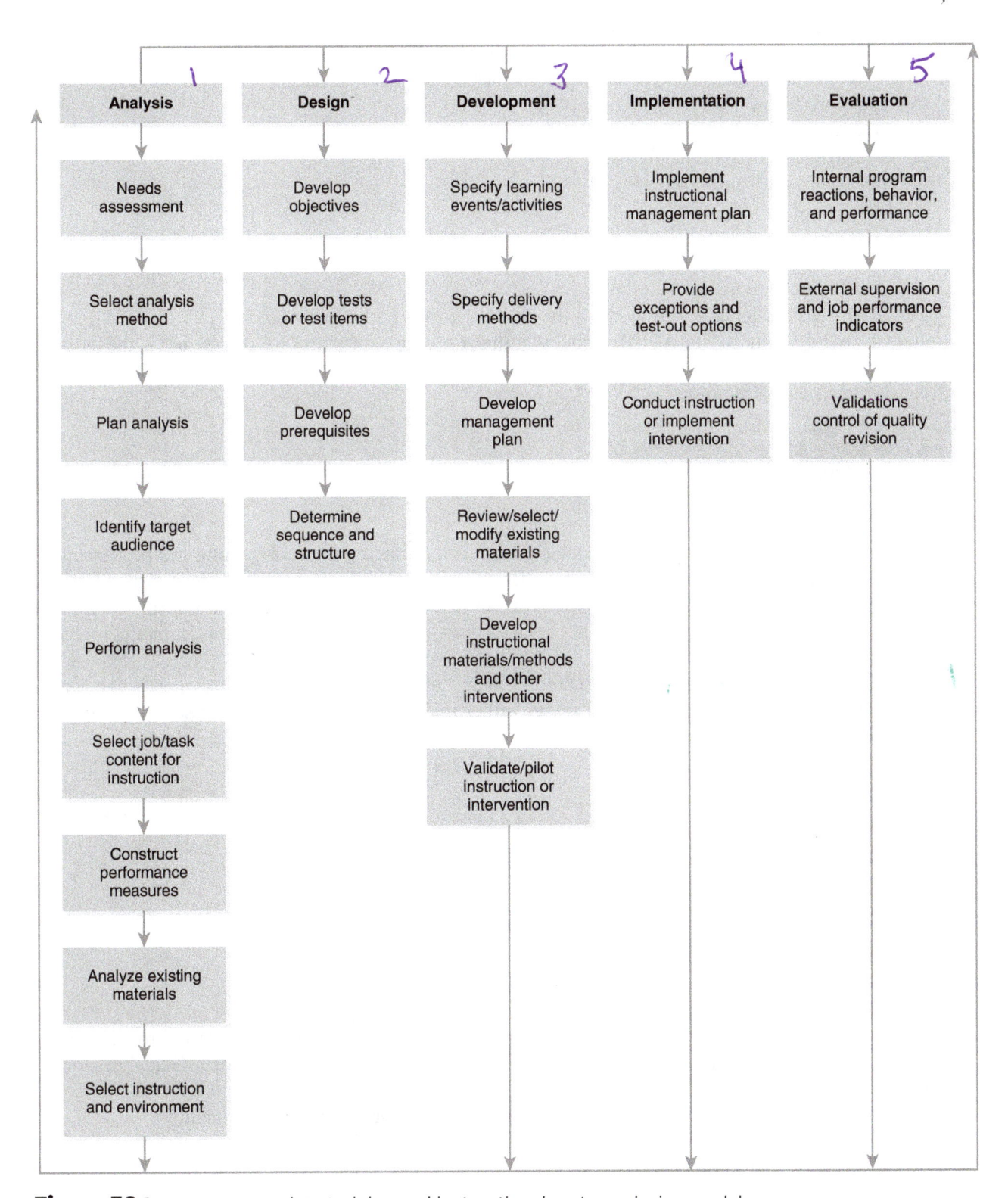

Domain 8: Training, Education, and Communication

1 Analysis	2 Design	3 Development	4 Implementation	5 Evaluation
Needs assessment	Develop objectives	Specify learning events/activities	Implement instructional management plan	Internal program reactions, behavior, and performance
Select analysis method	Develop tests or test items	Specify delivery methods	Provide exceptions and test-out options	External supervision and job performance indicators
Plan analysis	Develop prerequisites	Develop management plan	Conduct instruction or implement intervention	Validations control of quality revision
Identify target audience	Determine sequence and structure	Review/select/modify existing materials		
Perform analysis		Develop instructional materials/methods and other interventions		
Select job/task content for instruction		Validate/pilot instruction or intervention		
Construct performance measures				
Analyze existing materials				
Select instruction and environment				

Figure 36 Systems approach to training and instructional systems design models

Selecting the media to be used for presenting instructional content should be done only after a planning process that includes content analysis, audience analysis, and other steps. OSHA's publication training guidelines follow a model that consists of:
1. Determining if training is needed
2. Identifying training needs
3. Identifying goals and objectives
4. Developing learning activities
5. Conducting the training
6. Evaluating program effectiveness
7. Improving the program

The ADDIE instructional design model is the generic process traditionally used by instructional designers and training developers. The ADDIE model is at the very core of instructional design and is the basis of instructional systems design (ISD). There are various adaptations of the ADDIE model but it generally consists of five cyclical phases:
1. Analysis
2. Design
3. Development
4. Implementation
5. Evaluation

These processes represent a dynamic, flexible guideline for building effective training and performance support tools. Most current ISD models are variations of the ADDIE process. Rapid prototyping is a commonly accepted improvement to this model. This is the idea of reviewing continual or formative feedback while creating instructional materials. This model strives to save time and money by catching problems while they are still easy to fix.

3. **Answer: A.** Media used for any purpose takes advantage of the two senses people use most when learning: sight and hearing. The highest retention comes with actual experience. The retention scale, in increasing order, is as follows:

1. Words, spoken or written
2. Auditory aids
3. Still pictures
4. Motion pictures
5. Live television
6. Displays
7. Familiarization
8. Demonstration
9. Simulations
10. Actual experience

While training often relies on the participants' listening skills, most learning takes place through sight rather than through the other senses. Retention increases as more senses are activated. Guidelines for media selection include:

- Select media that do not conflict with the specific training or job task environment.
- Select media that effectively support the learning objectives.
- Select media that support the training strategy.
- Select media that allow individualization of training when appropriate.
- Select media that will support anytime anywhere training.
- Select media with time and dollar resources in mind.
- Select media that are effective and cost-efficient.

4. **Answer: D.** According to authors Mager, Peterson, Knowles, and many others, a facilitator's actions have a major impact on how a learner reacts to the training environment. Usually, adults tend not to model behavior that is punished. To avoid conflicting values, safety training objectives should be relevant to the work environment.

5. Answer: **A**. The benefit of a lecture (**Table 17**) is that information can be imparted to a large group in a relatively short time. However, this leaves little time or opportunity for interaction between trainee and instructor.

Table 17 Lecture Strategy

Advantages	Limitations	Uses	Types of Objectives
Presents much information in a short time. Provides for instructor control. Good for introducing and summarizing new information. Can be entertaining.	Does not develop reasoning skills. Makes learners dependent on instructor. Is instructor-paced. Tends to be overused. Can be boring.	Introduce new material. Summarize lesson. Establish instructor's expertise and leadership. Excellent for reflective observers. Enhanced by media.	Best for knowledge-level objectives, acquisition of facts.

6. Answer: **C**. The facilitator of adult learning is a guide to adults who are involved in an educational journey. Being technically proficient is not enough; a trainer must possess personality characteristics, interpersonal skills, and positive behaviors. A trainer's attitude is a major motivational condition that has a great impact on creating a conducive learning environment.

   Dr. Knowles' theory of **andragogy** is an attempt to develop a theory specifically for adult learning. Knowles emphasizes that adults are self-directed and expect to take responsibility for decisions. Adult learning programs must accommodate this fundamental aspect. Andragogy makes the following assumptions about the design of learning:
   1. Adults need to know why they need to learn something.
   2. Adults need to learn experientially.
   3. Adults approach learning as problem solving.
   4. Adults learn best when the topic is of immediate value.

   In practical terms, andragogy means that instruction for adults needs to focus more on the process and less on the content being taught. Strategies such as case studies, role-playing, simulations, and self-evaluation are most useful. Instructors adopt a role of facilitator (**Table 18**) or resource rather than lecturer or grader.
   - Six Characteristics of Adult Learners:
     1. Are autonomous and self-directed
     2. Have a foundation of life experiences and knowledge
     3. Are goal oriented
     4. Are relevancy oriented
     5. Are practical in nature
     6. Need to be shown respect
   - Four Adult Learning Needs:
     1. Need to know why (application to immediate challenges)
     2. Need to apply experience (opportunity to share and discuss)
     3. Need to be in control of their learning (flexible environment, voice concerns)
     4. Want to learn things that will make them more effective and successful

   Adults have four basic training needs:
   - Adults need to know why they are learning a particular topic or skill, because they need to apply learning to immediate, real-life challenges.
   - Adults have experience that they apply to all new learning.
   - Adults need to be in control of their own learning.
   - Adults want to learn things that will make them more effective and successful.

   Modified from Knowles, M.S. "The Adult Learner: A Neglected Species." Houston: Gulf Publishing Co., 2011.

   To help meet these needs, training should include precise behavioral guidelines and procedures that the trainees are required to follow.

Table 18 Guided (Facilitated) Discussion Strategy

Advantages	Limitations	Uses	Types of Objectives
Encourages participation. Shows respect for participants' knowledge. Stimulates interest. Allows instructor to check for understanding. Useful in many situations.	Can be dominated by one individual or faction. Susceptible to drift or "mission creep." Can be difficult to focus on objectives. Can degenerate into a lecture or chaos. Does not give trainer complete control.	Can be used as an icebreaker. Can be used to generate ideas. Can be used to solve problems. Can be used for review. Best to use with small groups, or a large group divided into small groups. Useful for both active participants and reflective observers.	Best for comprehension and problem-solving objectives.

7. Answer: **A**. When presenting new material to trainees, trainers should refrain from asking them to validate the training program content. However, questions concerning the training environment, instructor's skill, and presentation are valid questions.

8. Answer: **B**. **Reliability** is a measure of how well a test item discriminates the knowledge level of participants.

   Evaluations for training purposes are *not* norm-referenced. Norm-referencing means that each trainee's score depends on how well or how poorly other trainees perform.

   Evaluations for training purposes should always be criterion-referenced. This means performance is measured against a pre-set standard. The evaluation tool should always be developed before training begins.

   Evaluations are used to determine how well the trainee learns the material. The difficulty index is simply a measure of how many trainees answered the question correctly. A test can be reliable, but not valid, and test scores from a test will follow a normal bell curve.

9. Answer: **A**. This type of communications has several problems:
   - Information flows only in one direction. The lack of feedback means the sender will not know if the message has been received and/or understood. This is the major drawback to one-way communications.
   - The receiver may not understand the message.

10. Answer: **D**. Cohesiveness is defined as a member's desire to remain in a group. The advantages of building and maintaining group cohesiveness are that the group develops a "we" concept; each person feels a part of the group; and cohesiveness acts as a bonding agent. It does not start with or maintain a standardized structure. In team training, consensus is reached when everyone agrees to support the conclusion or outcome.

11. Answer: **C**. Two-way, face-to-face communications are the best way to convey messages on the job.

12. Answer: **A**. At the bottom of Maslow's "Hierarchy of Human Needs" are the physiological or survival needs of food, water, and physical well-being (see **Figure 37**). According to the **progression principle**, as soon as these survival needs are met, one attempts to satisfy the next level of needs, those of security, protection, and stability in day-to-day life activities. If these are met, one moves on to social needs, etc. The first three needs in the model are called lower-order needs and are concerns for a person's desire for social and physical well-being. The top two needs in the pyramid are higher-order needs that satisfy psychological development and growth. Maslow's needs are often used as the most elementary model in the complex study of humans' needs and desires. The chart below shows how needs are satisfied in life and in business.

    Today, organizations have discovered that many of the physiological needs have to be satisfied by methods other than a paycheck.

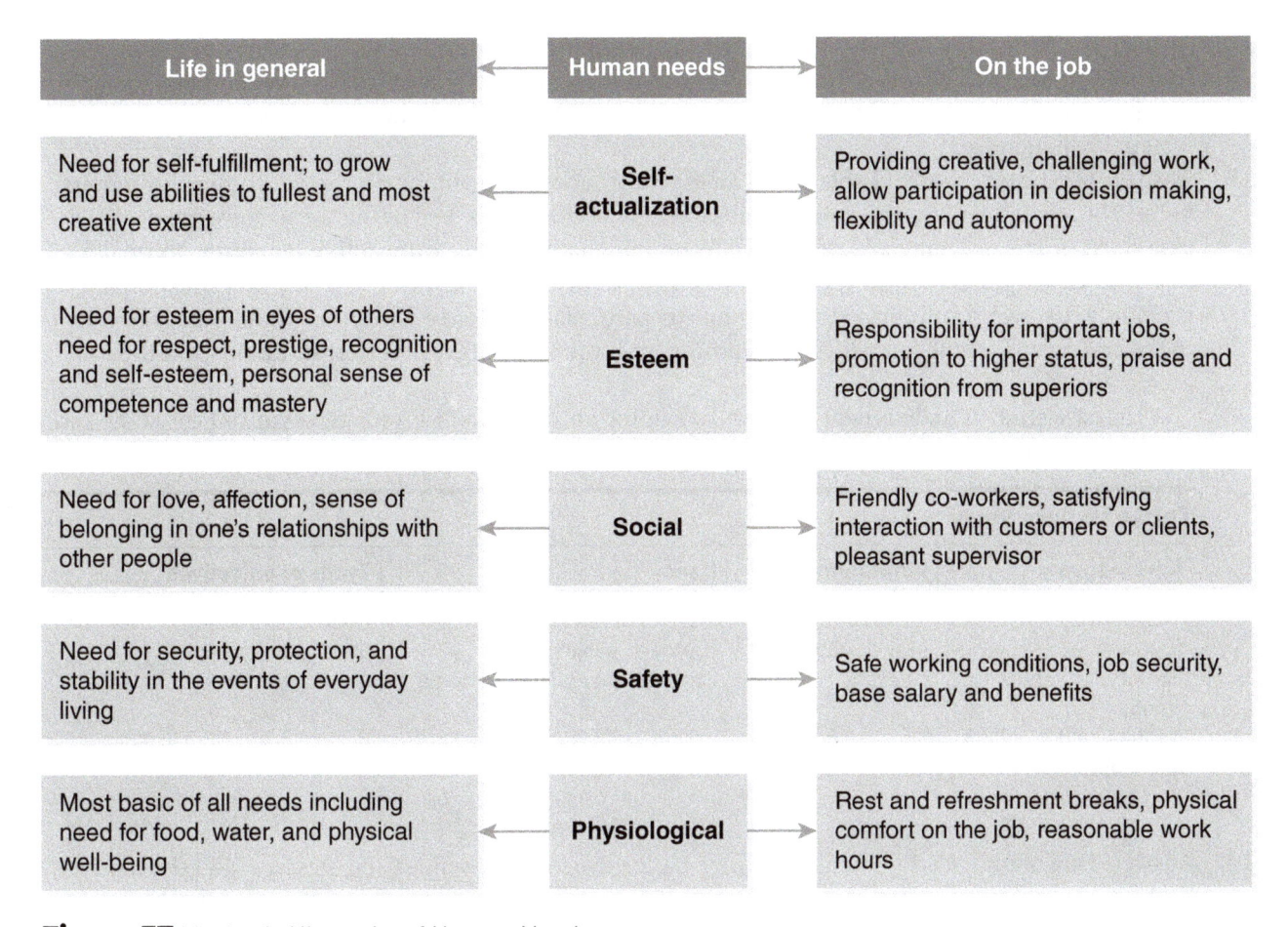

Domain 8: Training, Education, and Communication

Life in general	Human needs	On the job
Need for self-fulfillment; to grow and use abilities to fullest and most creative extent	Self-actualization	Providing creative, challenging work, allow participation in decision making, flexiblity and autonomy
Need for esteem in eyes of others need for respect, prestige, recognition and self-esteem, personal sense of competence and mastery	Esteem	Responsibility for important jobs, promotion to higher status, praise and recognition from superiors
Need for love, affection, sense of belonging in one's relationships with other people	Social	Friendly co-workers, satisfying interaction with customers or clients, pleasant supervisor
Need for security, protection, and stability in the events of everyday living	Safety	Safe working conditions, job security, base salary and benefits
Most basic of all needs including need for food, water, and physical well-being	Physiological	Rest and refreshment breaks, physical comfort on the job, reasonable work hours

Figure 37 Maslow's Hierarchy of Human Needs

13. Answer: **A**. According to the NSC, communication is defined as "sharing information and/or ideas with others and being understood."
14. Answer: **D**. The instructor should follow the lesson plan and ensure that trainees meet course objectives. Training must meet the trainees' expectations, without overkill.
15. Answer: **A**. When dealing with human behavior, trainers are not dealing with the same degree of certainty as if working with a safety situation. The known fact that people differ greatly has been referred to as the "personal equation" or as "individual differences." The behavior of one person will always vary somewhat from another person's.
16. Answer: **C**. One of the most valuable group techniques is the conference method. The strength of the conference method is in individual knowledge and experience of participants. The number of members should be kept small to allow maximum exchange of ideas. The establishment of goals and objectives is crucial to the success of this method. But more than anything else, this teaching method hinges on the capability of the facilitator or instructor. The facilitator logs objectives and keeps information and opinions flowing during sessions. After the conference, the facilitator distributes recommendations and informs members of actions taken as a result. Shortfalls associated with this method can occur if the facilitator fails to ensure that the conference does not become a whine session or management does not follow up on recommendations, resulting in lack of group support for future efforts.

17. Answer: **A**. During any training situation when attempting to change habits or procedures, trainees will have questions about why it is necessary and why the recommended way is best. When trainees are permitted to share ideas, evaluate the material, and become involved, their overall acceptance of course material will increase.
18. Answer: **C**. The case study (**Table 19**) is an especially effective technique for safety and health training because it often illustrates the multicausal aspects of accidents, as well as the tragic consequences. The case study is an excellent problem-solving technique that facilitates **interactive learning**. Normally, case studies are presented to a group that has the goal of evaluating mistakes made in a situation and providing real-world solutions. The technique is particularly effective when the group is allowed to come to the conclusion that it can benefit by learning from the mistakes of other organizations and thus prevent accidents.

    The case study is an excellent tool for developing analytical skills. A major disadvantage of the case study is that a pre-existing case may not actually relate to a specific training situation.

Table 19 Case Study

Advantages	Limitations	Uses	Types of objectives
Interactive Relevant Explores complex issues Applies new knowledge Can be entertaining	Time consuming May not be relevant	Develop analytic and problem-solving skills Enhanced by pictures/media	Best for knowledge-level objectives, problem solving

19. Answer: **D**. Communications consist of three basic elements: the sender, the message, and the receiver. When communicating, whether orally or in writing, people must always provide for feedback. This is the only way to ensure that the message was received.
20. Answer: **A**. Role-playing (**Table 20**) is ideally suited for human relations education or training. It allows students to become participants in a "drama" or "play" that depicts interaction of humans during stressful or error-provoking situations. The technique is not suited for problem solving or technical training.

Table 20 Role-Play Strategy

Advantages	Limitations	Uses	Types of objectives
Creates a learner-centered environment Employs learner creativity Elicits empathy Addresses complex issues Can be entertaining	Participants may be resistant Risk of embarrassing participants Easily distracted, difficult to maintain control Requires intense focus on the objective Requires a skilled facilitator	Useful as a cap-stone exercise to bring together learned concepts Promotes understanding of others' perspective Excellent for active participants	Excellent for affective and problem-solving exercises

Domain 8 Quiz 2 Questions

1. Which is the least interactive training method?
   A. Demonstration
   B. Technical speech
   C. Guided discussion
   D. Individualized instruction

2. A student's ability to remember the task learned last is a Law of Learning known as the:
   A. Law of Frequency.
   B. Law of Recency.
   C. Law of Effect.
   D. Law of Readiness.

3. One example that is not a communication barrier is student:
   A. bias.
   B. mood.
   C. negative reinforcement.
   D. nonverbal actions that conflict with the training subject.

4. What is the most important consideration during the planning stage of an occupational health and safety training program?
   A. Training objectives
   B. Training methods
   C. Instructor qualifications
   D. Training program content

5. What is the most crucial factor when performing instructor duties for a health and safety training session?
   A. Dressing for the occasion
   B. Knowing lesson content
   C. Using numerous visual aids
   D. Using a well-prepared lesson plan

6. The training method used primarily to find new, innovative approaches to issues is:
   A. a meeting.
   B. brainstorming.
   C. a case study.
   D. role-playing.

7. The least likely section(s) to be included in a lesson plan developed for a health and safety training session is/are the:
   A. introduction.
   B. objectives.
   C. training aids.
   D. student survey.

8. What is the primary benefit of safety training?
   A. Reduced costs
   B. Improved performance
   C. Fewer incidents/accidents
   D. Reinforcement of organizational operation goals

9. On-the-job training (OJT) is used primarily because:
   A. it is cost effective.
   B. more than one person can be trained at a time.
   C. it requires a minimum amount of time for total training.
   D. it allows workers to be productive during the training period.

10. What training is required to get a new, but experienced worker qualified as a power truck operator?
    A. Send the employee to a formal school.
    B. Accept the previous company's worker qualification.
    C. Require the employee to attend the new company's initial training program.
    D. Ensure that the operator has the knowledge and skills required to operate power trucks, including relevant company procedures.

11. Who is in the best position to provide effective safety training of industrial work groups?
    A. Supervisors
    B. Senior management
    C. Safety manager
    D. Training professionals

12. Which of the following best describes the training required for the general hazardous waste site worker?
    A. 40 hours of training on-site, with at least 2 days field experience under a trained supervisor
    B. 24 hours training on-site, and two days hands-on
    C. 24 hours training off-site, one day hands-on
    D. 40 hours of training off-site, with at least 3 days field experience under a trained supervisor

13. When is the least effective time to present a safety training session?
    A. After an accident
    B. After the company announces it is downsizing
    C. After the monthly accident data shows an increase in the incident rate
    D. After a plant explosion

14. When performing a training needs analysis, what is the fundamental question that a safety professional must ask?
    A. Will this organization's management commit to implementing this training?
    B. Will this organization's employees implement what they learn during training?
    C. Will this organization accept the learning objectives?
    D. Will training resolve this organization's needs?

15. Which is an example of a well-constructed training objective?
    A. Students will understand the safety policy
    B. General industry training standards
    C. Each student can demonstrate the proper Energy Isolation Procedures
    D. Supervisors will be motivated to deliver safety training

16. While communicating health and safety information with workers, the main objective is to:
    A. teach workers to understand what is being said.
    B. provide a vehicle for suggestions.
    C. teach workers to write and read well.
    D. provide a safety message that will be understood and accepted by all workers.

17. The greatest potential for accidents is known to be in which employee class?
    A. New employees
    B. Experienced employees
    C. Administrative employees
    D. Disabled employees

18. Considering interactive computer-assisted training, or distance learning, which attribute is least valuable?
    A. Works well for organizations with small workforces
    B. Works well for organizations that cannot remove large groups from their jobs at one time
    C. Allows instructors to interact with each other without restrictions
    D. Allows trainees to work at their own pace

19. For training to be effective, training objectives should be established and measured. Which statement about training objectives least affects performance outcomes?
    A. Training objectives should be reasonable and practical.
    B. Training objectives must be measurable.
    C. Training objectives should be obtainable.
    D. Training objectives must be written.

20. You are facilitating a one-hour training session and arrive five minutes before the start of class to find that your presentation did not synchronize with the company server. Participants are taking their seats and you do not have access to the presentation. What is the best course of action?
    A. Cancel the training session.
    B. Reschedule the training session for a later time.
    C. Get into your facilitator toolkit and begin the training.
    D. Ask a participant familiar with the topic to deliver the training.

Domain 8 Quiz 2 Answers

1. Answer: **B**. A lecture or a technical speech is one-way communication and the least interactive between the instructor and learner. The methods listed below are standard instructional strategies:
   - Lecture
   - Demonstration
   - Guided discussion
   - Individualized instruction
   - Role-play
   - Learner discovery method

2. Answer: **B**. The "Laws of Learning" are as follows:

   Law of Recency: People tend to recall and use that which they learned last or most recently. It is easier to remember a subject after a recent seminar, or how to solve a complex technical problem on the job, than to recall a simple trigonometry problem from high school.

   Law of Frequency: The more often a mental connection is made, the stronger it becomes. Repetition is helpful in skill and attitude development and habit formation.

   Law of Effect: People like to do things that bring pleasure and enjoyment. They learn easily and quickly those things that are pleasant experiences and they remember these things longer.

   Law of Readiness: People must be in a receptive frame of mind if learning is to be effective. Learning a particular thing must be seen as a benefit to them. Everyone learns more easily if they see the value and have a desire to learn.

Law of Disuse: When knowledge or a skill is not used, it becomes fuzzy or rusty, making it more difficult to recall or use. Knowledge is the first to suffer from disuse, and a skill may become rusty, but both are often quickly regained with a little practice.

Law of Primacy: People learn things that are important to them and have special meaning to their lives. These are primary to them and will often ease the difficulty in learning complex skills or knowledge.

Law of Intensity: The more involved students become with learning, the more they learn and the better they recall knowledge. Active learning from reading and/or performing a skill are far superior to passive learning from watching a movie or listening to a lecture. Learning is an individual effort that greatly intensifies with individual participation.

3. Answer: **C**. Communication barriers consist of:
   - Knowledge: Trainees believe that they already know all that is needed.
   - Bias: People's pre-existing attitudes may cause them to tune out the information.
   - Mood: An individual's frame of mind/disposition may prevent hearing information.
   - Nonverbal actions: Inconsistent body language confuses the transfer of information.

4. Answer: **A**. The establishment of training objectives is key to good planning. No other single element has as much bearing on the success of the training program. The primary purpose of a training objective is to describe the intended outcome of the instruction.

5. Answer: **D**. The use of a lesson plan will provide standardization to a presentation and avoid omission of essential material. The lesson plan also helps the instructor conduct the class according to a timetable and should provide for student participation or involvement.

6. Answer: **B**. Brainstorming (**Table 21**) is a technique of utilizing group interactions that encourages each participant to present ideas on a specific issue. The method is normally used to find new, innovative approaches to issues. There are four ground rules:
   - Ideas presented are not criticized.
   - Freewheeling creative thinking and building on ideas are positively reinforced.
   - As many ideas as possible should be quickly presented.
   - Combining several ideas or improving suggestions is encouraged.

Table 21 Brainstorming

Advantages	Limitations	Uses	Types of objectives
Interactive Relevant Creative Can be entertaining	Time consuming Requires skilled facilitator	Problem solving Troubleshooting Enhanced by pictures/media	Best for knowledge-level objectives, problem solving

7. Answer: **D**. There are many formats for lesson plans. However, the most widely used format includes the following areas:

Title: Indicates subject matter being taught. It should be very clear and concise.

Objectives: Indicate session purpose or goals. Specifically, it should indicate what students are expected to know or be able to do at the conclusion of the session or lesson.

Aids: A list of all training aids such as videos, equipment, charts, etc., should be incorporated to develop important points in the lesson.

Introduction: The introduction to the class should develop group interest. This essential component provides students with the scope and importance of the subject.

Presentation: This is the plan of action. It is the guide for conveying ideas, information, or skills all students should learn. It should also indicate the method of presentation, such as lecture, demonstration (**Table 22**), guided discussion, etc.

Domain 8: Training, Education, and Communication 185

Application: If possible, application examples should be illustrated either by student experience or by an actual illustration by the instructor.

Summary: The summary restates the main points of the lesson and helps strengthen weak points in the instruction. Its importance cannot be overstated.

8. Answer: **B**. According to the NSC, the goal of effective training is learning that leads to improved on-the-job performance.
9. Answer: **D**. According to the NSC, OJT is widely used because it allows the worker to produce during the training period.

Table 22 Demonstration/Practice Strategy

Advantages	Limitations	Uses	Types of objectives
Provides hands-on experience/practice. Incorporates multiple senses and learning styles. Proficiency evaluated through demonstrated performance.	Requires significant preparation. Is time consuming. May increase safety risks. May require a cadre of instructors.	Useful for any hands-on skills. Useful for troubleshooting. Works well only with small groups. Excellent for active participants.	Best with application-level/psychomotor objectives. Useful for problem solving with equipment (troubleshooting).

10. Answer: **D**. CFR1910.178, Powered Industrial Trucks, requires anyone changing equipment or the workplace location to meet the requirements outlined in the Refresher Training requirements (para 1910.178 (l)(4)).
11. Answer: **A**. Supervisors are in the best position to provide realistic and effective training for industrial workers. They have detailed knowledge of work processes and control workflow. Work group members are attached to the group and are loyal to the members, including the leader. Group members and their leader have a high degree of confidence and trust in each other. Thus, the more important a value seems to the group, the greater likelihood that an individual will accept it.
12. Answer: **D**. The US OSHA standard 1910.120, Hazardous Waste Operations and Emergency Response (HAZWOPER), requires training for waste site workers, occasional workers, and site supervisors. The standard requires general workers to be provided 40 hours of hands-on instruction off site, combined with at least 3 days of field experience under the supervision of a trained supervisor. Additionally, these workers must complete 8 hours of refresher training every 12 months. Training under this standard also applies to TSDF workers and emergency responders. 29 CFR 1910.120, states in paragraph (e)(5) that "Trainers shall be qualified to instruct employees about the subject matter that is being presented in training." In addition, 29 CFR 1910.120(e)(5) explains that the qualifications of the instructors may be shown by academic degrees, completed training courses, and/or work experience. At this time, OSHA does not have any specific requirements to certify an instructor. The subjects that trainers should be able to convey to employees at hazardous waste operations who need training are summarized in paragraphs (e), (p), and (q) of the HAZWOPER standard. OSHA Regulations 29 CFR 1910.120 Appendix E or 29 CFR 1926.65 Appendix E, *Training Curriculum Guidelines - (Non-mandatory)*

Training 1910.120(q)(6). Training shall be based on the duties and function to be performed by each responder of an emergency response organization. The skill and knowledge levels required for all new responders, those hired after the effective date of this standard, shall be conveyed to them through training before they are permitted to take part in actual emergency operations on an incident. Employees who participate, or are expected to participate, in emergency response shall be given training in accordance with the following paragraphs:

First responder awareness level. First responders at the awareness level are individuals who are likely to witness or discover a hazardous substance release and who have been trained to initiate an emergency response sequence by notifying the proper authorities of the release. They would take no further action beyond notifying the authorities of the release. First responders at the awareness level shall have sufficient training or have had sufficient experience to objectively demonstrate competency in the following areas:

- An understanding of what hazardous substances are, and the risks associated with them in an incident
- An understanding of the potential outcomes associated with an emergency created when hazardous substances are present
- The ability to recognize the presence of hazardous substances in an emergency
- The ability to identify the hazardous substances, if possible
- An understanding of the role of the first responder awareness individual in the employer's emergency response plan, including site security and control, and the U.S. Department of Transportation's *Emergency Response Guidebook*
- The ability to realize the need for additional resources, and to make appropriate notifications to the communication center

First responder operations level. First responders at the operations level are individuals who respond to releases or potential releases of hazardous substances as part of the initial response to the site for protecting nearby persons, property, or the environment from the effects of the release. They are trained to respond in a defensive fashion without actually trying to stop the release. Their function is to contain the release from a safe distance, keep it from spreading, and prevent exposures. First responders at the operational level shall have received **at least eight hours** of training or have had sufficient experience to objectively demonstrate competency in the following areas in addition to those listed for the awareness level and the employer shall so certify:

- Knowledge of the basic hazard and risk assessment techniques
- Know how to select and use proper personal protective equipment provided to the first responder operational level
- An understanding of basic hazardous materials terms
- Know how to perform basic control, containment, and/or confinement operations within the capabilities of the resources and personal protective equipment available with the unit
- Know how to implement basic decontamination procedures
- An understanding of the relevant standard operating procedures and termination procedures

Hazardous materials technician. Hazardous materials technicians are individuals who respond to releases or potential releases for the purpose of stopping the release. They assume a more aggressive role than a first responder at the operations level in that they will approach the point of release in order to plug, patch, or otherwise stop the release of a hazardous substance. Hazardous materials technicians shall have received **at least 24 hours of training** equal to the first responder operations level and in addition have competency in the following areas and the employer shall so certify:

- Know how to implement the employer's emergency response plan
- Know the classification, identification, and verification of known and unknown materials by using field survey instruments and equipment
- Be able to function within an assigned role in the incident command system
- Know how to select and use proper specialized chemical personal protective equipment provided to the hazardous materials technician
- Understand hazard and risk assessment techniques
- Be able to perform advance control, containment, and/or confinement operations within the capabilities of the resources and personal protective equipment available with the unit
- Understand and implement decontamination procedures
- Understand termination procedures
- Understand basic chemical and toxicological terminology and behavior

Hazardous materials specialist. Hazardous materials specialists are individuals who respond with and provide support to hazardous materials technicians. Their duties parallel those of the hazardous materials technician, but require a more directed or specific knowledge of the various substances they may be

Domain 8: Training, Education, and Communication 187

called upon to contain. The hazardous materials specialist would also act as the site liaison with federal, state, local, and other government authorities in regard to site activities. Hazardous materials specialists shall have received **at least 24 hours** of training equal to the technician level.

On-scene incident commander. Incident commanders, who will assume control of the incident scene beyond the first responder awareness level, shall receive **at least 24 hours** of training equal to the first responder operations level and in addition have competency in the following areas and the employer shall so certify:

- Know and be able to implement the employer's incident command system
- Know how to implement the employer's emergency response plan
- Know and understand the hazards and risks associated with employees working in chemical protective clothing
- Know how to implement the local emergency response plan
- Know of the state emergency response plan and of the Federal Regional Response Team
- Know and understand the importance of decontamination procedures

Those employees who are trained in accordance with paragraph (q)(6) of this section shall receive annual refresher training of sufficient content and duration to maintain their competencies, or shall demonstrate competency in those areas at least yearly.

13. Answer: **B**. There are three things that will keep a person from listening: Word barriers (words such as death, liar, layoff, IRS, etc.); emotional barriers (bias, boredom, envy, fatigue, etc.); and distractions.
14. Answer: **D**. According to *Developing Safety Training Programs,* the basic question is: Will training solve the problem? The other questions are secondary. Training is most appropriate for new skills or knowledge.
15. Answer: **C**. According to *Developing Safety Training Programs,* a learning objective must identify what the student will be able to do at the end of the training program. Learning objectives are determined in the design phase. The outline of the training program is determined after the learning objectives are established.
16. Answer: **D**. The bottom line is that any training or education effort must provide a message that will be understood and acted on by the workers.
17. Answer: **A**. According to the NSC, although statistical data differ, it is generally agreed that new employees are significantly more prone to work-related accidents.
18. Answer: **C**. According to the NSC, the valuable attributes of interactive computer-assisted training, sometimes called computer-based training (CBT) or distance learning, are as follows:
    - Workers can work at their own pace.
    - Records of all training can be automatically kept.
    - Correct answers are required before a student can proceed.
    - Workers receive training as time is available.
    - Instructors can guide workers step by step through the entire lesson plan.
    - This method works extremely well for organizations with a small workforce or that cannot remove large groups from their jobs at any one time.

    When someone completes coursework away from an actual training facility, it is generally called distance learning. This is an umbrella term for many types of learning, including online training and training available through the mail. Before implementing CBT or any type of training, a needs analysis should be completed to ensure that the best method is being selected.
19. Answer: **D**. Training objectives should, above all, be reasonable, measurable, and obtainable. It is very desirable, but not imperative, that the objectives and goals for any program be written, so as not to be misplaced or relegated to a low priority. When writing training objectives, use action verbs such as *add, answer, compare, lineup* etc. Avoid words such as *understand, know, comprehend,* and *notice,* as these are actions that are difficult to measure.

    To gain a competitive edge, training must involve more than basic job skills. Included now are advanced skills and understanding of customers and entire manufacturing systems. The training is linked to strategic business goals and specific objectives, and uses an instructional process that ensures effective training and compares favorably with training programs found in other companies.

20. Answer: **C**. First, facilitators should arrive early—at least 30 minutes before the start of training—to get set up (mentally and technologically), check the learning environment, verify that materials are in order, and greet participants as they arrive. It is always a good idea to carry a backup memory stick with a copy of the presentation. To be an effective trainer/facilitator, one must have a go-to facilitator toolkit. While multimedia presentations are great tools, death by PowerPoint is the result of this technology being overused as a crutch for poor facilitation skills. Some of the best presentations delivered by skilled facilitators have been done spontaneously due to technical difficulties. On the other hand, such disruptions can be disastrous for a one-dimensional, inflexible, or novice instructor. Facilitators should *always* have a backup plan.

One of the pitfalls of instruction is that trainers tend to develop training programs that accommodate the way the trainer learns best, not the way the participants learn best. The key to accommodating learning styles is that instructional strategies and media should be selected as a means to help the learner and not as a convenience for the instructor. The best training stimulates multiple senses in the learner and should be a blend of various learning strategies:

- Lecture
- Brainstorm
- Case study
- Demonstration
- Role-play
- Guided discussion
- Self-directed/distance learning
- Learner discovery/individualized instruction
- Interactive computer-based training (CBT)
- Activity-based/hands-on/demonstration
- E-learning/m-learning
- Hybrid/blended

Many people recognize that each person prefers different learning styles and techniques. Learning styles group the common ways that people learn. Everyone has a mix of learning styles. Some people may find that they have a dominant style of learning, with far less use of the other styles. Others may find that they use different styles in different circumstances. There is no right mix. Nor are styles fixed. Participants can develop ability in less dominant styles, as well as further develop styles they already use well. Considering learning styles helps trainers to:

- Recognize that everyone learns differently, and the need for a variety of instructional strategies and media
- Recognize that trainers *also* have preferred learning styles
- Be learner focused, not instructor focused
- Be creative and include exercises or instructional strategies or media that help adults learn the information appropriate for the learning objectives
- Make real-time adjustments and employ alternative instructional methods best suited to the learners so they can accomplish the learning objectives
- Empathize with training participants

By recognizing and understanding learning styles, skilled trainers can use a variety of techniques best suited to the audience and learning objectives. This improves the speed and quality of training.

The ANSI Z490-2009 Criteria for Accepted Practices in Safety, Health and Environmental Training is a well-constructed standard specific to SH&E training.

Competency is having the skills, knowledge, and abilities to perform the task as determined by the employer. A competent training professional is a person prepared by education, training, or experience to develop and implement various elements of a training program. This role is also known in the Z490 standard as a training professional.

A trainer is the person who delivers a training event.

Trainer criteria for safety, health, and environmental trainers shall be specified during training development. Criteria shall include subject-matter expertise and training delivery skills.

Domain 9: Law and Ethics

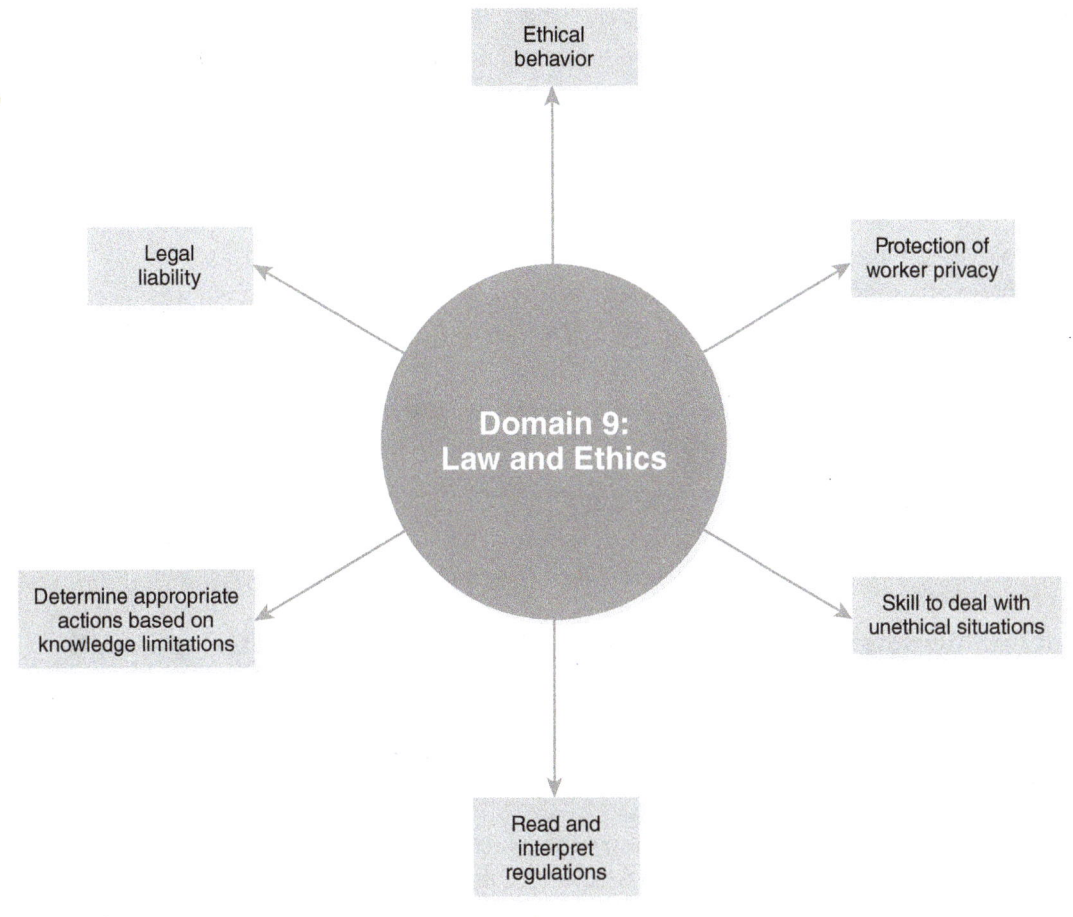

Modified from ASP® Exam Blueprint (ASP10), November 10, 2019

Domain 9 Quiz 1 Questions   16 questions

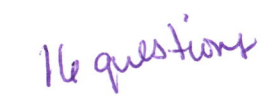

1. Two ways to modify insurance rates based on modifying the manual rate to reflect the insured's safety record are the prospective experience rating and the retrospective rating. Which of the following identifies the retrospective rating?
    A. Past experience
    B. Experience during the policy period
    C. Projected losses
    D. Manual premiums are not modified.

2. To adjust workers' compensation insurance rates, a company must use the:
    A. experience modification rate.
    B. incident rate.
    C. workers' compensation modification rate.
    D. accident rate.

3. An accident including a company vehicle that impacted an overpass support structure involved a company's driver. All company vehicle records are requested by the NTSB. According to 49CFR, what must be provided?

   A. Only the records deemed necessary by the safety supervisor
   B. Records are not required.
   C. All information requested by the NTSB
   D. Only records the insurance company deems necessary

4. Which principle involves the "fellow servant" rule?

   A. The employer must establish a "two-man" rule.
   B. Employees will not be responsible for each other.
   C. Rules will be established for more than one worker.
   D. The employer will not be responsible for injuries caused by another worker.

5. An agreement or contract in which one party agrees to hold the other free from responsibility for any liability or damage that might arise from the transaction involved is called a/an:

   A. strict liability.
   B. hold harmless agreement.
   C. negligence.
   D. exclusive remedy.

6. Which of the following identifies the four mandatory elements for any legal contract?

   A. Consent, legal tender, parties, consideration
   B. Management, labor, money, contract
   C. Agreement, consideration, purpose, legal tender
   D. Agreement, consideration, purpose, competent parties

7. Safety professionals may need to have insurance protection, depending on business status. Of numerous types of coverage, one specific to safety consultants and trainers is professional liability that covers all of the following except:

   A. errors and omissions.
   B. fire damage.
   C. libel and slander.
   D. negligence.

8. An Associate Safety Professional (ASP) must accept responsibility for his or her continued professional development by acquiring and maintaining competence through continuing education, experience, professional training, and:

   A. monitoring safety websites.
   B. maintaining a presence on social networks.
   C. keeping current on relevant legal issues.
   D. writing a regular Internet blog.

9. An ASP works with a large safety and occupational health staff. The ASP has been asked to perform hygiene sampling, even though the ASP has had no formal training or education on sampling. According to the BCSP Code of Ethics, what should the ASP do first in this situation?

   A. The ASP does not have an ethics concern under BCSP professional conduct guidelines and should perform the sampling.
   B. The ASP may conduct the sampling but should advise the BCSP that a possible ethics violation occurred.
   C. The ASP should perform the sampling but should contact the BCSP after completion to verify if an ethics violation occurred.
   D. The ASP should not perform the sampling because doing so may violate the BCSP Code of Ethics.

10. Employee unions can impact safety:
    A. negatively, when there is insistence on engineering control as a substitute for disciplinary action.
    B. negatively, when union leaders have a role in safety training.
    C. positively, when employees bargain for safety incentive programs based upon reducing accident rates.
    D. positively, when workers have more direct involvement in reducing workplace hazards.

11. As an ASP, you are working as a consultant for a company and identify a condition that poses serious risk to the employees. You notify the client of serious safety concerns and he tells you that he does not have the resources to fix the condition. The most ethical response to this situation is to:
    A. report the situation to the regulating government agency.
    B. keep good documentation of this situation.
    C. discuss the situation with the client to find a solution.
    D. claim that you have informed the client and your responsibility has ended.

12. You are conducting a safety inspection of a manufacturing plant in southwest Missouri. The site visit is designed to fulfill two purposes: to mentor a university safety degree intern, and to determine regulatory compliance of the facility. During the inspection, you observe an employee, without eye protection, working at a bench installing parts. This is not a hazardous operation, but it is being conducted in a posted "eye protection" area. Which is the best course of action?
    A. Contact the immediate supervisor and discuss the situation.
    B. Test the safety intern's skills by letting her handle the situation.
    C. Confront the employee and determine why eye protection is not being used.
    D. Note the discrepancy and discuss it later when the CEO and the supervisor are both present.

13. A local safety conference planning committee has asked you speak about fall protection engineering on a construction safety expert panel. Your experience with fall protection is with maintenance employees in an aerial lift and cherry picker operators. You should:
    A. attend the conference for professional development and decline to speak on the panel.
    B. agree to speak on the panel only if the panel is not taking questions from the audience.
    C. decline to speak on the panel and notify the BCSP.
    D. decline to attend the conference so as to avoid any conflict of interest.

14. You are working for the general contractor and assisting subcontractors with job safety analysis on a multiemployer job site. The electricians identified a new pipefitter task that would assist the plumbers with installing water lines. The pipefitters stated that the union agreement precluded them from assisting the plumbers. What is the best course of action to resolve the issue of task responsibility?
    A. Assign the responsibility to all trades.
    B. Negotiate the tasks with the union representatives.
    C. Assign the task responsibility to only the pipefitters.
    D. Notify the general site management to resolve the issue and communicate the policy to the appropriate parties.

15. You are conducting activity-based trenching competent person training in a representative trench that is 15 feet deep in class C soil. All trainees and protection systems have been removed. A trainee notifies you and his project manager that he has left his paycheck in the trench. Which is the best advice for the decision-makers?
    A. Inform the trainee of the risks, direct the trench competent person to escort the trainee into the trench to retrieve the item, and stand by as the entry attendant.
    B. Advise the project manager of the risks for workers entering an unprotected trench, and work with the team to find an acceptable solution.
    C. Direct the equipment operator to close the trench and inform the project manager that trainees' personal items are not the trainer's responsibility.
    D. Advise the trainee to enter the trench during the next break to retrieve the item and be careful not to collapse the trench or be witnessed.

16. **Professional ethics refers to:**
    A. a set of principles and standards that guide the actions of professionals that are often referenced in civil or criminal cases involving professional conduct.
    B. the laws that the professional must comply with or face possible civil and criminal charges.
    C. a set of bylaws established for members of an organization to follow.
    D. voluntary rules regarding what is expected of members of professional associations.

17. **Management has increased work hours and is pushing for more productivity. As an ASP, you are concerned about some of the safety risks associated with this production schedule. You should:**
    A. report your concern to the U.S. Department of Labor (DOL).
    B. tell workers to launch a work slowdown.
    C. inform/communicate increased hazards due to increased production and verify that the risk is acceptable.
    D. not challenge the management; accept the production schedule.

18. **As a salaried safety professional for a large company, you are obligated to be a faithful agent to your employer. You have recently purchased a substantial financial interest as a limited partner in a medium-sized safety consulting firm. Your employer recently acquired a new business that had hired your consulting firm to perform a safety compliance audit and you were assigned the task. After disclosing the conflict of interest to your boss, she permits you to perform the work. Is this an acceptable resolution?**
    A. Yes; the conflict of interest has been addressed in accordance with your employer's code of ethics.
    B. No, because this situation does not avoid circumstances where compromise of conduct or conflict of interest may arise related to safety responsibilities.
    C. Yes, as there is not a conflict of interest if the issue was fully disclosed to your employer.
    D. No, because the situation cannot allow you to be honest, fair, and impartial and act with responsibility and integrity.

19. **You are part of an interview team to fill a new facility safety manager position. The candidate claims to be an ASP but is not listed on the BCSP website as a credential holder. You should:**
    A. notify the BCSP and impart all the pertinent information.
    B. tell the person to stop using the ASP designation.
    C. do nothing, if the person is qualified in other areas.
    D. notify the corporate attorney to pursue legal action.

20. **You are conducting an audit in a supervisor's area and he is a friend of yours. You identify significant hazards in his department, and the supervisor tells you he will fix the hazards by the end of the day. Which is the best course of action?**
    A. Write everything in the report, and note the conversation with supervisor.
    B. Write the report and note that the hazard was corrected.
    C. Omit the hazard finding from the report, since he said he would fix it by the end of the day.
    D. Notify the supervisor's boss of the hazard and ask her to verify that the hazard has been abated.

21. **When advising decision-makers, the safety professional should:**
    A. always seek an outside opinion before deciding.
    B. consult the local ASSP chapter for guidance when needed.
    C. offer advice that is most appealing to the decision-maker.
    D. limit advice and recommendations to one's knowledge.

Domain 9 Quiz 1 Answers

1. Answer: **B**. Because past experience modifies future rates, this plan is known as **prospective experience rating** to distinguish it from **retrospective experience rating**, which further modifies the manual rate to reflect experience during the policy period.

2. Answer: **A**. The insurance industry uses EMR for workers' compensation insurance as a means of determining equitable premiums. These rating systems consider the average incident losses for a given firm's type of work and amount of payroll and predict the dollar amount of expected losses due to work-related injuries and illnesses.

    Modification rates charged by private carriers are usually affected by risks beyond the insured's control, products produced or services provided, and potential for catastrophic accidents.

3. Answer: **C**. According to CFR (1998), "The Safety Board may issue a subpoena, enforceable in Federal district court, to obtain testimony or other evidence. Authorized representatives of the Board may question any person having knowledge relevant to an accident/incident, study, or special investigation. Authorized representatives of the Board also have exclusive authority, on behalf of the Board, to decide the way in which any testing will be conducted, including decisions on the person that will conduct the test, the type of test that will be conducted, and any individual who will witness the test."

4. Answer: **D**. *[handwritten: No longer exists   Good Samaritan Rule]*

    Fellow Servant Rule: A defense which, prior to the enactment of workers' compensation laws, could be used by an employer to protect him/herself when sued by an employee for damages from injury caused by one or more fellow employees.

    Assumption of Risk: The worker knew he/she was involved in a risky or hazardous occupation.

    Contributory Negligence: The worker contributed to his/her injury. These were two other pre-workers' compensation defenses for employers.

    The principle of **foreseeability** involves liability for actions that a normal person would have known to exist and would have taken precautions to prevent. These actions result in injury or damage when hazards were foreseeable. Foreseeability is a fundamental legal principle used in product liability cases.

5. Answer: **B**. A **hold harmless (*indemnity*) agreement** is used between two parties to establish that the indemnitee is protected from any unforeseen liabilities, losses, claims, or damages during the indemnitee's involvement in an activity. A hold harmless agreement is developed to prevent lawsuits by assigning liability in a contract. Hold harmless means that if there is a problem and a suit later, one party shields or "holds harmless" the other. A hold harmless clause is a statement in a legal contract stating that an individual or organization is not liable for any injuries or damages caused to the individual signing the contract. An individual may be asked to sign a hold harmless agreement when undertaking an activity that involves risk for which the enabling entity does not want to be legally or financially responsible. *[handwritten: lawsuit always holds up]*

    Strict liability is the concept whereby the plaintiff need not show negligence or fault to prove liability.

    Negligence is the failure to exercise a reasonable amount of care or to carry out a legal duty, so that injury or property damage occurs to another. An example would be a landlord who did not provide adequate security, and the renter was robbed.

    Exclusive remedy: State workers' compensation statutes gave employees a definite remedy for injuries and diseases arising out of or suffered in the course of their employment. In exchange for a definite recovery, the workers' compensation remedy is exclusive, that is, with just a few exceptions, a worker's right of recovery against the employer is limited to the benefits provided by the workers' compensation law. The employee may not sue for tort.

    The **attractive nuisance** doctrine applies to the law of torts, in the United States. It states that a landowner may be held liable for injuries to children trespassing on the land if the injury is caused by an object on the land that is likely to attract children. A backyard swimming pool is an example.

Tort is a wrongful act or a failure to exercise due care that results in damage or injury in the broadest sense. A manufacturer or distributor would not have to label a large-bladed hunting knife because the product involves an **obvious peril**, sometimes called an obvious hazard, that is well known to the public.

The term **res ipsa loquitur** (the thing speaks for itself) is involved in accidents where the damage-producing agent was under the sole control of the defendant and the accident would not have happened if the defendant had exercised proper control.

6. Answer: **D**. A legal contract must have four parts:
   - Agreement
   - Consideration
   - Purpose
   - Competent parties
7. Answer: **B**. Safety consultants and trainers professional liability insurance covers errors and omissions, libel and slander, negligence, oral and written publication of information that causes damage, and infringement upon copyrighted materials. Safety consultants commercial general liability covers bodily injury/property damage, fire damage, and medical expenses.
8. Answer: **C**. According to the BCSP Code of Ethics, an ASP should accept responsibility for his or her continued professional development by acquiring and maintaining competence through continuing education, experience, professional training, and keeping current on relevant legal issues.
9. Answer: **D**. According to the BCSP Code of Ethics, an ASP should undertake assignments only when qualified by education or experience in the specific technical fields involved.
10. Answer: **D**. Unions are important participants in a safety culture. They want to eliminate injuries that harm their members. To do that, unions favor changes to the workplace that make it safer. Unions have challenged the reliance of some employers upon the discipline of individual workers for safety-related behaviors. Unions assert that the disciplining of individuals for errors is far less effective than a program of pre-incident planning, risk assessment, and engineering controls. A fail-safe device or design makes the errors less likely to cause injuries. The desirable investment in workplace design change that the union prefers would render the machine quieter, the floor safer, and the equipment guards impregnable to removal or evasion. This emphasis shifts the issues away from discipline of errant people to the needs for engineers to devise built-in constraints on people's capacity for accepting risk or making foolish judgments.

    Unions' effectiveness in collective bargaining for safety issues varies with economic situations, and with the urgency felt by an individual local bargaining team to assert itself on safety issues. If the union is able to win concessions on safety issues, the enhanced union-management effort probably increases the likelihood that workers will support the culture and act with greater awareness of safety. If work teams are used, the training of work teams for safety should include the support of union leadership such as the local president or shop steward for the safety program.
11. Answer: **C**. Professional responsibility is to advise the client of the risks of serious injuries and help the client to find a solution.
12. Answer: **A**. The first action should be to contact the supervisor who has control of the workplace and discuss the infraction. Further action may include some of the solutions presented in the other answer options.
13. Answer: **A**. According to the BCSP Code of Ethics, certified professionals should undertake assignments only when qualified by education or experience in the specific technical fields involved. They should accept responsibility for their continued professional development by acquiring and maintaining competence through continuing education, experience, professional training, and keeping current on relevant legal issues. They should issue public statements only in an objective and truthful manner and only when founded upon knowledge of the facts and competence in the subject matter. They should not misrepresent or exaggerate their degree of responsibility in or for the subject matter of prior assignments.
14. Answer: **D**. It is important for a safety professional to realize when issues are beyond his/her control. For management-versus-labor operational conflicts, it is best to direct the issue to management for resolution.

Domain 9: Law and Ethics   195

[Handwritten note at top: "Inform decision makers my prime responsibility"]

15. Answer: **B**. Your primary responsibility is to inform the decision-makers of the risk exposure to workers entering an unprotected trench. Then help the decision-makers explore solutions to achieve an acceptable level of risk. Entering an unprotected 15-foot-deep excavation is a clear violation of the regulations and advising the contractor to enter an unprotected trench, actively or tacitly, is unethical. After communicating the risks of entering an unprotected trench, a fair resolution may be attempting to retrieve the trainee's item, such as by using remote retrieval, or placing the protection systems back in the trench. If an option is technically, legally, or theoretically acceptable, then another good measure is to determine if it is balanced. The decision to tell the trainee, "Tough—it is your own fault," is perhaps not balanced or fair. Nor is exposing workers to unacceptable risk for production gains.

16. Answer: **A**. Ethics refers to a set of principles and standards that guide the actions of professionals and are often referenced in civil or criminal cases involving professional conduct. A basic definition of ethics is moral principles or practice. Professional ethics require consideration of additional areas, including professional values, culture, acceptable standards of behavior, and legality. Professionals will likely face ethical dilemmas during their career. Some day-to-day ethical dilemmas are simple to determine the correct course of action; others are not as clear.

17. Answer: **C**. Informing/communicating to upper management the increased hazards due to increased production and verifying that the risk is acceptable is the best solution.

18. Answer: **B**. Most employer codes of ethics require you to disclose to your employer any conflicts of interest. Once you disclose a conflict of interest, your employer has the option to require you to resolve the conflict of interest by ending the relationship/situation that causes the conflict of interest, or can elect to allow the situation to continue. As per the BCSP and many other professional codes of conduct, certified professionals must avoid any perceptions of conflicts of interest even when their own company's code of ethics is satisfied.

19. Answer: **A**. If you have difficulties finding an individual or question an individual's certification status, please contact our office at bcsp@bcsp.org or at +1 317-593-4800. To report unauthorized use, use the BCSP complaint form. Individuals who have used BCSP credentials without authority are listed in the directory when you click on Unauthorized Use. The Unauthorized Use Directory is a listing of individuals who have claimed to hold BCSP credentials but do not. The BCSP receives inquiries from a variety of sources, including other credential holders, employers, and membership organizations. The BCSP pursues all cases in which there is clear evidence of the unauthorized use and the individual clearly has responsibility, control, or knowledge of the use. Evidence may be a business card, résumé, letter, website, or other publication. The BCSP may take a variety of actions as a result of verified and unauthorized use of BCSP credentials or marks. Such actions may include but are not limited to:
    - Publish name on the BCSP website: If it is determined that an individual uses a BCSP credential or mark without authorization, in most cases a penalty will be imposed that includes publishing the individual's name in a directory on the BCSP website and the period for which the penalty will be in place. If a person is found in violation of the Unauthorized Use Policy and a penalty is imposed, the individual will not be allowed to apply for, pursue, or regain the credential or mark for a period of five (5) years, or such other period as the BCSP determines is appropriate.
    - Cease and desist agreement: If a person uses a BCSP credential or mark without authorization, the BCSP may consider an alternative resolution of allowing the individual to enter into a cease and desist agreement with the BCSP. If the BCSP determines that the said person fails to comply with the agreement, the person will be subject to all penalties pursuant to the Unauthorized Use Policy, and may also be subject to civil penalties in the event that the BCSP is required to enforce the cease and desist agreement or take other action to protect its registered marks by filing a lawsuit against the person.

20. Answer: **A**. The best course of action is to note the hazard in the report along with the conversation with the supervisor about the planned corrective actions. The BCSP Code of Ethics states:
    - Be honest, fair, and impartial; act with responsibility and integrity. Adhere to high standards of ethical conduct with balanced care for the interests of the public, employers, clients, employees, colleagues, and the profession. Avoid all conduct or practice that is likely to discredit the profession or deceive the public.

- Issue public statements only in an objective and truthful manner and only when founded upon knowledge of the facts and competence in the subject matter.
- Avoid deceptive acts that falsify or misrepresent academic or professional qualifications. Do not misrepresent or exaggerate the degree of responsibility in or for the subject matter of prior assignments. Presentations incident to the solicitation of employment shall not misrepresent pertinent facts concerning employers, employees, associates, or past accomplishments with the intent and purpose of enhancing a prospective employee's qualifications and work history.

21. Answer: **D**. The best answer of those listed is to make recommendations only if you are sure that the result will ensure a safer work area. Making recommendations about areas in which you lack skill has the potential to be incorrect.

Introduction

This section of the workbook contains 600 questions divided into six self-assessment examinations designed for self-study and facilitated professional development workshops. After each subsection of the workbook, there are fully developed explanations supporting the correct answer choice. In many cases, information about all the selections offered as possible answers will be included to assist in developing a better understanding of the subject. These sections are designed to allow the safety professional to measure progress during the extended program of self-study that is normally required to pass the certification exams.

Knowing how to take the examination will help improve your score. The examination uses multiple-choice items with only one correct answer and three incorrect answers. Remember, the goal is to get as many items correct as possible. There is no penalty for selecting an incorrect answer. However, only correct answers count toward reaching the passing score.

- Read the items carefully.
- Psychometricians design multiple-choice questions so that all the possible answer choices are plausible. Use deductive and inductive reasoning to eliminate detractor answer choices.
- Understand the problem.
  - Consider the context.
  - What is given? What is wanted?
- Use examination time wisely.
  - Conduct multiple passes, solving the "easy" problems first and saving the challenging problems for the end.
- Complete all items.
  - Blank answers are scored as wrong answers.

To replicate the exam environment of a timed exam, allocate 90 minutes to each of the 100-question practice exams. The objectives are to:

- Determine how many correct answers you can achieve, given 90 minutes for 100 questions
- Identify and close knowledge gaps
- Improve reading, comprehension, and decision-making skills

Self-Assessment Exam 1 Questions

1. **A random sample implies:**

   A. that any object, person, or thing has an equal chance of being selected.
   B. samples that are separated by layers.
   C. a patterned response (every fourth instance or situation, etc.).
   D. that a sample confined to a particular location and the location is representative.

2. **A truck displays the following placard. This indicates that the product on board is:**

   A. an acid.
   B. a caustic.
   C. flammable.
   D. More information is needed.

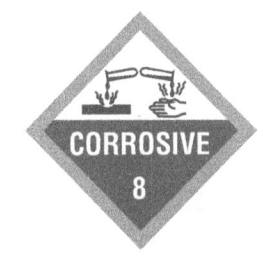

   Pictogram
   Copyright © 2019 by SPAN International Training, LLC

3. **The pressure that water exerts on a diver during descent increases by one atmosphere for every 33 feet of depth. This is explained by:**

   A. water becomes denser linearly with depth.
   B. water exerts more force/unit area with depth.
   C. the force of gravity increases with depth.
   D. the mass of the water increases with depth.

4. Of the following, which is considered an aromatic hydrocarbon?

   A. Methane
   B. Naphthalene
   C. Butane
   D. Propane

5. Activated carbon is used as a sample collecting and/or filtering medium. What properties of activated carbon make this an effective medium?

   A. Self-cleaning over a short period of time
   B. Small surface area
   C. High absorbency of the carrier gas only
   D. Extremely porous with a nonpolar surface

6. Which of the following is *not* a characteristic of a centrifugal fan?

   A. High volume with a low pressure drop
   B. Low space requirement
   C. Often used with particle-laden air
   D. Low to medium noise

7. Convert 400 ppm of carbon tetrachloride to mg/m^3, given the following information: MW = 153.8, VP = 90 mm, SG = 1.59.

   A. 1518 mg/m^3
   B. 1600 mg/m^3
   C. 2516 mg/m^3
   D. 3100 mg/m^3

   $$ppm = \frac{mg/m^3 \times 24.45}{MW}$$

8. For protecting Light Hazard Occupancy, what is the maximum travel distance allowed for a fire extinguisher?

   A. 75 feet
   B. 25 feet
   C. 35 feet
   D. 50 feet

9. In some industrial occupancies, fire doors are provided to allow compartmentalization of the facility and prevent the spread of fire and smoke. If these doors are equipped with self-closing devices they must be inspected regularly to assure operation. All of the following are valid inspection items *except*:

   A. check lubrication on guides and bearings.
   B. check to insure fusible links are painted to prevent rust.
   C. check that binders are not bent, thus obstructing the door.
   D. check to insure chains or wire ropes have not stretched.

10. The *primary* cause of fire sprinkler system failure is:

    A. improper maintenance of the sprinkler system.
    B. sprinkler heads clogged with rust and residue.
    C. lack of water pressure.
    D. closed water supply shut-off valves.

11. **Determine the WBGT index where the indoor globe temperature is 85°F and the wet bulb temperature is 74°F.**

    A. 109.2°F
    B. 84°F
    C. 77.3°F
    D. 34°C

    WBGT = 0.7WB + 0.3GT

12. **What is the requirement for sound-level meter calibration?**

    A. Monthly
    B. Quarterly
    C. Before each survey
    D. Before and after each survey

13. **Of the solid airborne contaminants listed below, which *most likely* has the largest average particulate size?**

    A. Silica dust
    B. Asbestos fibers
    C. Zinc fumes
    D. Fiberglass fibers

14. **The safest method to determine electrical current through a circuit is to use which of the following devices?**

    A. Standard volt-ohm meter
    B. Megger meter
    C. Glavometer
    D. Split core ammeter

15. **The recommended treatment for skin exposure to liquid oxygen is to:**

    A. immerse the affected body part in warm water.
    B. immerse the affected body part in hot water.
    C. immerse the affected body part in ice water.
    D. apply dry heat until feeling returns.

16. **Safety Data Sheets (SDS) must contain all of the following *except*:**

    A. protective equipment requirements.
    B. fire and explosion data.
    C. the manufacturer's part number.
    D. health hazard data.

17. **Communications regarding any form of warning, such as warning signs or hazardous materials, must be in:**

    A. English and Spanish.
    B. English.
    C. The Hazcom Standard does not specify language.
    D. all the languages spoken in a workplace.

18. **A temporary change in the threshold of hearing is called a(n):**

    A. Occupational Noise Correction Factor (ONCF).
    B. Temporary Threshold Shift (TTS).
    C. Permanent Threshold Shift (PTS).
    D. Reduction Hearing Index (RHI).

19. Selecting the appropriate PPE when handling hazardous materials is critical to worker safety. When handling containers that may be contaminated with a corrosive, such as an acid, which type of glove listed below would be appropriate?
    A. Neoprene
    B. Polyvinyl alcohol
    C. Latex
    D. Polyvinyl

20. There are three component parts of every noise issue. These components parts are:
    A. shock, alternating, and sound status.
    B. vibration source, path, and diminution system.
    C. noise source, path, and receiver.
    D. resonance level, transmission path, and attenuation source.

21. The HAZWOPER standard, OSHA 29 CFR 1910.120, specifically states that site safety and health training programs for waste sites must provide:
    A. training for all site workers and supervisors.
    B. training for spill response.
    C. training on personal protective equipment.
    D. All of the responses listed are correct.

22. Training for welders on the fire characteristics of a liquid hazardous material would include all of the following *except*:
    A. auto-ignition temperature.
    B. TLV.
    C. LEL.
    D. UFL.

23. When posting a Danger tag, under 29 CFR 1910.145, all of the following are correct *except*:
    A. the signal word shall be readable at a minimum distance of 7 feet or greater.
    B. the meaning shall be offered in wording, pictographs, or both.
    C. the tags shall be attached as close as practicable to the hazard.
    D. employees must be informed of the meaning of the signs.

24. What is the appropriate sequence for hazard control?
    (1) Use a guard for the hazard; (2) use engineering controls; (3) train workers
    A. 3,2,1
    B. 1,2,3
    C. 2,1,3
    D. 1,3,2

25. What is the *best* course of action for an employee to take when a supervisor orders a shutdown on a construction project due to safety violations that are nonexistent?
    A. Shut down the project as ordered.
    B. Advise the next level of management.
    C. Resign the position.
    D. Write a letter of protest to the CEO.

26. During an industrial inspection, an enclosed parts-cleaning operation using a spray gun is observed. The operation results in one-half pint of methylene chloride (MW = 84.94 and SG = 1.336) being released each hour. You measure concentrations of 60 ppm methylene chloride, which is above the TLV of 50 ppm. How much dilution ventilation is required to lower the concentration to half the TLV? You may assume a K factor of 4.

   A. 50,710 cfm
   B. 25,350 cfm
   C. 8452 cfm
   D. 4225 cfm

27. The *best* field instrument to measure air velocity in the opening of a paint spray booth is a:

   A. rotating vane anemometer.
   B. thermal anemometer.
   C. smoke tube.
   D. pitot tube.

28. Monitoring of industrial effluents generally includes which of the following?

   A. chlorine, pH, metals, and temperature.
   B. BOD, TSS, pH, and LANL.
   C. enzymes, pH, and TSS.
   D. BOD, TSS, metals, and temperature.

29. In ventilation hood design, the function of the slot in a slot hood is to:

   A. increase capture velocity.
   B. provide greater static pressure per horsepower.
   C. obtain proper air distribution.
   D. decrease capture velocity.

30. A volatile liquid at any given temperature under any equilibrium condition will exert a pressure that is defined as:

   A. vapor pressure.
   B. partial pressure.
   C. universal fluid pressure (UFP).
   D. the pressure of equilibrium.

31. Regarding friction, the *most correct* statement would be:

   A. There is no difference between static friction force and kinetic friction force.
   B. Surface area is used in the determination of frictional forces.
   C. Kinetic friction does not depend on speed.
   D. Normal force is used in the calculation of static friction.

32. How many states have OSHA-approved State Plans?

   A. 15
   B. 30
   C. 25
   D. 50

33. Characteristics of carbon disulfide, CS_2, would include all of the following *except*:

   A. it is nonflammable.
   B. it is a systemic poison.
   C. it is absorbed through the skin.
   D. it is used as a solvent, disinfectant, and insecticide.

34. In some combustible gas indicators (CGIs), an electrical circuit consisting of a series of resistors is used to measure the mixture of the combustible gas to air. The resistors are balanced and one leg of the circuit, called a hot wire, is exposed to the suspect atmosphere. If a combustible mixture is present, a catalytic combustion increases the wire resistance and causes an imbalance. The circuit is called a:

   A. combustible resistor circuit (CRC).
   B. Wheatstone bridge.
   C. combustible balancing circuit.
   D. hot wire detector (HWT).

35. To qualify as a Star site in general industry for the OSHA Voluntary Protection Program (VPP), a company's Days Away Restricted or Transferred (DART) rate must be:

   A. at least 25% below the national average.
   B. at or below the national average for at least 1 of 3 years.
   C. at least 50% below the national average for 3 years.
   D. at or above the national average for 1 out of the previous 3 years.

36. A means of egress, as defined by the National Fire Protection Association (NFPA), is defined as a continuous path of travel from within a building to the outside. Which of the following choices is *not* included as part of this definition?

   A. The exit
   B. The exit mechanism
   C. The exit access
   D. The exit discharge

37. Which of the following classes of organic chemicals can potentially form highly explosive organic peroxides?

   A. Anhydrides
   B. Alkyds
   C. Ethers
   D. Aniline

38. Exit doors, according to the Life Safety Code, must conform to all of the following *except*:

   A. doors should be properly marked.
   B. doors should swing in the direction of exit.
   C. doors can be held open if equipped by fusible links.
   D. doors cannot be locked.

39. The NFPA has established three main classes of occupancy in the Sprinkler Standard. According to this standard, which of the following correctly identifies these three classes?

   A. Low Hazard, Ordinary Hazard, and High Hazard
   B. Low Hazard, Ordinary Hazard, and Extra Hazard
   C. Low Hazard, High Hazard, and Ultra High Hazard
   D. Class A, Class B, and Class C

40. Fatalities and substantial property losses associated with airborne particles and explosions are likely caused by:

   A. combustible dust/powders.
   B. fertilizer mixing with oil.
   C. ionizing radiation.
   D. spontaneous combustion.

41. Dilution ventilation is *primarily* used to control:
    A. a contaminant at its source.
    B. fumes from lead fusing.
    C. low-toxicity vapors.
    D. asbestos fibers during remediation projects.

42. Firefighting standpipe systems that are to be used only by trained fire departments are called:
    A. Class I.
    B. Class II.
    C. Class III.
    D. Combined.

43. *Intrinsically* safe equipment may be used in a flammable or explosive atmosphere because it is capable of:
    A. containing internal explosions.
    B. not producing any ignition sources.
    C. operating below the auto-ignition temperature.
    D. shutting down the equipment serviced.

44. NFPA 20 details performance criteria for the installation of firefighting booster pumps. Any new industrial fire pump with the U.L. or FM label will comply with this standard. Which of the following statements is *most* correct concerning flow rates and pressures?
    A. The pump must develop 150% of rated pressure at churn without cavitating.
    B. The pump must deliver 150% flow at 65% pressure.
    C. The pump must deliver 150% pressure at 100% flow.
    D. The pump must deliver 150% pressure at the rated flow.

45. A flammable liquid with a flash point at or above 200°F is classified by the NFPA as a:
    A. Class I liquid.
    B. Class III liquid.
    C. Class IB liquid.
    D. Class IIIB liquid.

46. A major purpose of hoods on grinders and cutting wheels is to:
    A. shield the operator if the wheel should disintegrate.
    B. cover at least 75% of the wheel.
    C. prevent the operator falling into the wheel.
    D. None of these responses is correct.

47. The acronym AQL represents:
    A. atypical quotient level.
    B. average quality level.
    C. acceptable quality level.
    D. associate quantity level.

48. In comparing morbidity and mortality data for epidemiological studies, which of the following would be the *best* expression?
    A. The variable of age is adjusted with a SMR (Standard Mortality Ratio).
    B. Cross-sectional studies are allowed to use World Death Rates (WDR) for comparison.
    C. Data is compared to World Mortality Data Bank figures.
    D. Morbidity data is sometimes linked with etiological data.

49. Employees experienced several slips and falls in a newly constructed area of a warehouse. This has been occurring for several weeks and the problem has finally been corrected by installing skid-resistant material on the walkways. When and/or by whom should this problem have been identified?

   A. After the first incident
   B. By a company insurance "safety expert"
   C. By maintenance personnel
   D. During review of the building design plans

50. The acronym LTPD is used in sampling strategies and stands for:

   A. Lot Tested Permissible Defect.
   B. Lot Total Percent Defective.
   C. Labile Total Percent Defective.
   D. Labrification Total Permissible Defect.

51. An OSHA-mandated hearing conservation program requires all the following *except*:

   A. employees must be provided with appropriate hearing protection.
   B. employees must be trained and retrained annually.
   C. employees must receive an audiogram within 6 months.
   D. employees must be given time off to allow the auditory ossicles to recover.

52. If variations in noise levels are occurring at a rate more often than once per second, the noise is considered _____ under OSHA's noise standard.

   A. impulse.
   B. continuous.
   C. impact.
   D. impulse and impact.

53. Are exposures above the Threshold Limit Value (TLV) permitted?

   A. Yes, if not exceeded by more than 12%
   B. Yes, if not exceeded by more than 18%
   C. Only if below the TLV-C
   D. Exposures above the TLV are never allowed.

54. The *most* effective design for noise control barriers is:

   A. baffles.
   B. airtight enclosures.
   C. absorbent materials.
   D. partial enclosures.

55. When designing a ventilation system, which work operation would require the system to have the greatest capture velocity?

   A. Grinding
   B. Solvent evaporation from open surface tanks
   C. Spray booths
   D. Hot work

56. The *most* serious heat related illness is:

   A. heat cramps.
   B. heat exhaustion.
   C. heatstroke.
   D. heat syncope.

57. A disease that could cause numbness of the fingers could be associated with:

A. silicosis.
B. dermatitis.
C. Asperger syndrome.
D. Raynaud's syndrome.

58. The *most* common cause of melanomas on the skin is:

A. chemical exposure.
B. exposure to sunlight.
C. arc welding.
D. arc flash.

59. All of the following terms are associated with pulmonary function testing during a normal industrial physical *except*:

A. Maximal Voluntary Ventilation (MVV).
B. Forced Vital Capacity (FVC).
C. One-second Forced Vital Capacity (FEV1).
D. Tidal Volume (TV).

60. The greatest exposure risk from current X-ray equipment is from:

A. alpha.
B. high voltage.
C. beta.
D. RF.

61. Another term for specific gravity in modern scientific usage is:

A. relative density.
B. volumetric mass density.
C. Baft density.
D. None of the responses listed are used.

62. Loss of consciousness can occur if a person is exposed to levels of CO_2 that are equal to or exceed:

A. 4%.
B. 6%.
C. 9%.
D. 1100 ppm.

63. The *most* commonly used safety precaution to eliminate or lessen the accumulation of static electricity when transferring flammable liquids is:

A. bonding and grounding.
B. electron flow detection systems.
C. fill pipe extensions.
D. increasing the conductivity of the liquid.

64. Which of the following statements is *most* correct concerning the affliction of frostbite?

A. It causes uncontrolled shivering.
B. Frostbitten skin is soft, puffy, and darker than normal.
C. A "pins and needles" sensation is followed by numbness.
D. Typical characteristics are irregular heartbeat and respiration.

65. What is the maximum burst pressure required for LPG hoses?

A. 1250 psig
B. 750 psig
C. 500 psig
D. 250 psig

66. In general industry, which of the following would *not* be considered a major type of machine guards?

   A. Fixed
   B. Swing-away
   C. Interlocked
   D. Automatic

67. The minimum riser height and maximum tread run for fixed industrial steps as recommended by OSHA and ANSI are:

   A. 6½ in and 11 in.
   B. 7 in and 11 in.
   C. 8 in and 12 in.
   D. 5 in and 14 in.

68. A health hazard associated with arc welding of stainless steel is the production of fumes containing:

   A. nickel and chromium.
   B. carbon and nickel.
   C. copper, nickel, and acid gases.
   D. fluorides, nickel, and chromium.

69. Pressure testing is generally considered to be a/an _____ test.

   A. destructive
   B. baetyl
   C. elemental
   D. rachitogenic

70. Static electricity is described as high current flow and with very low voltages. This is:

   A. false.
   B. false, as both voltage and current flows are high.
   C. true.
   D. true, since static electricity involves no current flow.

71. A typical electrical distribution transformer used inside a plant, when compared to the primary side, has voltages that are:

   A. lower.
   B. higher.
   C. the same.
   D. variable.

72. The *most* economical way to protect an elevated water tank from the damaging effects of corrosion is to:

   A. install a glass-lined system.
   B. line the tank with a fiberglass liner.
   C. ground and bond all components.
   D. install cathodic protection.

73. When wire rope is used for lifting or hoisting, inspection would include all the following *except*:

   A. corrosion.
   B. lubrication.
   C. nondestructive testing.
   D. kinking.

74. Which organization is responsible for publishing *The Fire Protection Handbook?*

    A. OSHA
    B. NIOSH
    C. NFPA
    D. NIH

75. The 3 in the diagram indicates:

    A. health.
    B. fire.
    C. reactivity.
    D. storage.

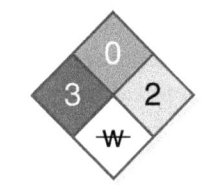

Figure 38 Hazard Diamond
© Standard Studio/Shutterstock.

76. A combustible solvent that is sprayed into a fine mist during an industrial parts-cleaning operation attains a:

    A. greater toxicity.
    B. reduced UEL.
    C. lowered flash point.
    D. LEL remains unchanged.

77. The NFPA standard under which a Private Fire Brigade most aptly falls would be:

    A. NFPA 1500.
    B. NFPA 600.
    C. NFPA 101.
    D. NFPA 10.

78. All of the following are correct regarding reverse jet baghouse fabric filtration devices *except*:

    A. baghouses exhibit very low efficiency.
    B. baghouses are expensive and require a large area.
    C. baghouses require the control of moisture in the dust.
    D. baghouses require costly preventive maintenance.

79. All the following require an equipment-grounding conductor *except*:

    A. a double reverse delta electrical system.
    B. a double-insulated hand tool.
    C. a circuit that is protected with circuit breakers.
    D. a system with a wye connected transformer.

80. The standard material for chain slings utilized in lifting and moving material is:

    A. proof coil chain.
    B. steel and bronze alloy chain.
    C. alloy steel chain.
    D. annealed, high-strength, pure steel chain.

81. Under the Commercial Motor Vehicle Safety Act of 1986, a commercial driver's license, or CDL, is required when:

    A. transporting passengers.
    B. towing a trailer with a gross weight of 6000 lbs.
    C. operating a vehicle with a total length of 35 feet.
    D. operating a single vehicle with a GVW of 26,000 lbs.

82. Who has the responsibility to determine if a material is hazardous, as outlined under OSHA 29 CFR1910.1200?

    A. The manufacturer or importer of the chemical is responsible.
    B. All employees have this responsibility.
    C. Only unionized employees have this responsibility.
    D. The employer is legally obligated to make this determination.

83. The statement, "Lock-out/tag-out programs only apply to electrical or high-pressure utility systems in general industry" is:

    A. true.
    B. false.
    C. false; it only applies to electrical systems.
    D. true, unless OSHA-approved audits are performed annually.

84. License renewal for powered industrial truck operators occurs once every _____ or if an operator has been observed operating the PIT in an unsafe manner.

    A. year
    B. 6 months
    C. 2 years
    D. 3 years

85. The definition of ergonomics is very broad and involves many disciplines. Which of the following simple phrases provides the *best* description of ergonomics?

    A. The measurement of the human body in the work environment (form versus function)
    B. Modification of the work task to obtain optimum production
    C. Designing the job to fit the person
    D. Fitting the person to the job

86. When designing large parking lots that feed busy arterial roadways, the technique that provides the largest margin of safety is:

    A. ensuring that one entrance/exit is at least 40 feet wide.
    B. arranging for a crosswalk at the intersection for workers.
    C. having separate entrances/exits that favor right-hand turns.
    D. providing several two-way exits to facilitate rapid movement.

87. The *best* earth ground for an electrical installation as required by the National Electrical Code is:

    A. a metal underground water pipe and connection to a driven electrode.
    B. a single connection to the structural building support steel on a slab-mounted building.
    C. a made electrode consisting of a single 7-foot copper electrode installed at the transformer.
    D. connection to another service on the same property that has an Ufer grounding system installed.

The following three questions refer to the following information:

Table 23 Above Ground Fuel Tank Requirements

Tank Capacity in Gallons	Minimum Distance in Feet from Property Line	Minimum Distance in Feet from Nearest Public Way or Nearest Important Building
0 to 275	10	5
751 to 12,000	15	5
12,001 to 30,000	20	5
30,001 to 50,000	30	10

(Continues)

Table 23 Above Ground Fuel Tank Requirements *(Continued)*

Tank Capacity in Gallons	Minimum Distance in Feet from Property Line	Minimum Distance in Feet from Nearest Public Way or Nearest Important Building
50,001 to 100,000	50	15
100,001 to 500,000	80	25
500,001 to 1,000,000	100	30

88. Determine the distance a 60,000-gallon aboveground fuel tank can be located from a plant property line if filled to capacity (Table 23).

    A. 20 feet
    B. 30 feet
    C. 50 feet
    D. 80 feet

89. A 100,000-gallon fuel tank can be placed no less than what distance from an inhabited building within the plant boundaries (Table 23)?

    A. 5 feet
    B. 10 feet
    C. 15 feet
    D. 20 feet

90. Is a fuel tank located more than 50 feet from a property line required to be equipped with a fire protection system (Table 23)?

    A. Yes, it is a requirement.
    B. No, it is not a requirement.
    C. It is required only if taller than 50 feet.
    D. This tank must be located exactly 50 feet from the property line.

91. The purpose of electrical circuit breakers is to:

    A. prevent excessive fault current and to be used as a method of disconnect when labeled SWD.
    B. serve as a safety system that will disconnect circuits from a source of electrical energy that proves to be hazardous.
    C. prevent overheating of conductors or insulation.
    D. immediately interrupt electrical current flow whenever the current circuit breaker rating is exceeded.

92. Determine the total area of a flat piece of metal that has been cut into the shape illustrated below.

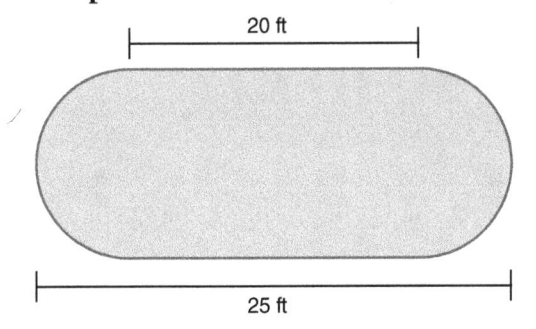

Figure 39 Flat Metal Shape

    A. 100 ft²
    B. 60 ft²
    C. 19.6 ft²
    D. 119.6 ft²

93. A metal bar weighs 125 pounds on land. In water it weighs 75 pounds submerged. What is the specific gravity of the bar?

   A. 0.025
   B. 0.25
   C. 2.50
   D. 22.5

94. Aside from ensuring that the site of a new process facility meets all building codes, SH&E professionals can also help determine the:

   A. location of future facilities.
   B. building design size and type.
   C. availability of local labor.
   D. hazard to the local community.

95. The Hazen-Williams empirical formula for determining friction loss in hydraulic calculations that involve fire sprinkler systems is required by NFPA 13. Which of the following factors has the greatest impact in determining friction loss when using this formula?

   A. Coefficient of pipe roughness
   B. Quantity of fluid flowing
   C. Internal pipe diameter
   D. Hydraulic gradient

96. Special carts were designed to accommodate both male and female employees. The coefficient of friction for both carts is 0.12. Assume a push of 100 feet once per 8-hour shift and the handles are 40 inches in height from the floor and weigh 105 pounds. Determine the weight that could be carried by 90% of the male workforce.

Sustained Forces Involved in Pushing Tasks in Kg

Height in inches	% of workforce	One 100-ft push every (Minutes)				8 hrs	Height in inches	% of workforce	One 100-ft push every (Minutes)				8 hrs
		1	2	5	30				1	2	5	30	
40	90	9	10	12	13	14	36	90	9	9	11	12	13
	75	11	12	14	15	17		75	10	10	13	14	15
	50	13	15	17	19	20		50	11	12	14	16	17

   A. 258 lbs
   B. 153 lbs
   C. 173 lbs
   D. 133 lbs

$F = \mu N$

97. **Determine the height of the antenna tower at radio station SPAN ham radio station if a shadow strikes the ground 10 feet from the transmitter wall. Note: The building wall is 12 feet tall.**

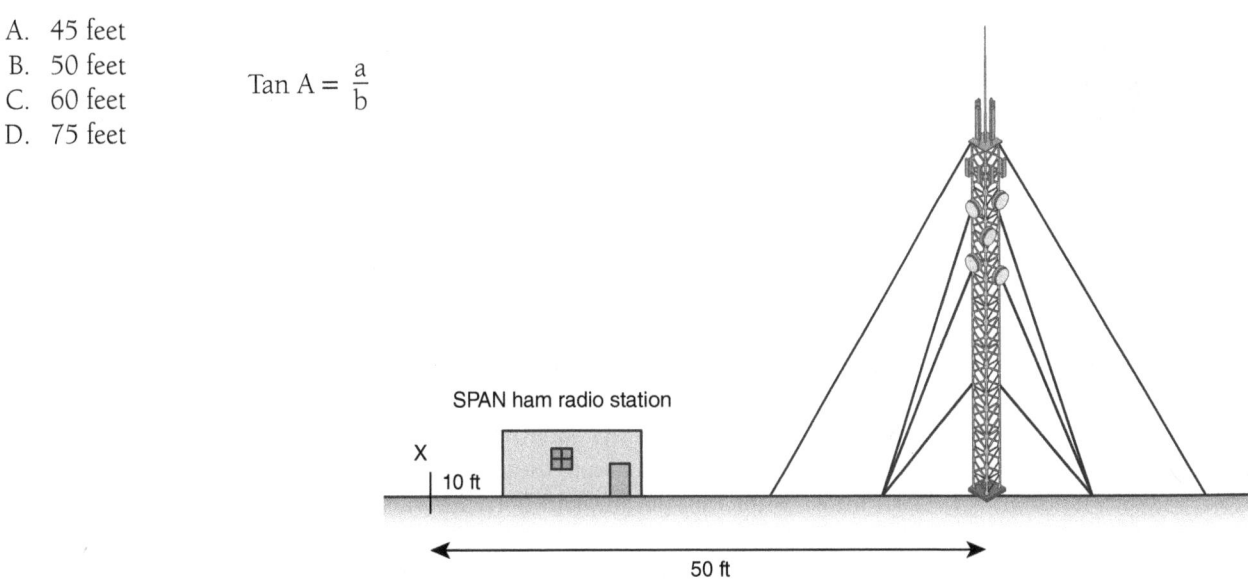

    A. 45 feet
    B. 50 feet
    C. 60 feet
    D. 75 feet

    $$\text{Tan } A = \frac{a}{b}$$

    Figure 40 SPAN Ham Radio Station

98. **Workplace injuries and deaths are now behind violence in frequency during recent years. Which of the following is *not* a legal basis for providing workplace security?**

    A. Company policy
    B. City ordinance
    C. State statute
    D. Federal code

99. **Which of the following is *not* a characteristic of integrated performance assurance, safety and health, and quality assurance programs?**

    A. Require common intangible asset control
    B. Serve common underlying objectives
    C. Share common success and failure measures
    D. Use common approach to achieve objectives

100. **Drug testing of a company's over-the-road transport drivers is required by the DOT at what rate?**

    A. 10% annually
    B. 25% annually
    C. 50% annually
    D. 100% annually

Self-Assessment Exam 1 Answers

1. Answer: **A**. The random sample, as the name implies, allows everyone in a universe to have an equal chance of selection. The term *universe* in statistical work implies ALL of the data. Stratified samples are separated by layers. Systematic samples are patterned response (every third car accident, person etc.). Cluster samples are confined to a particular location and assume the location will be representative.
2. Answer: **D**. This is the corrosive placard. A pH of less than 7.0 indicates the contents are acidic. A pH of more than 7.0 would indicate an alkaline cargo. A pH of 7 is considered neutral. More information is needed, as both acids and bases are corrosive.
3. Answer: **B**. Pressure is defined as a force per unit area. As the weight of water increases with the increasing depth, the pressure or force per unit area also increases.
4. Answer: **B**. Naphthalene is an organic compound with the formula $C_{10}H_8$. It is the simplest polycyclic aromatic hydrocarbon, and is a white crystalline solid with a characteristic odor that is detectable at concentrations as low as 0.08 ppm by mass. As an aromatic hydrocarbon, naphthalene's structure consists of a fused pair of benzene rings. It is best known as the main ingredient of traditional mothballs.

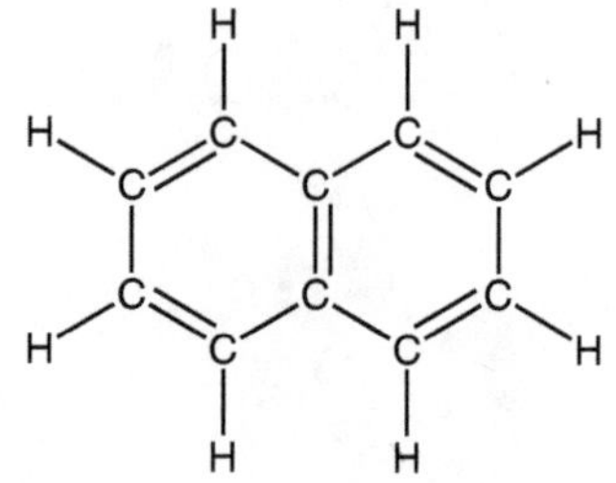

Figure 41 Naphthalene $C_{10}H_8$

5. Answer: **D**. Activated carbon is extremely porous and has a nonpolar surface. It adsorbs molecules to its surface readily. When bathed in a nonpolar solvent such as carbon disulfide, the adsorbed molecules are easily removed and dissolved into the solvent.
6. Answer: **A**. High volume and low pressure drop are characteristics of axial flow fans, which are most commonly used for general ventilation or dilution ventilation work. Centrifugal fans are used against low to moderate static pressures such as are encountered in heating and air conditioning work. These fans have low space requirements and are quiet. The paddle wheel or long shaving wheel is used with a medium tip speed for buffing exhaust, woodworking exhaust, or when a heavy dust must pass through the fan.
7. Answer: **C**.

$$ppm = \frac{mg/m^3 \times 24.45}{MW}$$

$$mg/m^3 = \frac{ppm \times MW}{24.45}$$

$$mg/m^3 = \frac{400 \times 153.8}{24.45}$$

$$mg/m^3 = 2516$$

8. Answer: **A**. NFPA 13 5.2: Light hazard occupancies shall be defined as occupancies or portions of other occupancies where the quantity and/or combustibility of contents is low and fires with relatively low rates of heat release are expected. Light hazard occupancies include occupancies having uses and conditions similar to the following:
    a) Animal shelters
    b) Churches
    c) Clubs
    d) Eaves and overhangs, if of combustible construction with no combustible material beneath
    e) Educational
    f) Hospitals, including animal hospitals and veterinary facilities
    g) Institutional
    h) Kennels

i) Libraries, except large stack rooms
j) Museums
k) Nursing or convalescent homes
l) Offices, including data processing
m) Residential
n) Restaurant seating areas
o) Theaters and auditoriums, excluding stages and prosceniums
p) Unused attics

The maximum travel distance to a fire extinguisher regardless of the rating for Class A hazards is 75 feet.

9. Answer: **B**. Fusible lead links should not be painted because the paint affects the temperature at which the links will melt.
10. Answer: **D**. Sprinkler systems are very reliable and function flawlessly about 95% of the time. When failures do occur, about 35% of the time the main cause of failure is closed water-supply valves. The main cause of leaking sprinkler heads is overheating caused by placement of sprinkler heads too close to heat-generating processes or utilities.
11. Answer: **C**. Apply indoor formula and solve.

    WBGT = 0.7 WB + 0.3 GT

    WBGT = (0.7 × 74) + (0.3 × 85)

    WBGT = 51.8 + 25.5

    WBGT = 77.3°F

12. Answer: **D**. In accordance with most manufacturers' recommendations and in keeping with good practice, calibrations should be done at the start of measurements and after completion to insure that all readings are accurate.
13. Answer: **A**. Silica dust has the largest particulate size and zinc fumes have the smallest size of the materials listed.
14. Answer: **D**. A split core ammeter has fingers that enclose the conductor under test without opening or tapping the circuit. This is much safer than other methods.
15. Answer: **A**. For skin contact with liquid oxygen, remove any clothing that may restrict circulation to the frozen area. Do not rub frozen parts, as tissue damage may result. As soon as practical, place the affected area in a warm water bath with a temperature not exceeding 105°F (40°C). Never use dry heat. Call a physician as soon as possible. Frozen tissue is painless and appears waxy with a possible yellow color. It will become swollen, painful, and prone to infection when thawed. If the frozen part of the body has been thawed, cover the area with a dry sterile dressing with a large bulky protective covering, pending medical care.
16. Answer: **C**. The Hazard Communication Standard (HCS) requires chemical manufacturers, distributors, or importers to provide Safety Data Sheets (SDSs) (formerly known as Material Safety Data Sheets or MSDSs) to communicate the hazards of hazardous chemical products. As of June 1, 2015, the HCS will require new SDSs to be in a uniform format, and include the section numbers, the headings, and associated information under the headings below:

    Section 1, Identification includes product identifier; manufacturer or distributor name, address, phone number; emergency phone number; recommended use; restrictions on use.

    Section 2, Hazard(s) identification includes all hazards regarding the chemical; required label elements.

    Section 3, Composition/information on ingredients includes information on chemical ingredients; trade secret claims.

    Section 4, First-aid measures includes important symptoms/effects, acute, delayed; required treatment.

    Section 5, Firefighting measures list suitable extinguishing techniques, equipment; chemical hazards from fire.

    Section 6, Accidental release measures lists emergency procedures; protective equipment; proper methods of containment and cleanup.

Section 7, Handling and storage lists precautions for safe handling and storage, including incompatibilities.

Section 8, Exposure controls/personal protection lists OSHA's Permissible Exposure Limits (PELs); Threshold Limit Values (TLVs); appropriate engineering controls; personal protective equipment (PPE).

Section 9, Physical and chemical properties lists the chemical's characteristics.

Section 10, Stability and reactivity lists chemical stability and possibility of hazardous reactions.

Section 11, Toxicological information includes routes of exposure; related symptoms, acute and chronic effects; numerical measures of toxicity.

Section 12, Ecological information

Section 13, Disposal considerations

Section 14, Transport information

Section 15, Regulatory information

Section 16, Other information, includes the date of preparation or last revision.

Hazard Communication Safety Data Sheets, U.S. Department of Labor. Retrived from https://www.osha.gov/Publications/HazComm_QuickCard_SafetyData.html

The specific part number of the manufacturer is not required.

17. Answer: **B**.

OSHA 29 CFR 1910.1200 requires that all information be presented in English (other languages can be used in addition to English).

DANGER is a signal word intended for immediate hazards that will result in severe personal injury or death.

WARNING is a signal word intended for immediate hazards that could result in severe personal injury or death.

CAUTION is a signal word intended for minor personal injury or property damage.

18. Answer: **B**. A temporary depression of the hearing is called a *temporary threshold shift*, or TTS. When people are exposed to a high level of noise, they almost always exhibit a transient attenuation in their ability to hear. This temporary threshold shift usually vanishes a few hours after the exposure. One theory has held that a *permanent threshold shift* (PTS) is simply the result of a large number of TTSs, each superimposed on the last. According to that theory, avoidance of any demonstrable TTS should result in no PTS.

19. Answer: **A**. Glove materials such as butyl rubber or neoprene are generally best for handling acids like hydrochloric acid. Latex allergies are common and need to be considered when selecting gloves for employees.

20. Answer: **C**. Every noise problem is comprised of three components:
    - Source of sound energy
    - Path of sound energy
    - Receiver of sound energy

21. Answer: **D**. OSHA 1910.120 requires an extensive safety and health plan that includes a safety and health training plan. Extensive requirements are outlined in the HAZWOPER standard on the various levels and complexity of training. Training for responding specialists, such as Hazmat teams, is required but generally the responsibility for this training would fall upon the specialists' employer, rather than the owner of the cleanup contract.

22. Answer: **B**. The Threshold Limit Value (TLV) as defined by the American Conference of Governmental Industrial Hygienists (ACGIH) refers to "airborne concentrations of substances and represent conditions under which it is believed that nearly all workers may be repeatedly exposed day after day without adverse health effects." Certainly information about TLVs should be included in welder training; however, this question asked about the fire characteristics of hazardous chemicals. TLVs mainly concern health effects and are not indicators of flammability TLV® Chemical Substances Introduction, American

Conference of Governmental Industrial Hygienists (ACGIH). Retrived from https://www.acgih.org/tlv-bei-guidelines/tlv-chemical-substances-introduction. Selection A, auto-ignition temperature, is defined by the National Fire Protection Association (NFPA) as "the lowest temperature at which a flammable gas or vapor-air mixture will ignite from its own heat source or a contacted heat source without the necessity of spark or flame." Modified from National Fire Protection Association (NFPA), Glossary of terms. Selection C, the Lower Explosive Limit, is defined as "the minimum concentration of combustible gas or vapor in air below which propagation of flame does not occur on contact with a source of ignition." Selection D, Upper Flammable Limit, is defined as "the maximum concentration of vapor or gas in air above which propagation of flame does not occur." EPA (1995).

23. Answer: **A**. The required difference for readability is "5" feet. The use of both written text and pictographs will ensure understanding in a culturally diverse workforce. Additionally, signs should be in positive, concise, easy-to-read terms, should warn against potential hazards, and should not vary in design at the same location and in the identical situation.

24. Answer: **C**. Engineering is always the first and most successful method of dealing with a problem. The second choice is to guard the hazard, and the last method is to educate the human element. Some safety texts break down "guarding the hazard" into (1) incorporation of safety devices and (2) providing warning devices. Guarding the hazard is also classified as administrative controls. "Educating personnel" may also be subdivided into (1) developing and implementing operating procedures and employee training programs and (2) using personal protective equipment. Lock-out/tag-out (LOTO) is considered an administrative control. Another example of an administrative control is to require employees to rest for 10 minutes after working for a set period of time in a high-temperature environment. Remember that although engineering is the first choice to fix a problem, interim measures such as PPE may have to be used until the engineering fix is completed.

25. Answer: **A**. The selection of an answer is very difficult because there is individual preference when approaching these problems. However, the preferred answer in this case would be to elevate the problem up the management chain until an executive that supports your decision is found. However, your supervisor must be informed of this concern and plan to notify higher management.

26. Answer: **C**.

$$Q = \frac{403 \times 10^6 \times SG \times ER \times K}{MW \times C}$$

$$Q = \frac{403 \times 1{,}000{,}000 \times 1.336 \times 0.0083 \times 4}{84.94 \times 25}$$

$$Q = \frac{17{,}875{,}146}{2124}$$

$$Q = 8416 \text{ cfm}$$

Note: Remember, the solvent is being applied at an hourly rate, thus the need for the "60" minutes in the equation. We also reduced the TLV to 25 instead of 50. The "K" factors are **safety factors** and range from 3 to 10 and depend on:
a) The toxicity of the material (lower TLV = higher "K")
b) The evolution rate of the contaminant (usually nonuniform)
c) The effectiveness of ventilation (location in airflows)
It is anticipated that questions on the professional exams requiring this type of calculation will provide "K" factors or safety factors; you simply apply the formula. Don't forget the "length of release," 60 minutes in this problem.

27. Answer: **B**. The *thermal anemometer* is the instrument of choice where the exhaust opening is large and the air velocities are low, as in spray booths or chemical hoods. The thermal anemometer is a fairly recent addition to air measuring instrument inventory. The device has a heated probe (usually about 150°F) and senses velocity by the amount of heat removed from the probe. Its reading is direct, very accurate, and can be used in low-airflow conditions. It is also mildly resistant to particulate matter in the airstream. The

rotating vane anemometer is useful for measuring the airflow through large supply and exhaust openings where the air velocities are relatively high.

28. Answer: **D**. Most effluents are monitored for biochemical oxygen demand, total suspended solids, the amount of metal content, and temperature. Effluents must comply with the EPA's National Pollution Discharge and Elimination System (NPDES) permit.

29. Answer: **C**. Slot hoods are commonly used to provide uniform exhaust airflow, such as over the surface of a tank. Points to remember:
    - The function of the slot is solely to obtain proper air distribution.
    - Slot velocity does not contribute to capture velocity.
    - The calculation of capture velocity involves exhaust volume and slot length, not slot velocity.

30. Answer: **A**. Vapor pressure is defined as the pressure exerted by the vapor that is in equilibrium with the liquid at a given temperature. It is the ability of the liquid to evaporate or give off vapors.

31. Answer: **C**. Consider any given object being pushed by a force seen. At first, the object does not move; it stays in equilibrium. It is being opposed by the force of static friction. Static friction is the result of the contact of the object and the surface on which it rests. As you continue to apply additional force, the block begins to move; the block is no longer in equilibrium. When just enough force is applied to break out of the static condition, the limit of static friction has been reached. Once the object is in motion, it can be kept in motion by a force smaller than that which was required to initiate movement; this is known as kinetic friction.
    - Static friction is the force parallel to the surface of contact when there is no motion between the two surfaces.
    - Kinetic friction is the force parallel to the surface of contact when there is motion between the two surfaces.

    Both static and kinetic friction are dependent on the surface of the two materials (i.e., a rough surface would have a higher coefficient of friction than would smooth steel, the surface would be slicker when wet than when dry, etc.). Neither static nor kinetic friction is affected by the amount of surface area in contact. Under normal conditions, speed does not affect kinetic friction.

    The maximum frictional force on an object resting on another surface is proportional to all forces perpendicular to the surface in contact and the coefficient of static friction.

32. Answer: **C**. *The Occupational Safety and Health (OSH) Act* covers most private-sector employers and their workers, in addition to some public-sector employers and their workers in the 50 states and certain territories and jurisdictions under federal authority. Those jurisdictions include the District of Columbia, Puerto Rico, the Virgin Islands, American Samoa, Guam, Northern Mariana Islands, Wake Island, Johnston Island, and the Outer Continental Shelf Lands as defined in the *Outer Continental Shelf Lands Act*. OSHA covers most private-sector employers and workers in all 50 states, the District of Columbia, and the other United States (US) jurisdictions either directly through federal OSHA or through an OSHA-approved State Plan. State Plans are OSHA-approved job safety and health programs operated by individual states instead of federal OSHA. Section 18 of the OSH Act encourages states to develop and operate their own job safety and health programs and precludes state enforcement of OSHA standards unless the state has an OSHA-approved program.

    OSHA approves and monitors all State Plans and provides as much as 50% of the funding for each program. State-run safety and health programs must be at least as effective (ALAE) as the federal OSHA program. Twenty-five states, plus two territories, Puerto Rico and the Virgin Islands, have OSHA-approved State Plans. Twenty-two State Plans (21 states and one U.S. territory) cover both private and public sector workplaces. The remaining five State Plans (four states and one U.S. territory) cover state and local government workers only.

33. Answer: **A**. Carbon disulfide is an extremely flammable liquid. It has a flash point of 22°F and an auto-ignition temperature of 212°F. The flammable range of CS_2 extends from 1% to 44% by volume.

    It is a major fire and explosion hazard that has been ignited by hot lightbulbs, steam lines, static electricity, etc. It is widely used as a solvent for waxes, resins, and rubbers. It is used for desorbing contaminants from sorbent tubes and in the manufacture of rayon, cellophane, and carbon tetrachloride. The health hazards are widely known and as of this writing the NIOSH exposure limit is 1 ppm with STEL of 10 ppm and an IDLH of 500 ppm.

34. Answer: **B**. The question describes a Wheatstone bridge electrical circuit.
35. Answer: **B**. To qualify for VPP Star, both your 3-year TCIR and your 3-year DART rate must be below at least 1 of the 3 most recent years of specific industry national averages for nonfatal injuries and illnesses at the most precise level published by the U.S. Department of Labor's Bureau of Labor Statistics (BLS). The Total Case Incidence Rate (TCIR) is a number that represents the total nonfatal recordable injuries and illnesses per 100 full-time employees. This rate is calculated for an individual worksite, all worksites within an applicant/participant's Designated Geographic Area (DGA), or all worksites of an employer for a specified period of time (usually 1 or 3 years). Days Away, Restricted, and/or Transfer Case Incidence Rate (DART rate) is the rate of all injuries and illnesses resulting in days away from work, restricted work activity, and/or job transfer. This rate is calculated for an individual worksite, all worksites within an applicant/participant's Designated Geographic Area (DGA), or all worksites of an employer for a specified period of time (usually 1 or 3 years).
36. Answer: **B**. The Life Safety Code includes the term *exit* in an overall definition of means of egress. A means of egress is a continuous path of travel from any point in a building or structure to the open air outside at ground level and consists of three separate and distinct parts: (1) the way of exit access; (2) the exit; and (3) the means of discharge from the exit.
37. Answer: **C**. During storage, practically all ethers form ether peroxides. When the ether peroxide mixture is heated or concentrated, the peroxide may detonate. Isopropyl ether is believed to be considerably more susceptible to peroxide formation than other ethers. These peroxides can sometimes be seen as crystal growth in the ether solution.
38. Answer: **C**. The Life Safety Code requires that exit doors be kept normally closed to serve their function of stopping the spread of smoke, or if open, must be closed immediately in case of fire. Ordinary fusible link–operated devices to close doors in case of fire are designed to close in time to stop the spread of fire, but do not operate in time to stop the spread of smoke. At relatively low temperatures, the smoke accumulation could continue with fatal effects.
39. Answer: **B**. The NFPA has three main classifications for occupancy (**Table 24**).

Table 24 NFPA classifications for occupancy

Class	Comments	Examples
Low Hazard	Fires with low rates of heat are expected	Apartments, churches, single-family dwellings, hotels, public buildings, office buildings, and schools
Ordinary Hazard	Group 1 - combustibility is low, quantity is moderate, stock piles less than 8 ft.	Canneries, laundries, and electronic plants
	Group 2 - combustibility is moderate, quantity is moderate, stock piles less than 12 ft.	Cereal mills, textile plants, printing and publishing plants, and shoe factories
	Group 3 - combustibility is high, quantity is high. High rates of heat release are expected.	Flour mills, piers and wharves, paper manufacturing and processing plants, rubber tire manufacturing, and storage (paper, household goods, etc.)
Extra Hazard	Group 1 - small quantities of flammables, but severe fires.	Die casting, metal extruding, rubber production, sawmills, upholstering using plastic foams
	Group 2 - moderate amounts of flammables, very severe fires.	Asphalt saturating, flammable liquid spraying, open oil quenching, solvent cleaning, varnish and paint dipping

Data from NFPA 70E: Handbook for Electrical Safety in the Workplace; 2018 Edition.Jones, R. A., Mastrullo, K. G., et al. (2017). Quincy, MA: National Fire Protection Association.

40. Answer: **A**. The key word is airborne particles such as those in the explosion at a factory in Georgia that killed 14 workers and injured dozens. OSHA has promulgated a combustible dust standard.
41. Answer: **C**. Dilution ventilation lowers the concentration of a contaminant by adding air to the general work area. Since the air is added to the general work area, it will not effectively control exposure to a toxic

or highly toxic substance used in a specific location. Dilution ventilation costs more than local exhaust ventilation and is less efficient because it has to handle more air.

42. Answer: **A**. There are generally considered to be four classes of standpipe and hose systems.
    - Class I systems utilizing 2½-inch hose with 65 psi residual pressure (at the hydraulically most remote connection) are designed to be used by trained fire departments.
    - Class II systems utilizing 1½-inch hose are designed to be used by the building occupants for "first-aid" firefighting.
    - Class III systems have the features of both Class I and Class II and are equipped with both 2½- and 1½-inch hose or fittings for both.
    - Combined systems are Class I or III systems designed in connection with a sprinkler system.

    There is a great deal of controversy within the fire service and within the safety community concerning standpipe systems. The advent of fog nozzles for firefighting has caused the pressure ratings to increase in most cases to 100 psi or greater. Most fire and safety officials believe that untrained personnel cannot safely handle a 1½-inch hose at 100 psi and the rated flow of 100 gpm.

    Additionally, controversy often surfaces surrounding the advisability and effectiveness of occupants fighting a fire, instead of exiting. This is an interesting subject for additional study; the authors recommend referencing the NFPA *Fire Protection Handbook*.

43. Answer: **B**. Intrinsic safety is a protection technique for safe operation of electrical equipment in hazardous areas by limiting the energy available for ignition. Areas with dangerous concentrations of flammable gases or dust are found in applications such as petrochemical refineries and mines.

44. Answer: **B**. A new industrial fire pump must be capable of performing to three test criteria:
    - The pump cannot develop more than 140% of its rated pressure at shutoff or churn (working against a closed system).
    - The pump must deliver the rated flow at the rated pressure.
    - The pump must deliver 150% of the rated flow at 65% of the rated pressure.

    NFPA 20 requires an annual flow test of all firefighting booster pumps.

45. Answer: **D**. Flammable and combustible liquids are subdivided into classes as shown in **Table 25** (taken from NFPA 30 and 321, Basic Classification of Flammable and Combustible Liquids).

Table 25 NFPA Basic Classification of Flammable and Combustible Liquids

Class	Boiling Point	Flash Point
I		below 100°F
IA	below 100°F	below 73°F
IB	at or above 100°F	below 73°F
IC		at or above 73°F and below 100°F
II		at or above 100°F and below 140°F
III		at or above 140°F
IIIA		at or above 140°F and below 200°F
IIIB		at or above 200°F

46. Answer: **A**. Hoods on grinding and cutting operations serve a dual function: They protect the worker from the hazards of a bursting wheel, and provide for removal of the dirt, dust, and material generated during grinding or cutting operations.

47. Answer: **C**. Acceptable Quality Level (AQL). When a continuous series of lots is considered, the AQL is the quality level, which, for the purposes of sampling inspection, is the limit of a satisfactory process average. Reference MIL-STD-105.

Self-Assessment Exam 1 Answers   219

48. Answer: **A**. Each of the epidemiological studies provides a comparison with a control group, which is most often standardized data that is collected throughout the region or country. The SMR (Standardized Mortality Ratio) provides an adjustment for age in the data. The concept is often contested due to the different exposures experienced by the various age groups.
49. Answer: **D**. Many accident-producing situations can be discovered during the design review stages of construction, thus reducing the time required to prevent mishaps.
50. Answer: **B**. Lot Total Percent Defective or the preferred term *Lot Tolerance Percent Defective* is a term used in conjunction with sampling strategies. More information on strategies and terms relating to quality procedures for inspection may be obtained from MIL-STD-105 or the civilian version, ANSI/ASQC Z1.4.
51. Answer: **D**. The OSHA requirements include provisions for insuring that the employees are provided hearing protection and given a baseline hearing test (audiogram); in most cases the audiogram is required within 6 months. However, the requirement for removal of personnel from the industrial environment in order to protect hearing is only after a hearing threshold shift is detected. The **ossicles** (also called **auditory ossicles**) can become fatigued and cause a temporary hearing loss because they serve to transmit sounds from the air to the fluid-filled labyrinth (cochlea). Removal from the noisy environment will allow them to recover. When issuing hearing protection for the first time to an employee, safety professionals should ensure the employee knows when to use it and how to wear it.
52. Answer: **B**. If the occurrence of sound is greater than once per second, the sound is considered to be continuous and should be measured as continuous sound. Reference OSHA 29 CFR 1910.95.
53. Answer: **C**. Excursions above the TLV are permitted, provided that they are compensated by equivalent excursions below the TLV-TWA during the workday. The relationship between the TLV and the permissible excursion is not a hard-and-fast rule and in certain cases may not apply. The amount by which the TLV may be exceeded for short periods without injury to health depends upon a number of factors such as the nature of the contaminant, whether very high concentrations, even for short periods, produce acute poisoning, whether the effects are cumulative, the frequency with which high concentrations occur, and the duration of such periods. The TLV-C (ceiling) should not be exceeded at any time during the work exposure. When performing personal monitoring for exposure to an airborne chemical, the sampling device and sampling protocol must be designed so that the employee's TWA exposure can be inferred from the sampling results.
54. Answer: **B**. Airtight enclosures are the best choice for the noise protection. It is important to note that any small leak can cause significant noise penetration through the barrier. Therefore, it is advisable to design enclosures to keep leaks to the lowest level possible.
55. Answer: **A**. Grinding operations create large amounts of contaminants at very high initial velocities, thus demanding higher capture velocities to secure contaminants. All other operations listed generate contaminants with low velocities.
56. Answer: **C**. The symptoms of heatstroke include an elevated temperature and dry skin (not sweaty). Syncope is synonymous with partial or full loss of consciousness due to overexposure to heat.
57. Answer: **D**. A combination of cold and vibration often causes Raynaud's phenomenon or traumatic vasospastic disease. This is a condition, usually of the fingers and hands, characterized by pallor caused by a greatly diminished blood supply resulting from spasm of the blood vessel walls. In addition to white fingers, the victim may also experience numbness of the affected area. The disease is most prevalent among those who work with vibrating machinery in the cold. Typical occupations are chain saw operators, jackhammer operators, tamping tool operators, etc.
58. Answer: **B**. Exposure to sunlight is the most common occupational cause of melanoma skin cancer.
59. Answer: **D**. Tidal Volume (TV) is the volume of air or a gas inspired or expired during each respiratory cycle, and is normally not considered during standard pulmonary function evaluation. Generally, the ventilation tests conducted are those dealing with forced expiration and inspiration to determine airway obstruction and general efficiency of the ventilation function. The Maximal Voluntary Ventilation (MVV) determines the volume of air that a person can breathe with voluntary maximum effort for 10–15 seconds. This indicator is used to determine the suitability for respirator use. The Forced Vital Capacity (FVC) is a test of expiration as forceful and rapid as possible. The FEV1 measures the forced vital capacity during the first second. It is strongly recommended that a thorough review of this area be conducted prior to sitting for the Safety Fundamentals examination.

60. Answer: **B**. Today's X-ray machines have several levels of safety incorporated into the design process. The highest risk is not from radiation, but from the high voltages required to generate the X-rays.
61. Answer: **A**. Relative density, or specific gravity, is the ratio of the density (mass of a unit volume) of a substance to the density of a given reference material. Specific gravity usually means relative density with respect to water. The term "relative density" is often preferred in modern scientific usage. Specific gravity is the ratio of the weight of one volume of a substance to that of a similar volume of water. Therefore if a liquid has a specific gravity of 1.2, it is 1.2 times heavier than water.
62. Answer: **C**. It is generally accepted that inhalation for prolonged periods of carbon dioxide above 9% will result in loss of consciousness and death. Several deaths from CO_2 have occurred. The loss of life has occurred mainly in confined spaces such as silos during harvest, in aircraft following vaporization of dry ice, and in ship holds carrying vegetables, sugar, or fish, etc.
63. Answer: **A**. Electron flow detection systems are not in widespread use to prevent the accumulation of static electricity when transferring flammable liquids. However, bonding and grounding is widely used, as is the prevention of free fall of liquid through the vapor space by use of bottom fill devices or fill pipes that extend to the bottom of the tank. Another common static prevention device is the use of a relaxation time (usually 30 seconds) downstream of a high-static-producing device, such as a filter. Relaxation allows dispersion and dissipation of the static charge. See NFPA 77, Static Electricity, for more discussion. Additional interesting information can be obtained from the API Standard 2003, Protection Against Ignition Arising Out of Static, Lightning and Stray Currents.
64. Answer: **C**. Frostbite occurs when the skin and body tissue just underneath it freezes. The skin becomes very cold, then numb, hard, and pale. Frostbite typically affects smaller, more exposed areas of the body, such as fingers, toes, nose, ears, cheeks, and chin. The first symptoms of frostbite are a "pins and needles" sensation, followed by numbness. Frostbitten skin is hard, pale, and cold, and has no feeling. When the skin is thawed out, it becomes red and very painful. Severe cases may blister and suffer gangrene and result in hard, frozen skin, sometimes all the way to bone. Answer selections A, B, and D are all symptoms of hypothermia.
65. Answer: **A**. The maximum burst pressure rating specified is 1250 psig. Working pressure is 250 psig, which provides a safety factor of 5.
66. Answer: **B**. The major types of machine guards include fixed, interlocked, and automatic. There is wide use of swing-away guards, but they are generally considered a subdivision of fixed guards and would not be a major type of guard.
67. Answer: **A**. The minimum riser and maximum tread width specified by OSHA for fixed industrial stairs are 6½ and 11 inches, respectively.
68. Answer: **D**. Stainless steel welding results in fumes containing nickel and chromium. The electrodes used in this process often contain a large amount of fluorides, which are released into the air in large quantities.
69. Answer: **A**. Pressure testing must always be considered destructive testing and stringent safety precautions should be implemented.
70. Answer: **A**. Static electricity in most instances is characterized by high voltages and very low current values.
71. Answer: **A**. The secondary transformer side features the step-down voltages; therefore the secondary side is of lower voltage. This is generally true in distribution transformers; however, many step-up transformers exist in equipment where the secondary side will contain very high voltage potential.
72. Answer: **D**. Internal corrosion of unenclosed water (and to a lesser extent fuel) tanks caused by the electrolytic action of water on the tanks has been a major problem. Cathodic protection is the preferred protection for preventing corrosion. A charged sacrificial anode is used quite effectively to prevent the electrolytic action. The only maintenance required is infrequent replacement of the anode.
73. Answer: **C**. Normally, inspection of wire rope used for hoisting or lifting includes:
    - Lubrication
    - Kinking
    - Corrosion
    - Loose or broken wires
    - Wear of crown wires
    - High strands
    - Nicks

    Additionally, cross-section measurements are usually made at some prescribed interval.

74. Answer: **C**. The National Fire Protection Association publishes the *Fire Protection Handbook*.
75. Answer: **A**. The NFPA 704 System Hazard Diamond is a symbol system intended for use of fixed installations, such as on chemical processing equipment, storage and warehousing rooms, and laboratory entrances. It informs responders of general hazards in the area. In this diamond, the three is the health diamond.
76. Answer: **C**. The rapid vaporization of sprays and mists will lower ignition temperature well below the freestanding liquid's flash point. The reduction in droplet size that occurs when a material is sprayed will also reduce the LEL. If the droplet or particle size is really small, below about 10 microns, the material will act like a pure gas mixture.
77. Answer: **B**. NFPA 600 Private Fire Brigades and NFPA 1500 Fire Department Occupational Safety and Health both may be used as information sources for the establishment and maintenance of an active fire brigade; however, NFPA 600 is the best answer to this question. NFPA 101 is the Life Safety Code and NFPA 10 is the Standard for Portable Fire Extinguishers.
78. Answer: **A**. One of the large advantages of a baghouse is the 99% collection efficiency of all but the smallest particle sizes.
79. Answer: **B**. Double-insulated equipment does not require a grounding conductor because of extra protection provided by additional insulation. Double insulation does not provide absolute protection (e.g., a double-insulated tool could still cause severe electrical shock if dropped in water).
80. Answer: **C**. Alloy steel is the standard material for chain used to hoist, lift, or support loads. The alloy material includes bronze, stainless steel, and Monel metals. Monel is a group of nickel alloys, primarily composed of nickel (up to 67%) and copper, with small amounts of iron, manganese, carbon, and silicon. Stronger than pure nickel, Monel alloys are resistant to corrosion by many agents, including rapidly flowing seawater. Chain made from alloy material is cold worked, resulting in high resistance to abrasion and failure. On the other hand, common hardware chain, also called proof coil chain, can never be used for lifting or for any purpose where failure would result in human injury.
81. Answer: **D**. According to the Commercial Motor Vehicle Safety Act of 1986, a commercial motor vehicle driver's license (CDL) is required for operation of any single vehicle with a GVWR of 26,000 pounds or more. The following table lists some of the more common subdivisions of commercial driver's licenses adopted by individual states.

Subdivisions of Commercial Driver's Licenses

Class or Endorsement	Vehicle Description
Class A	Any combination of vehicles with a gross vehicle weight rating (GVWR) of 26,000 pounds or more, provided the GVWR of the vehicles being towed is more than 10,000 pounds
Class B	Any single vehicle with a GVWR of 26,000 pounds or more, or any such vehicle towing a vehicle with a GVWR of 10,000 pounds or less
Class C	Any single vehicle less than 26,000 pounds GVWR, or any such vehicle towing a vehicle with a GVWR of 10,000 pounds or less—if endorsement is required. Any combination of vehicles where the towing vehicle is less than 26,000 pounds GVWR and the towed vehicle has a GVW of 10,000 pounds or less, but together they are 26,000 pounds GVWR or more.
Endorsement "T"	Combination vehicles with double or triple trailers
Endorsement "N"	A tank vehicle designed to transport any liquid or gaseous material with a designed capacity of 1,000 gallons or more
Endorsement "P"	Any vehicle designed to transport 16 or more passengers, including the driver. Any school bus designed to transport 11 or more passengers, including the driver.
Endorsement "H"	Any vehicle used to transport hazardous materials in placardable amounts
Endorsement "X"	Any tank vehicle used to transport placardable amounts of hazardous materials

Data from Motor Fleet Safety Manual; 5th Edition Brodbeck, J. E. (2010). Itasca, IL: National Safety Council

82. Answer: **A**. Hazard Communication, U.S. Department of Labor. OSHA 1910.1200(d)(1) states: "Chemical manufacturers and importers shall evaluate chemicals produced in their workplaces or imported by them to determine if they are hazardous. Employers are not required to evaluate chemicals unless they choose not to rely on the evaluation performed by the chemical manufacturer or importer for the chemical to satisfy this requirement."

83. Answer: **B**. At one time, lock-out/tag-out was only widely applied to electrical systems. However, for some time it has also applied to any mechanical system that possesses potential energy which could be released accidentally, thus causing injury. When evaluating the operating/shutdown procedures, the most critical step is to ensure that the machine energies are reduced to zero and remain at zero during the maintenance cycle.

84. Answer: **D**:

    Refresher training and evaluation: (OSHA 29 CFR 1910.178(l)(4). Training Assistance, U.S. Department of Labor.)

    Refresher training, including an evaluation of the effectiveness of that training, shall be conducted to ensure that the operator has the knowledge and skills needed to operate the powered industrial truck safely. Refresher training in relevant topics shall be provided to the operator when:
    - The operator has been observed to operate the vehicle in an unsafe manner.
    - The operator has been involved in an accident or near-miss incident.
    - The operator has received an evaluation that reveals that the operator is not operating the truck safely.
    - The operator is assigned to drive a different type of truck.
    - A condition in the workplace changes in a manner that could affect safe operation of the truck.
    - Each operator's performance must be evaluated at least once every three years.

85. Answer: **C**. Ergonomics is an extremely complicated subject made up of many disciplines. One formal definition, "the study of human characteristics for the appropriate design of the work environment," certainly approaches the simple phrase "Design the job to fit the person." A good review of basic principles involved in the field of ergonomics is in order prior to taking the Comprehensive Examination.

86. Answer: **C**. When designing parking lots, one factor often overlooked is the safety of entering and exiting vehicles. The most widely recommended technique is to provide a separate entry and exit way. These separate lanes should be located where traffic flow can be controlled by a traffic light or a merge/acceleration lane. Right turns from and into the parking lot are highly preferred.

87. Answer: **A**. The National Electric Code (NEC) allows several types of grounding electrode systems in Section 250-81:
    a) Metal underground water pipes
    b) Building steel
    c) Concrete-encased electrodes (Ufer grounds)
    d) Ground rings

    Metal underground water pipes are discussed at NEC 250-81(a). The Code requires the water pipe system to be in contact with the earth for 10 feet or more. However, it must be supplemented by an additional system, usually a driven electrode, to ensure that the path to ground is continuous in case the pipe is removed or replaced with plastic pipe.

    Building steel may be used as a ground, according to NEC 250-81(b), if it is connected to a ground grid or the reinforcing steel in the concrete footing. The path must be continuous and connect to the complete outer supporting structure.

    Concrete-encased electrodes are permitted under NEC 250-81(c). These grounding systems are commonly referred to as "Ufer" grounds after the Arizona engineer of the same name who did extensive research in grounds in dry, poorly conducting soil. The ground is capacitively coupled to the ground by installing 20 feet or more of steel reinforcing bars or rods or #4 AWG wiring in concrete. As in the case of the water pipe, the Ufer ground also requires connection to a driven ground. Ground rings can be used in accordance with NEC 250-81(d) and consist of a large diameter rod (#2 AWG or larger) that encircles the facility at a depth of 30 inches. Again, this system is generally connected to several driven electrodes. If none of these systems is available, a made electrode can be installed and usually consists of an electrode installed for this purpose. These can consist of pipes, rods, etc. Generally, rods must be driven 8 or more feet or be supplemented by additional electrodes to ensure a proper low-resistance path to ground. Several other systems are discussed in the NEC with a maximum resistance to ground of 25 ohms or less. Good engineering practices dictate that workers strive for 5 ohms or less.

88. Answer: **C**. According to **Table 23**, it is 50 feet.
89. Answer: **C**. According to **Table 23**, it is 15 feet.
90. Answer: **B**. It is not required to be "more than" 50 feet (**Table 23**) from the property line.
91. Answer: **C**. The purpose of electrical circuit breakers is to prevent the overheating of circuit conductors or insulation. The reference is the National Electrical Code Article 240-1, which states in the fine print that "overcurrent protection for conductors and equipment is provided to open the circuit if the current reaches a value that will cause an excessive or dangerous temperature in conductors or conductor insulation." Circuit breakers offer no primary protection from electrical shock or fires started from overheated equipment, as they are simply too slow. Shown below are some approximate action times for a typical 20-amp circuit breaker.

Approximate Action Times for a 20-amp Circuit Breaker

Load	Action Time
100%	Indefinite
125%	1 hour
200%	2 min
300%	35 sec
600%	5 sec

A 20-amp breaker overloaded 600% equals 120 amps for 5 seconds. Most inspectors can recall industrial situations in which 120 amps of heating for 5 seconds has caused serious problems.

NFPA 70E: Handbook for Electrical Safety in the Workplace; 2018 Edition, Jones, R. A., Mastrullo, K. G., et al. (2017). Quincy, MA: National Fire Protection Association.

92. Answer: **D**.
    Step 1 Redraw the shape, separating the individual rectangles and circles.

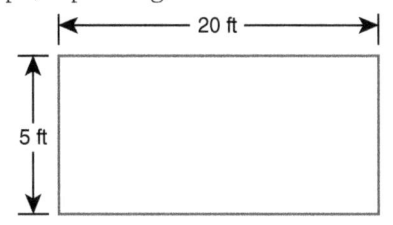

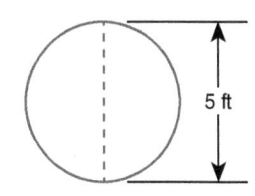

Figure 42 Flat metal shape 2

Step 2 Determine areas of the individual rectangles and circles.
First, figure the rectangle.
The radius of the circle is 2.5 feet, so the diameter is 5 feet, making the end length of the rectangle 5 feet.

$A = L \times W$

$A = 20 \text{ ft} \times 5 \text{ ft}$

$A = 100 \text{ ft}$

Then, figure the circle.

$A = \pi \times r^2$

$A = 3.14 \times (2.5 \text{ ft} \times 2.5 \text{ ft})$

$A = 19.6 \text{ ft}^2$

Step 3 Total the individual areas.
$$100 \text{ ft}^2 + 19.6 \text{ ft}^2 = 119.6 \text{ ft}^2$$

93. Answer: **C**. Specific gravity is the ratio of the metal bar's weight to an equal volume of water. Since the difference in weight on land and in water is 50 pounds, then an amount of water the same volume as the bar must weigh 50 pounds. But the bar weighs 125 pounds—so 125/50 = 2.5 times heavier than water. SG = 2.5.

94. Answer: **D**. The safety, health, and environment professional's duties are generally considered to include:
    - Safety
    - Loss control
    - Industrial hygiene
    - Environment

    Their inputs should always be limited to their areas of expertise. As part of the staff, safety professionals should work to keep safety at the management level and can best perform their function if they work in an advisory capacity to assist staff and management personnel.

95. Answer: **C**. Discussion: One can readily determine from the formula that factor D is raised almost to the fifth power and would therefore have the greatest impact on friction loss. That is, with steady-state conditions, should the diameter double, the friction loss would be reduced to about 1/32nd of the original value.

$$P_d = \frac{(4.52)(Q)^{1.85}}{(C)^{1.85}(d)^{4.87}}$$

Where P_d = pressure drop to friction
Q = Flow Rate
C = Coefficient of roughness
d = Internal pipe diameter

96. Answer: **B**.
From the table, 14 kg

$$\frac{14 \text{ kg}}{1} \times \frac{2.2 \text{ lbs}}{1 \text{ kg}} = 31 \text{ lbs}$$

$F = \mu N$
$31 = 0.12 \times N$
$N = \frac{31}{0.12} = 258$
$N = 258 - 105 = 153 \text{ lbs}$

97. Answer: **C**. Using ratio and proportion, 10 feet is to 12 feet as 50 feet is to "D_{2a}."
Note: The altitude to base ratio must stay the same between the two triangles.

$$\frac{D_{1a}}{D_{1b}} = \frac{D_{2a}}{D_{2b}}$$

$$\frac{12 \text{ ft}}{10 \text{ ft}} = \frac{D_{2a}}{50 \text{ ft}}$$

$$D_{2a} = \frac{50 \times 12}{10} = 60 \text{ ft}$$

Alternate Method:

Step 1   Label the diagram.

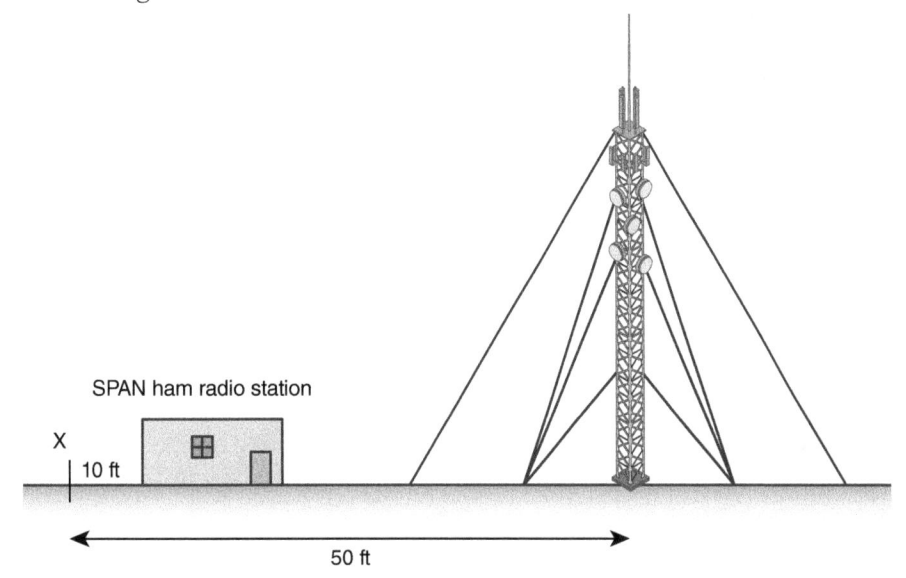

Figure 43 SPAN ham radio station

Step 2   Use calculated angle to determine antenna height.

$$\text{Tan } A = \frac{a}{b}$$

$$a = b \times \text{Tan } A$$

$$a = 50 \times \text{Tan } 50.2 = 60 \text{ ft}$$

$$\text{Tan } A = \frac{a}{b} \qquad \text{Tan } A = \frac{12}{10}$$

$$A = \text{Tan}^{-1} 1.2 = 50.2 \text{ degrees}$$

98. Answer: **A**. Legal requirements are based on laws, including 29 CFR.
99. Answer: **A**. Although industry generally separates the compliance, SH&E, and quality programs, these functions have many similarities, including:
    - Serving common underlying objectives, such as performance assurance or risk management
    - Using a common approach to achieve objectives, such as activity-specific evaluation or planning and oversight
    - Sharing common success and failure measures, such as cost, schedule, violations, or liabilities
    - The first step in establishing a good corporate quality plan is to determine customer requirements.
100. Answer: **B**. DOT regulations (Federal Motor Carrier Safety Administration (FMCSA)) contained in 49 CFR Part 382.305 require annual random testing of at least 25% of a company's entire fleet for random controlled substances. Additionally, drivers should be randomly tested prior to the start of safety-sensitive tasks. The minimum annual percentage rate for random alcohol testing is 10%. Other organizations, such as FTA, PHMSA, and FAA, require 25% of the subject population to be tested for random controlled substances.

Self-Assessment Exam 2 Questions

1. The analysis technique where individuals are interviewed about accidents, near misses, and hazardous conditions is known as:
   A. failure mode and effects analysis.
   B. operational hazard analysis.
   C. critical incident technique.
   D. sneak circuit analysis.

2. The key or first incident in event tree analysis is designated the:
   A. main failure event.
   B. primal event.
   C. top event.
   D. initiating event.

3. A methodology that can be implemented to increase the reliability of a system or process would be to:
   A. design parallel components.
   B. design series components.
   C. design redundancy into the system.
   D. All of the responses listed are correct.

4. An analysis system or a technique to determine human error is:
   A. THERP.
   B. PERT.
   C. MORT.
   D. FMEA.

5. A single-point failure can *best* be described as:
   A. a single failure that will seriously affect the safety of the system.
   B. a failure at a selected point in the system.
   C. a failure assigned one point on a scale of 10 when performing system safety analysis.
   D. a failure that is singular in nature and will affect the overall reliability of the system.

6. Which of the following statements is *false* concerning the Failure Modes and Effects Analysis (FMEA)?
   A. FMEA is a reliability tool.
   B. FMEA identifies multiple failures, human factors, and interfaces.
   C. FMEA identifies single-point failures.
   D. FMEA is normally considered to be inductive.

7. Which of the following were included in Heinrich's domino theory of accidents?
   A. Social, fault, unsafe act, accident, injury
   B. Safety, security, belonging, and self-esteem
   C. The three Es
   D. Man, machine, money, injury, accident

8. Several methods of securing line accountability for safety are widely accepted within the safety community. Of these, which of the following techniques will have the greatest significance and influence on a line manager or supervisor?
   A. Charge accidents to departments.
   B. Integrate safety into each supervisor's performance evaluation.
   C. Have safety affect each supervisor's income.
   D. Implement a combination of accountability measures.

9. **Which is the *least* important item concerning instituting management goals for the Occupational Safety and Health Program?**
    A. Management goals should be measurable.
    B. Management goals should be published.
    C. Management goals should be obtainable.
    D. Management goals should be reviewed frequently.

10. **An implied warranty is an inference by a dealer that a product is suitable for a specific purpose. The statement of warranty can be made in many ways and could include all of the following *except*:**
    A. advertising that it will satisfy that purpose.
    B. placing it for sale for that purpose.
    C. making it look like a product that will accomplish the purpose.
    D. indicating in the operating instruction that it will accomplish that purpose.

11. **Concerning the abatement date of an OSHA violation, employees have the right to:**
    A. appeal the abatement date.
    B. ignore the abatement date.
    C. speed up the abatement date.
    D. Employees have no rights concerning abatement dates.

12. **The number of days an employer has to contest an OSHA issued citation is:**
    A. 5 days from receipt.
    B. 3 working days from receipt.
    C. 15 days from receipt.
    D. 15 working days from receipt.

13. **There are several factors that are often used to determine when an organization should have the services of a full-time safety professional. Which of the following is generally accepted as the primary determining factor in assigning safety personnel?**
    A. The accident rate of the organization
    B. The gravity of accidents suffered by the organization
    C. The potential for accidents in the organization
    D. The type of industry and operation of the organization

14. **Epidemiological studies are *best* described as:**
    A. remote and widespread.
    B. differential or inferential.
    C. toxicological or geometric.
    D. descriptive or analytical.

15. **Stoichiometry is *best* defined as:**
    A. a compound with a low hydrogen-to-carbon ratio.
    B. a process of determining the Avogadro's number of a compound.
    C. calculations relating the amounts of reactants and products in chemical reactions.
    D. hydrocarbons with only single bonds between the carbons.

16. **What effect does leukemia have on the blood?**
    A. Overproduction of red blood cells
    B. Overproduction of white blood cells
    C. Inability to clot
    D. Excessive clotting

17. **Which of the following is *not* considered a common redundant design philosophy?**

    A. Derating
    B. Parallel
    C. Series
    D. Standby

18. **Which of the following would *best* describe an insurance company in business to establish a profit?**

    A. Stock
    B. Captive
    C. Paternal
    D. Mutual company

19. **Do NIOSH employees have right of entry like that of OSHA compliance officers?**

    A. Yes
    B. No
    C. Yes, if NIOSH employees have a federal warrant.
    D. No; NIOSH employees must have an OSHA escort.

20. **The basic elements of a contract include all the following *except*:**

    A. competent parties.
    B. legal consideration.
    C. mutuality of agreement.
    D. monetary duty.

21. **The entity responsible for defects in a product as it moves from manufacturer to consumer is:**

    A. the manufacturer.
    B. the distributor and the manufacturer.
    C. the wholesaler and retailer.
    D. any entity in the chain from raw material to finished product.

22. **With the current trend in product safety lawsuits, one possible defensive technique would be to maintain all design, manufacturing, and engineering records for a period lasting:**

    A. in perpetuity.
    B. 30 years.
    C. 10 years as required by OSHA.
    D. until the facility closes.

23. **OSHA's operational procedures provide for seeking a warrant if the employer challenges:**

    A. the right to enforce.
    B. the right of probable cause.
    C. the right of entry.
    D. the right to sample.

24. **Most errors causing downtime in a computer system occur due to:**

    A. computer software.
    B. computer hardware.
    C. insufficient grounding.
    D. power supply problems.

25. **All the following guidelines for instructing adults learners are true *except*:**

    A. explain the objectives (purpose) for the training session.
    B. acknowledge the learners' experience and expertise.
    C. do not allow participants to ask questions.
    D. do not talk down to learners.

26. **The generally accepted testing methods for cognitive knowledgellevel training are true-false, fill-in-blank, oral testing, or multiple choice. Which of the following statements correctly identifies characteristics of the associated testing format?**
    A. True-false: easy to grade, a problem with objectivity, a creative format
    B. Fill-in-blank: hard to grade, no problem with objectivity, a creative format
    C. Oral testing: easy to grade, no problem with objectivity, a creative format
    D. Multiple choice: easy to grade, no problem with subjectivity, difficult to measure ability to recall unprompted information

27. **The purpose for displaying safety posters in the workplace includes all of the following *except*:**
    A. demonstrating safety leadership.
    B. providing instructions on the use of safety equipment.
    C. helping maintain a high level of safety awareness.
    D. reminding employees of specific hazards.

28. **Often in safety and health training, programmed or instructional learning is used instead of more traditional methods. The technique of programmed learning is *best* described in which of the following statements?**
    A. Programmed learning is not suitable for complex and/or complicated undertakings.
    B. Programmed learning is very contentious because it attempts to control the actions of workers.
    C. Programmed learning is confined to CBT only.
    D. Programmed learning is an effective method for very short study sessions.

29. **When conducting pre-disaster emergency response planning, at the local level, coordination would be expected to occur with:**
    A. the public health department.
    B. the fire and EMS departments.
    C. the police and sheriff departments.
    D. local responders, company SMEs, and public officials.

30. **A major drive in human factors engineering is to engineer and connect things in a fashion that prevents errors and increases performance. In general, people make four types of errors or mistakes. Which of the following *best* describes the four types of errors?**
    A. Prospective, omission, transaction, reaction
    B. Transaction, reaction, interval, series
    C. Timing, commission, omission, sequence
    D. Inappropriate, detrimental, potential, response

31. **Ergonomics is the study of people's efficiency in their working environment. Which one of the following disciplines is *not* included in the broader definition of ergonomics?**
    A. Anthology
    B. Biomechanics
    C. Physiology
    D. Psychology

32. **All of the following may be barriers in communicating, with the exception of:**
    A. feedback.
    B. prejudice.
    C. knowledge.
    D. attitude.

33. Which of the following training approaches is *primarily* used to find new, inventive methodologies to problems?

   A. Holding a convention
   B. Conducting a case study
   C. Brainstorming
   D. Role playing

34. Conducting a needs assessment is important for all the following *except*:

   A. identifying the type of training necessary.
   B. identifying a need before developing a solution.
   C. saving time and money by ensuring that solutions effectively address problems they are intended to solve.
   D. identifying factors that will affect training before it is developed.

35. Early development of system safety techniques is credited to which one of the industries listed?

   A. Auto manufacturing
   B. Chemical manufacturing
   C. Nuclear power
   D. Aerospace

36. The term "multiplexing" means:

   A. the synthesis of signals for increased bandwidth.
   B. the transmission of small, compressed packets of information.
   C. a method of decreasing bandwidth and signal-to-noise ratio.
   D. the transmission of multiple signals on a single path.

37. If flammable products are kept in a storage facility where the possibility of explosion is high, what is the maximum travel distance to exits, with and without a fire sprinkler system installed, allowed by NFPA 101®, *Life Safety Code*®?

   A. 75 feet without and 150 feet with an approved fire sprinkler system
   B. 100 feet without and 150 feet with an approved fire sprinkler system
   C. 200 feet without and 200 feet with an approved fire sprinkler system
   D. 75 feet without and 100 feet with an approved fire sprinkler system

38. The public relations manager was injured when he was hit with a ball in a softball tournament at the company-owned and -maintained field. Participation in these tournaments is not required by company policies but is strongly encouraged. Would this accident be recordable under the provisions of the OSH Act?

   A. No, participation was not required.
   B. No, it is not, because of the remote location.
   C. Yes, it occurred on the employer's premises.
   D. Yes, it's required by informal policy.

39. The plant RN advised an employee with a strained wrist to use an elastic wristlet until the wrist had healed. How would this be recorded on the OSHA 300 log?

   A. All other illnesses
   B. Skin disorder
   C. Injury
   D. This medical situation is not recordable.

40. The t-distribution is like normal distribution. However, for the same area under the curve and the same standard deviation, the peak is _____ and the tails are _____.

   A. Higher, lower
   B. The same, higher
   C. Higher, higher
   D. Lower, higher

41. When presenting statistical data for comparison at a safety meeting, which of the following options would be the *best* choice for a visual delivery?

   A. Bar graph
   B. Table
   C. Pie charts
   D. Organizational chart

42. What is the *best* way to determine speech-level interference that would result due to a new process implemented in a manufacturing facility?

   A. Sound-level monitors
   B. An impact noise analysis
   C. The use of noise dosimeters
   D. Use of an octave band analyzer

43. When performing a standard hydrostatic test, the minimum pressure required by the ASME Code, based on the maximum working pressure of the vessel, would be:

   A. 50%.
   B. 150%.
   C. 175%.
   D. 200%.

44. In general industry the suggested maximum angle for a ramp is:

   A. 20 degrees.
   B. 25 degrees.
   C. 30 degrees.
   D. There is no maximum angle suggested.

45. The amount of electrical current passing through a person that would induce fatality is:

   A. 3 amps.
   B. 7 amps.
   C. 70–100 mA.
   D. 500–750 mA.

46. When using AWG #12 jacketed wire for a branch circuit, the maximum allowable current is:

   A. 15 amps.
   B. 20 amps.
   C. 30 amps.
   D. 50 amps.

47. According to OSHA, 29 CFR 1910.66, safety lanyards and lifelines are required to have a minimum breaking strength of:

   A. 2500 lbs.
   B. 3500 lbs.
   C. 4500 lbs.
   D. 5000 lbs.

48. A very serious hazard associated with crane operations is contact with overhead electrical power distribution lines. What is the OSHA requirement for foot separation between any part of a crane and power lines rated at less than 50 kV?

   A. 10
   B. 12
   C. 15
   D. The distance is left to the discretion of the crane operator.

49. OSHA requires a fixed ladder on a commercial building to be equipped with a cage. To be in full compliance with the law, the cage cannot extend any closer than _____ feet from the ground.

   A. 6 feet
   B. 7 feet
   C. 9 feet
   D. 10 feet

50. Three electrical appliances are connected to a 120-volt AC electrical branch circuit. Appliance A is consuming 1000 watts and runs intermittently; appliance B is consuming 500 watts and runs intermittently; and appliance C is consuming 700 watts and runs continuously. Which of the following protective devices is the *most* appropriate for this circuit?

   A. 15-amp breaker
   B. 25-amp breaker
   C. 30-amp fuse
   D. 40-amp fusetron

51. According to the *Fire Protection Handbook*, what are the piled and stacked storage heights that are safely allowed?

   A. 10, 12
   B. 12, 14
   C. 12, 15
   D. 15, 20

52. It is observed that an operation involving a mechanical power press requires guarding in accordance with the provisions of OSHA 1910.217. The press is equipped with an electrical main power disconnect switch that has provisions for locking out in the OFF position. However, the point of operation enclosure does not meet the OSHA standard. The plant has instead chosen to use an allowed "point of operation device" that requires the operator to use both hands to operate the controls. Using this method requires that the controls be placed at a safe distance from the point of operation so that the slide completes the downward travel or stops before the operator can reach into the point of operation with his or her hands. What is the safe distance if the total press cycle is 1 second in duration?

   A. 3.25 feet
   B. 5.25 feet
   C. 7.25 feet
   D. 9.25 feet

53. Is the statement "Personal protective equipment tends to increase worker efficiency and decrease personnel injury" valid?

   A. Yes, across all industries
   B. No, across all industries
   C. Yes, for the maritime industry
   D. No, for confined-space operations

54. **The amount of exposure to ionizing, which is regulated by the Nuclear Regulatory Commission (NRC), limits the occupational exposure to how many rems per year?**

    A. 0.05 rem
    B. 0.5 rem
    C. 5 rem
    D. 4000 millirem

55. **The *most* effective means of protecting an employee's eyes who is handling corrosives is:**

    A. safety glasses.
    B. safety goggles.
    C. a face shield.
    D. a face shield in addition to safety goggles.

56. **Of the floor surfaces listed, which would provide the greatest coefficient of friction against slips?**

    A. Wood
    B. Tread plate
    C. Ceramic tile
    D. Linoleum

57. **The *most* effective means of controlling dermatitis of employees in an industrial setting is to:**

    A. avoid contact.
    B. replace solvents.
    C. use PPE.
    D. eliminate the source.

58. **Aisles that are utilized by both fork-trucks and pedestrians must have a width of:**

    A. at minimum, 3 feet wider than the largest equipment.
    B. 22 inches wider than the greatest width of the load.
    C. 5 feet wider than the largest equipment to be utilized.
    D. at least enough space for sufficient safe clearances.

59. **In the operation of a part revolution clutch press requiring a two-hand control, the control buttons must be placed a minimum distance from the point of operation to protect the operator and prevent injury. These distances are based upon hand movement speed and which of the following?**

    A. Time and speed of the stroke
    B. Stroke speed and stroke stopping time
    C. Stopping time of the slide/ram mechanism
    D. Stroke and brake speed

60. **The probability of ignitable dust exploding is governed by:**

    A. oxygen content and dust accumulation.
    B. the dust particle size and impurities present.
    C. the type of ignition source and enclosure.
    D. All the responses listed are correct.

61. **The conditions necessary for a dust explosion or deflagration to occur include:**

    A. a high concentration of combustible dust suspended in air.
    B. confinement of the dust cloud.
    C. an ignition source with some type of oxidant.
    D. all the responses listed.

62. A highly exothermic redox reaction that occurs between two substances spontaneously at room temperature to produce a deflagration or an explosion is called (the reaction is between an oxidizer and an organic compound):

   A. pyrophoric.
   B. toxicologic.
   C. hypergolic.
   D. isotropic.

63. Flash point is defined as the _____ temperature that will produce a vapor concentration high enough to propagate a flame when a source of ignition is present.

   A. highest
   B. lowest
   C. absolute
   D. normal

64. When training personnel to erect and disassemble scaffolding, which of the following is true?

   A. Training must be conducted under the supervision of an OSHA-certified training instructor.
   B. A competent person must perform the training.
   C. The nature of any electrical hazards, fall hazards, and falling object hazards in the work area would not be included.
   D. Training is not required.

65. The Mine Safety and Health Administration (MSHA) requires certain training for each new underground miner. Which of the following *best* describes that training?

   A. Performance-based training
   B. 120 hours of on-the-job training
   C. 40 hours of prescribed training
   D. 8 hours of classroom education

66. Employees *most likely* to be involved in a production accident could be described as:

   A. employees new to the job or with less than one year of experience.
   B. employees with 10 or more years' experience.
   C. employees with administrative or clerical training.
   D. employees with functional and access needs.

67. Completion of the shipping documents for the conveyance of hazardous materials is the responsibility of the:

   A. carrier.
   B. customer.
   C. shipper.
   D. material manufacturer.

68. When an employee is walking across a production-line floor and sees a safety hazard that presents imminent danger to the workers in the area, that employee's first response should be to:

   A. warn surrounding employees and notify the area supervisor.
   B. fix the hazard.
   C. post a lock-out/tag-out sign until the hazard is corrected.
   D. do nothing, as it is not that employee's responsibility.

69. **Which of the following is the *most often* recommended fundamental safety training for plant workers?**
    A. First aid, supervisors' safety, and welding
    B. Welding, fork truck training, and back care
    C. Fire extinguisher training, first aid, and contingency
    D. Contingency, first aid, and vehicle operations

70. **Workers involved with permit-required confined space entry operations must receive training for all of the following situations *except*:**
    A. annual rescue team training on a representative space.
    B. after employees perform an entry or a change in shift occurs.
    C. whenever a change in permit space operations introduces a new hazard.
    D. whenever deviation from company procedures occurs or the employee requires retraining.

71. **Under the OSHA Hazard Communication Standard, which of the following is *not* a required training item?**
    A. Work area operations containing hazardous chemicals
    B. Location of hazardous chemical list and SDSs
    C. Plant emergency evacuation plan
    D. Details of the labeling system

72. **Most pressure vessels are required by ASME to have safety devices (i.e., relief valves, fusible plugs, etc.) to adequately protect against overpressure, chemical reaction, or other abnormal conditions. When discharge lines are provided to carry discharge away from safety valves, the area of the discharge pipe should be _____ the area of the valve outlet(s).**
    A. greater than
    B. less than
    C. equal to
    D. equal to or greater than

73. **An exceptional method of measuring variance in statistical analysis is:**
    A. the inverse square law.
    B. mode.
    C. mean deviation.
    D. standard deviation.

74. **The practice of safety sampling is usually completed when:**
    A. there is federal money available.
    B. the safety program needs new direction.
    C. it is mandated by NIOSH.
    D. a mature program has a low incident rate.

75. **Safety program audits are intended to achieve which of the following objectives?**
    A. Measurement of the safety plan's effectiveness
    B. Determination if the plan is being followed
    C. Determining whether accidents are being reported
    D. Extent of cost reduction

76. **The steps for continuous improvement safety processes are the same as in continuous quality improvement processes. Which of the following is *not* included in these processes?**
    A. Follow procedures
    B. Specify standards
    C. Measure compliance
    D. Provide feedback on improvement

77. **The turnout at plant safety meetings at a certain facility has a coefficient of correlation of −0.7 to −0.9; this indicates:**

    A. a strong positive correlation.
    B. a spurious correlation.
    C. no correlation.
    D. a strong negative correlation.

78. **Using the logic illustrated in this fault tree, calculate the Top Event probability of failure.**

    A. 10×12^{-8}
    B. 0.0002
    C. 11.99%
    D. 10×8^{-8}

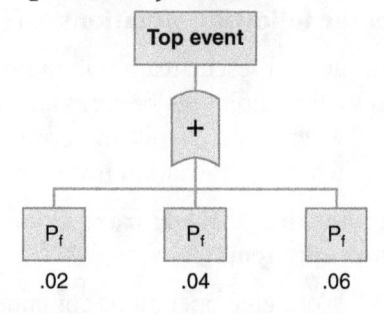

    Figure 44 Fault Tree Analysis Example 1

79. **Using the logic illustrated in this fault tree, calculate the Top Event probability of failure.**

    A. 4.8×10^{-8}
    B. 1.5%
    C. 0.9%
    D. 0.00001

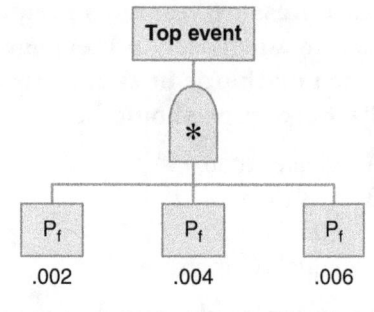

    Figure 45 Fault Tree Analysis Example 2

80. **The term "privity" best relates to:**

    A. group negligence.
    B. term insurance.
    C. a direct relationship.
    D. failure to exercise care.

81. **Warning labels are becoming an integral part of the manufacturing process. The labels are intended to warn users about potential product hazards and improper usage. Which fundamental legal principle is involved in *not* labeling a large-bladed hunting knife?**

    A. Res ipsa loquitur
    B. Obvious peril
    C. Foreseeability
    D. Tort

82. **Express warranty implies or states that a product will do all of the following *except*:**

    A. remain safe for the life of the product.
    B. perform in a specific manner.
    C. contain specific safety provisions.
    D. be suitable for a specific use.

83. **Three basic legal principles potentially used by plaintiffs in product liability cases include:**
    A. negligence, strict liability, res ipsa ioquitar.
    B. strict liability, express warranty, implied warranty.
    C. negligence, strict liability, breach of warranty.
    D. negligence, strict liability, tort.

84. **Because OSHA citations are categorized according to their potential impact on safety and health in the workplace, which of the following is *not* a violation category?**
    A. Local
    B. Willful
    C. Serious
    D. De minimis

85. **The leading cause of accidents in the wholesale and retail trade industry is:**
    A. falls to a lower level.
    B. highway accidents.
    C. personnel struck by objects.
    D. assaults and violent acts.

86. **New product development, according to Willie Hammer, includes six process phases. They consist of the concept phase, development go-ahead evaluation, product development, production go-ahead evaluation, production and operations, and support. During which phase will distributors, dealers, and field service personnel be included?**
    A. Concept phase
    B. Development go-ahead evaluation
    C. Product development
    D. Production go-ahead evaluation

87. **Which statement about static pressure in a ventilation system is *false*?**
    A. Static pressure is measured parallel to the direction of flow.
    B. Static pressure tends to collapse the duct in an exhaust system.
    C. Static pressure acts in all directions.
    D. Static pressure is a part of total pressure.

88. **Which occupational eye disorder causes the eye to become scratchy, red, and have a discharge?**
    A. Conjunctivitis
    B. Glaucoma
    C. Cataracts
    D. Nystagmus

89. **Low-voltage protection is offered by which class of hard hat?**
    A. A
    B. C
    C. E
    D. G

90. **Exposure to ionizing radiation in the United States is controlled by the Nuclear Regulatory Commission (NRC), which limits occupational exposure to _____ per year.**
    A. 0.05 rem
    B. 0.5 rem
    C. 5 rem
    D. 4000 millirem

91. What is the annual radiation dose limit for adults?

    A. 0.01 gray
    B. 0.02 gray
    C. 0.05 gray
    D. 0.08 gray

92. The diagram shown below illustrates a parallel component arrangement where the failure of one, two, or three components would not result in output failure (all four components must fail to produce output failure). Assuming the failure rate is the same for all components, which of the following formulas should be used for computing the probability of failure for this system?

    A. $C^2 - F^4$
    B. $C_1 + C_2 + C_3 + C_4$
    C. $F(e^{-t/m})$
    D. $F_1 \times F_2 \times F_3 \times F_4$

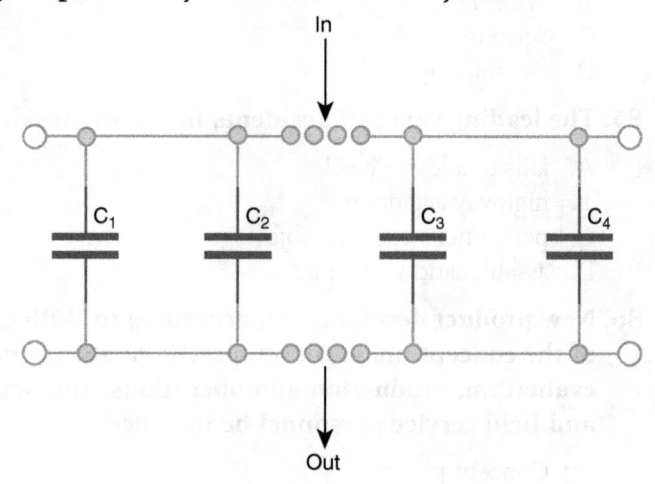

    Figure 46 Parallel Component Arrangement: Probability of Failure

93. Which of the following factors does *not* affect how individuals behave regarding workplace safety?

    A. Attitudes toward safety
    B. Views regarding team effort
    C. Recognition for personal efforts
    D. Moral standards

94. The *most* common colors involved in color blindness are:

    A. red-green.
    B. red-blue.
    C. green-blue.
    D. red-yellow.

95. The National Institute for Occupational Safety and Health in 1985 recommended criteria for defining lifting capacity, developing a revised lifting equation. The NIOSH 1991 lifting equation does *not* contain a:

    A. coupling multiplier.
    B. frequency multiplier.
    C. distance multiplier.
    D. speed multiplier.

96. What is the RWL, given the following conditions: Weight to be lifted = 12 kg; distance between body and hand grip on object to be lifted = 36 cm; vertical position at the beginning of the lift = 64 cm; vertical position at end of the lift = 20 cm; frequency of lift = once every 5 minutes for 3 hours. Note: Hand coupling is effective and this job does not require any twisting movement.
    A. 6.3 kg
    B. 7.7 kg
    C. 10.4 kg
    D. 12.1 kg

97. Treatment of hazardous wastes to eliminate their toxicity and/or their hazardous characteristics can be achieved using a wide spectrum of technologies that represent which of the following?
    A. Chemical treatment
    B. Mechanical treatment
    C. Physical treatment
    D. All the responses listed above

98. Interactive computer-assisted training, or distance learning, has which less-valuable component?
    A. It works well for organizations with small workforces.
    B. It works well for organizations that cannot remove large groups from their jobs at one time.
    C. It allows instructors to interact with each other without restrictions.
    D. It allows trainees to work at their own pace.

99. Student reaction to instruction being presented is greatly impacted by instructor behaviors. Which of the following statements is *false* concerning how a student will react to an instructor's actions or reactions?
    A. Observers learn by watching and imitating others; they tend to behave as they have seen others behave.
    B. Observers will more likely imitate a model who is passionate about his/her topic.
    C. Observers will more likely imitate a model when they see the model being rewarded for his/her actions.
    D. Observers will more likely imitate a model when they see the model being punished for his/her actions.

100. Successful communications include:
    A. sender and message.
    B. sender and receiver.
    C. message and receiver.
    D. sender, message, and receiver.

Self-Assessment Exam 2 Answers

1. Answer: **C**. Critical incident technique involves a set of procedures for collecting direct observations of human behavior and using the data to solve practical problems and to develop broad psychological principles. The theory is that a randomly selected sample of critical incidents should permit a deduction to be made concerning the existence of similar incidents.
2. Answer: **D**. The initial event in any event tree, as the name implies, is the *initiating event*.
3. Answer: **D**. Parallel and series design as well as redundancy are all appropriate methods for increasing the reliability of a system.
4. Answer: **A**. The Technique for Human Error Rate Prediction (THERP) is a detailed procedure for analyzing a task and applying tables of human reliability estimates. THERP provides human reliability data for probabilistic risk assessment studies; namely, to predict human error probabilities and to evaluate the degradation of human-computer systems likely to be caused by human errors alone or in connection with equipment malfunctioning, operational procedures, or other system and human characteristics that influence complex system (i.e., joint human-machine) behavior. The basic assumption of THERP is that the operator's actions can be regarded in the same way as the success or failure of a piece of

equipment. The theory is that the reliability of the operator can be assessed in essentially the same way as an equipment item. The operator's activities are broken down into task elements and estimates of the probability of an error for each task element are made, based on data or expert judgment.

5. Answer: **A**. A single point failure is generally defined as "a single failure that will seriously affect the safety of the system." An example would be the failure of the brake line on an automobile not equipped with redundant braking components. Another example might be the failure of the engine on a single-engine aircraft or failure of the only fuel pump on the engine. Single-point failures are almost always considered weak links in the system or process. However, this may not be the case when high-reliability components are used. The tree below shows a few single-point failures present in a gas furnace.

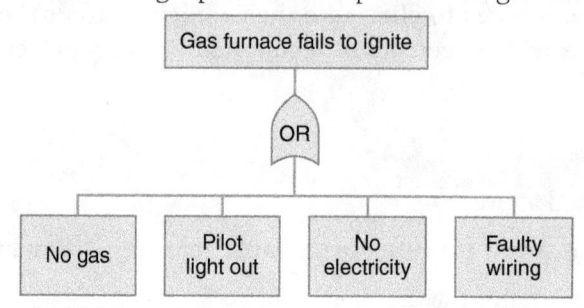

Figure 47 Single-Point Failure Present in Gas Furnace

6. Answer: **B**. The failure modes and effects analysis (FMEA) is a systematic evaluation of different ways each individual component can fail and the effects of that failure on the overall system or process. It is generally considered a reliability tool. It does an excellent job of identifying single-point failures and is an inductive analysis. The FMEA does not do a good job of identifying failures in complex systems requiring multiple operational interfaces, or multiple failures, and it does not address human factors.
Note: If the FMEA is done on a higher level than individual components, that is, at a functional level to include groups of components, it can be deductive. This "functional FMEA" asks what the cause of the subsystem- or assembly-level failure might be. It does not assign probability or reliability calculations and is gaining popularity as a deductive system safety tool.

7. Answer: **A**. The correct answer is social, fault, unsafe act, accident, injury.

8. Answer: **D**. The authors believe all of the actions listed will likely make line supervision take notice. However, a combination of efforts is required to maintain accountability.

9. Answer: **B**. This is a difficult question because the selections all provide reasonable characteristics of safety program management goals. However, the least desirable is selection D. Safety program management goals should probably be written, but they do not have to be published. Other descriptions include specific, realistic, and time bounded. Setting goals is a key component of the behavioral approach to safety.

10. Answer: **C**. Implied warranty is the implication by a dealer that the product will serve a specific purpose. The implication must be made by:
    - Placing it for sale for that purpose
    - Advertising it for that purpose
    - Indicating that it will operate for that purpose in books or manuals

11. Answer: **A**. The employees have the rights under 29 CFR 1903.17 to appeal the abatement date of an OSHA violation.

12. Answer: **D**. OSHA allows an employer 15 working days from the date of receipt to contest an OSHA citation.

13. Answer: **C**. All reasons cited here, and a long list of others, have been used at one time or another to justify the assignment of safety professionals. The prime factor in assignment of safety and health professionals to an organization should be the potential for harm within that organization. Although a supervisor has primary responsibility for safety in his or her department, the safety professional can help by acting in most situations in an advisory capacity.

14. Answer: **D**. Epidemiological studies may be classified as descriptive or analytic. In descriptive epidemiology, surveys are conducted to uncover the nature of a population affected by a particular disease, e.g.; sex, age, ethnic origin, occupation, etc. Any conclusions made from descriptive studies are then evaluated using analytical techniques, usually mathematical statistics.
15. Answer: **C**. Stoichiometry, pronounced "stoy-key-ah'-meh-tree," is derived from the Greek *stoicheion*, meaning element. Literally, stoichiometry means to measure the elements. However, the term is generally used more broadly in chemistry to include a wide variety of measurements and relationships involving substances and mixtures of chemicals. So, the definition in answer C, "calculations relating the amounts of reactants and products in chemical reactions." most closely describes stoichiometry. To do stoichiometry, one must interpret the coefficients of balanced chemical equations as the numbers of moles of reactants and products. A mole ratio is then developed to determine the amount of reactant reacted or product produced, given an amount of another reactant or product. This allows the limiting or excess reactants to be determined and theoretical yields determined.
16. Answer: **B**. Leukemia is the name given a wide range of diseases that result in widespread and uncontrolled creation of white blood cells. Most of these cells will never reach maturity and there will be a severe overaccumulation of diseased cells.
17. Answer: **A**. *Series redundancy* is employed as a redundant design in many systems as blocking devices. Many devices in series, each operated from a different source and involving a different parameter, must be activated before an accident can occur. The more items in series, the lower the probability of failure. *Parallel redundant* components perform the same function at the same time. This type of redundancy is often applied to equipment that is in continuous operation. *Standby systems* increase system reliability by having a redundant or idling standby unit that can take over if an operational unit fails. Emergency electrical generators fall into this category. Derating (or detuning) is the operation of a device at less than its rated maximum power in order to prolong its life.
18. Answer: **A**. Any insurance company may be in business to turn a profit or it may be a nonprofit organization. However, the stock insurance company is always profit motivated and it is generally believed that this motivation is evident in the organization's internal policies.
19. Answer: **A**. The OSH Act provides NIOSH with the same right of entry as OSHA representatives if they are undertaking health studies of alleged hazardous conditions and developing criteria for new standards.
20. Answer: **D**. The elements of a contract include competent parties, subject matter, legal consideration, mutuality of agreement, and mutuality of obligation.
21. Answer: **D**. The entire production chain from raw material to finished product can be held liable for a defective product.
22. Answer: **A**. To protect against product liability claims, a company should retain product records as long as possible. Of particular importance are all records pertaining to the consideration of product safety during production phases.
23. Answer: **C**. The Supreme Court case Marshall vs. Barlow dealt with OSHA's Right of Entry and resulted in the removal of the Right of Entry statement from the compliance officer's credentials. As a result of this case, some employers began to require OSHA to obtain a warrant to enter their workplace.
24. Answer: **A**. Computer software causes many times more errors than any other single item listed. Some estimates run as high as 100 to 1. Although recent development techniques have reduced the amount of computer software errors, the ratio still remains high. This does not mean the overall error rate is high, simply that the ratio of software to hardware is high. Most computer downtime is actually for preventive maintenance, updating equipment or software, and housekeeping functions.
25. Answer: **C**. The following are the guidelines for teaching adults:
    a) Explain the purpose of the training session.
    b) Describe the organization of the session.
    c) Demonstrate a fundamental respect for the learners.
    d) Acknowledge the learners' experience and expertise.
    e) Allow choices when possible.

f) Avoid body language that is degrading.
g) Do not talk down to learners.
h) Maintain a high degree of decorum and mutual respect.
i) Admit mistakes.
j) Ensure that everyone can see and hear and has comfortable seating.

26. Answer: **D**. Multiple-choice answers are easy to grade, can be statistically analyzed, can be objectively graded, and do prompt an answer. True-false questions are not creative. Fill-in-blank questions can have objectivity problems. Oral testing is subjective.

27. Answer: **A**. A safety poster does not demonstrate active caring and safety leadership of the company management.

28. Answer: **D**. Programmed or instructional learning is an excellent tool for learning just about anything. However, the development of programmed or instructional learning textbooks or computer programs is very expensive in both time and money. The newer programmed or instructional learning techniques involve interactive computer products. These products combine the features of video and small computers to produce a product that leads the student step by step through the learning process. The older instructional learning methods use the textbook approach that is presented in a series of numbered pages called *frames*, each frame consisting of three parts: explanation of a concept; questions based on the concept; and a "book" answer to the concept. Should the student answer the question incorrectly, some programmed lessons lead the student to another more detailed explanation of the concept.

  A programmed text or computer program is extremely useful to persons who must study for short periods of time due to hectic schedules. An additional advantage of this system is that effective studying is possible even when students feel tired or preoccupied because it provides a lot of repetition and forces readers to stay focused. Unlike conventional learning programs, programmed learning is excellent for studying when spare moments present themselves. Short periods spent on programmed learning are just as effective as longer sessions.

29. Answer: **D**. Disaster plans should be drawn up in advance and include neighboring companies, community agencies such as police and fire departments, industry, medical agencies, and governmental agencies.

30. Answer: **C**. The most common classification of errors, broken down into four distinct actions, is:
    - *Errors of omission* involve failure to perform some specific act.
    - *Errors of commission* involve failure to perform some specific action correctly.
    - *Errors of sequence* involve failure to perform some specific act in the proper sequence. Some references classify this as a subcategory under errors of commission.
    - *Errors of timing* involve failure to perform some specific act within the allowed time, or too fast, too slow, etc. Again, some references consider this a subcategory of errors of commission.

    Hint: Errors **COST** money, through **c**ommission, **o**mission, **s**equence, and **t**iming.

31. Answer: **A**. The field of ergonomics is extremely broad and encompasses many disciplines, including:
    - Bio-engineering
    - Industrial engineering
    - Anatomy
    - Anthropometry
    - Biomechanics
    - Physiology
    - Psychology
    - Sociology
    - Systems engineering, etc.

    However, an *anthology* is a collection of literary works chosen by the compiler. It may be a collection of poems, short stories, plays, songs, or excerpts that has no application to ergonomics.

32. Answer: **A**. Communication barriers consist of:
    - Knowledge: The trainee may think that he/she knows all that is needed.
    - Prejudice: A preconceived opinion that is not based on reason or actual experience

- Attitude: An expression of favor or disfavor toward a person, place, thing, or event. Attitude can be formed from a person's past and present. Attitude is also measurable and changeable, as well as influencing the person's emotion and behavior.
- Nonverbal actions: Trainees may say one thing while doing the opposite.

33. Answer: **C**. Brainstorming is a technique of group interactions that encourages each participant to present ideas on a specific issue. The method is normally used to find new, innovative approaches to issues. There are four ground rules:
    - Ideas presented are not criticized.
    - Freewheeling creative thinking and building on ideas are positively reinforced.
    - As many ideas as possible should be presented quickly.
    - Combining several ideas or improving suggestions is encouraged.

34. Answer: **A**. According to the NSC, a needs assessment helps to:
    - Distinguish between training and nontraining needs
    - Identify the problem or need before designing a solution
    - Save time and money by ensuring that solutions effectively address problems they are intended to solve
    - Identify factors that will impact training before its development

    The needs assessment is considered the first step in the training process. After the needs assessment, training goals are developed and during that process the trainee will determine what knowledge is needed to eliminate the problem. Remember, if the goal is to tell time, then trainees should be taught how to tell time, not how to build a watch.

    Another use for a needs analysis is any time a safety professional identifies a problem area and has to recommend a solution, he/she should perform a needs analysis to confirm the recommendation.

35. Answer: **D**. The aerospace industry is generally credited with development of several basic elements of system safety in use today. This results from the fact that government contract regulations required that systems safety methods be developed. The famous System Safety Criteria Document is a Military Specification (MIL-STD-882).

36. Answer: **D**. Multiplexing is defined as the transmission of multiple signals over a single transmission path (e.g., data and voice at the same time).

37. Answer: **D**. Section 29 of the NFPA 101®, *Life Safety Code*®, provides guidance on the maximum travel distance to exits. In the preceding question the content hazard was classified as an ordinary hazard and the distance to an exit could not exceed 200 feet, or 400 feet if equipped with an approved automatic fire sprinkler system. However, any area used for storage of high-hazard materials shall have an exit within 75 feet of the point where persons might be present. This distance can be extended to 100 feet when fire sprinkler protection is provided. Travel distances vary with different occupancies. A review of the *Life Safety Code*® is certainly in order prior to the examination.

38. Answer: **A**. Generally, injuries and illnesses that result from an event or exposure on the employer's premises are considered work-related. The employer's premises consist of the total establishment, including the primary work facility and other areas considered part of the employer's general work area. If the injury or illness results solely from voluntary participation in a wellness program or in a medical, fitness, or recreational activity such as blood donation, physical examination, flu shot, exercise class, racquetball, or baseball, it is **not** recordable.

39. Answer: **D**. According to the 1904.7, "Using any non-rigid means of support, such as elastic bandages, wraps, non-rigid back belts, etc. (devices with rigid stays or other systems designed to immobilize parts of the body are considered medical treatment for recordkeeping purposes) is considered first-aid." OSHA, 1904.7(b)(5)(ii)(F)

40. Answer: **D**. A t-distribution has a lower peak and higher tails and is commonly used to examine for differences between groups.

41. Answer: **A**. Bar charts are one of the simplest and most effective ways to display data to an audience.

42. Answer: **D**. Speech occurs in the 500–2000 Hz range. Identifying noise levels in this frequency range requires an octave-band analyzer. Octave-band analyzers are used to determine where noise energy lies in the frequency spectrum.

43. Answer: **B**. The ASME Code calls for 150% of the maximum *operating* pressure.
44. Answer: **C**. The suggested maximum angle for a ramp is 30 degrees.

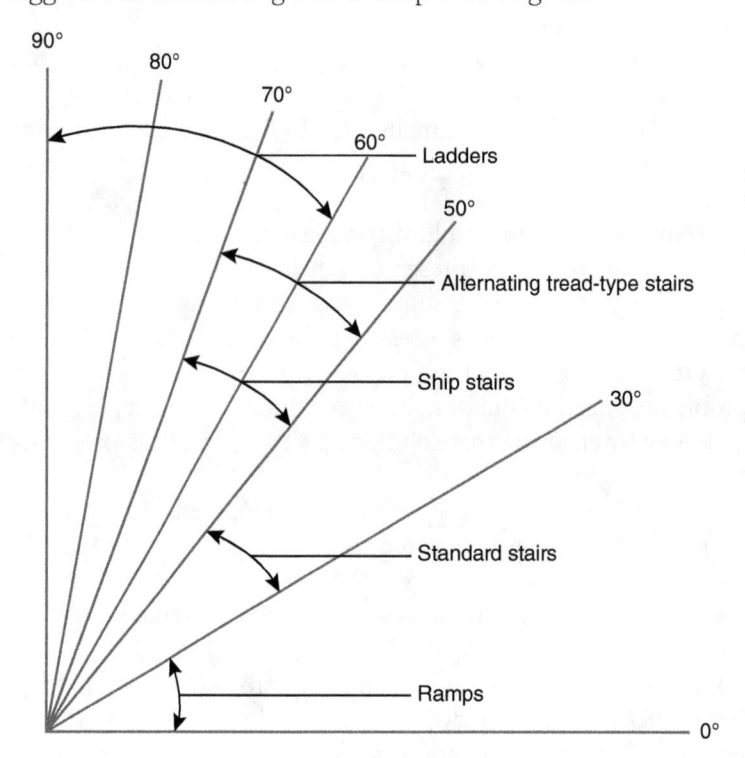

Angle	Type
≤ 30°	Ramps
30° – 50°	Standard stairs
50° – 70°	Ship stairs
50° – 70°	Alternating tread-type stairs
60° – 90°	Ladders

Figure 48 Suggested maximum angle for a ramp

45. Answer: **C**. The range of 70–100 mA is widely accepted as enough current to produce a fatality.
46. Answer: **B**. Number 12 gauge wire is the smallest presently allowed by the NEC for branch circuits rated at 20 amps.
47. Answer: **D**. OSHA 1910.66, App. C requires lifelines and lanyards to be capable of supporting a minimum dead weight of 5000 pounds.
48. Answer: **A**. OSHA 1926.550 requires a 10-foot separation between the crane and all power lines rated at 50 kV or less. Above 50 kV, the requirement is 10 foot plus 0.4 in. for each 1 kV over 50, or twice the length of the line insulator (but never less than 10 feet).
49. Answer: **B**. According to the OSHA 1910.27 standards, "Cages shall extend down the ladder to a point not less than 7 feet or more than 8 feet above the base of the ladder." Modified from OSHA 1910.27. Retrived from https://www.osha.gov/laws-regs/regulations/standardnumber/1926/1926.1053
50. Answer: **B**. Computation of branch circuit loads is fairly complex. However, in the past, exam questions have been straightforward and can usually be solved by this simple rule. Continuous loads are multiplied by a factor of 1.25 and added to the total of the noncontinuous loads to determine total load. No circuit breaker made is rated for 100% continuous load (By code, continuous is more than 3 hours). The most the manufacturer will list the breaker for is 80% of the listed rating for continuous loads. This means that

loading the circuit to more than 19.8 amperes is in violation of the manufacturer's listing for the breaker and voids the UL listing that most municipalities require for electrical equipment. Therefore the 25-amp breaker would be the choice.

700 × 1.25 = 875 Watts

1000 Watts

500 Watts

875 Watts

2375 Watts

P = IV

$I = \frac{P}{V} = \frac{2375}{120} = 19.8$ Ampere

Information on branch circuit calculations is contained in National Electrical Code *Article 220*.

51. Answer: **C**. According to the *Fire Protection Handbook*, 12 feet for piled and 15 feet for rack storage does not need to be adjusted.
52. Answer: **B**. OSHA 1910.217, "Mechanical Power Press," requires 63 inches (5.25 feet) per second of stopping time from "point of operation devices" to ensure safety of the operator.
53. Answer: **B**. Personal protective equipment does decrease injuries; however, efficiency is almost always affected. The employer is responsible and accountable for ensuring that employees wear the proper PPE while on the job.
54. Answer: **C**. The limit for ionizing radiation in the United States is established by the Nuclear Regulatory Commission as 5 rem per year.
55. Answer: **D**. Open frame safety glasses would offer little protection against the toxic effects of a high concentration of corrosives. Safety goggles and a face shield offer the best protection.
56. Answer: **A**. Wood offers the highest coefficient of friction and thus provides the most resistance to slips.
57. Answer: **D**. Of the choices listed, the authors believe all the answers would provide protection in reducing dermatitis. However, elimination of the hazard or source causing the dermatitis is the best solution.
58. Answer: **D**. Forklift operators should always be aware of conditions in their workplace, including pedestrian traffic. Forklift traffic should be separated from other workers and pedestrians where possible. OSHA requires that permanent aisles and passageways be free from obstructions and appropriately marked where mechanical handling equipment is used.

    Where mechanical handling equipment is used, sufficient safe clearances shall be allowed for aisles, at loading docks, through doorways, and wherever turns or passage must be made. Aisles and passageways shall be kept clear and in good repair, with no obstruction across or in aisles that could create a hazard. Permanent aisles and passageways shall be appropriately marked.
59. Answer: **C**. When a two-hand control is used to guard the point of operation on a part revolution clutch press, controls (buttons) must be located a safe distance from the point of operation hazard. This is to prevent the operator from placing his or her hand under the slide (ram) while it is in motion. Therefore, calculation of the safe distance takes into account maximum possible hand movement speed and the **stopping time of the slide or ram** measured from the time the operator's hand is removed from one of the two hand controls. The stopping time includes operating time of the control mechanism (switch), air exhaust from the clutch/brake (if necessary), and ram braking time.
60. Answer: **D**. Any activity that creates dust should be investigated to see if there is a risk of that dust being combustible. Dust can collect on surfaces such as rafters, roofs, suspended ceilings, ducts, crevices, dust screens, and other equipment. When the dust is disturbed, and under certain circumstances, there is the potential for a serious explosion to occur. The buildup of even a very small amount of dust can cause serious damage.

Essentially, a combustible dust is any fine material that has the ability to catch fire and explode when mixed with air. Combustible dusts can be from:
- Most solid organic materials (such as sugar, flour, grain, wood)
- Many metals
- Some nonmetallic inorganic materials
- Some of these materials are not "normally" combustible, but they can burn or explode if the particles are the right size and in the right concentration.

61. Answer: **D**. While the destructiveness of a dust explosion depends primarily on the rate of pressure rise, other factors are maximum pressure developed, duration of excess pressure, degree of explosion volume confinement, and oxygen concentration.

62. Answer: **C**. Hypergolic refers to a fuel that will ignite with an oxidizer but does not require an outside ignition source. Hypergolic is the explosive reaction of constituents usually associated with rocket propellants. A common hypergol, hydrazine, is used in combination with liquid oxidizers extensively in the space program.

63. Answer: **B**. The flash point of a volatile material is the lowest temperature at which it can vaporize to form an ignitable mixture in air. Measuring a flash point requires an ignition source. At the flash point, the vapor may cease to burn when the source of ignition is removed.

    The flash point is not to be confused with the auto-ignition temperature, which does not require an ignition source, or the fire point, the temperature at which the vapor continues to burn after being ignited. Neither the flash point nor the fire point is dependent on the temperature of the ignition source, which is much higher.

    An excellent reference is the National Fire Protection Association *Fire Protection Handbook*, 20th edition.

64. Answer: **B**. OSHA requires a competent person to provide training on the nature of fall hazards, correct procedures for erection, maintenance, and disassembly, proper use, placement, and care in handling, etc. Additionally, all erection and disassembly must be done under the supervision of a competent person.

65. Answer: **C**. Throughout the history of the Mine Safety and Health Administration (MSHA), the organization has stressed the importance of training for miners. The training is expressly prescribed, "Every new underground miner shall receive no less than 40 hours of prescribed training." MSHA then lists the prescribed training, complete with format. This is in contrast to the performance-based training required by recent legislation (i.e., the OSHA Hazard Communication Standard).

66. Answer: **A**. According to the NSC, although statistical data differ, it is generally agreed that new employees are significantly more prone to work-related accidents.

67. Answer: **C**. It is the shipper's responsibility to properly complete appropriate shipping documents, including classification of material.

68. Answer: **A**. All employees have the responsibility for life safety, hence notifying other workers in potential danger and then notifying the area supervisor to abate the problem would be the best response.

69. Answer: **C**. The three most often recommended fundamental training courses for general industrial workers are first aid, fire extinguisher, and contingency. Contingency means emergency procedures.

70. Answer: **B**. Training is required before an employee is assigned a role in confined space entry or a change in duty occurs, per OSHA's Confined Space Standard, 1910.146.

71. Answer: **C**. The OSHA Hazard Communication Standard requires employees to be provided with the following information and training:

Hazard Communication Standard requirements:
- Any operations in a work area where hazardous chemicals are present
- The location and availability of a written hazard communication program, to include a list of chemicals, and material safety data sheets
- Training on methods and observations that may be used to detect the presence or release of a hazardous chemical in a work area
- The physical and health hazards of chemicals in a work area
- The measures employees can take to protect themselves from these hazards, including specific procedures such as work practices, emergency procedures, and personal protective equipment

- The details of the Hazard Communication Program, including an explanation of the labeling system and the material safety data sheet, and how employees find and use information. Modified from OSHA 29 CFR 1910.1200
72. Answer: **D**. According to the ASME B31 series, *Pressure Piping*, sectional areas of a discharge pipe shall not be less than the full area of the valve outlets discharging. The discharge pipe shall be as short as possible and arranged to avoid undue stresses on the valve or valves. It is recommended that individual discharge lines be used for each valve, but if two or more valves are combined, the discharge piping shall be designed with sufficient flow area to prevent a blowout of steam or other fluids.
73. Answer: **D**. The standard deviation is the root square deviation about the mean. Standard deviation is often used in measuring variance. The standard deviation places great emphasis on extreme values because all individual deviations are squared.
74. Answer: **D**. Safety sampling or searching for increased factors of safety is usually only done after a safety program is well established and has proven to be effective. When undertaking observational human research, legal and ethical requirements emphasize the importance of informed consent.

$$s = \sqrt{\frac{\Sigma(x^2)}{n-1}}$$

where $(x = X - \bar{X})$

75. Answer: **B**. Audits are performed to determine if the plan is being followed. Audits can be performed by subprofessional safety personnel, such as quality control or assurance personnel, who know little about the rationale behind requirements since they are tasked only with seeing if the rules are being followed.

    Program evaluation is properly described as the measurement of results against accepted criteria. An appropriate parameter for evaluating the status of a safety program is an experience modifier.
76. Answer: **A**. Most behavior-based safety experts define the "continuous improvement safety process" as consisting of:
    - Specifying standards
    - Measuring compliance
    - Providing feedback on improvements

    Injuries and property damage caused by unsafe actions are best reduced by systematically reinforcing positive behavior.
77. Answer: **D**. A result near 1 indicates that the values have a strong linear relationship. A result near 0 indicates the values are only slightly related. A value near −1 indicates that the values are very closely related but in a negative way (an increase in one is related to a decrease in the other). In safety work, a correlation of less than + or − 0.6 is discounted. A coefficient of correlation of −0.7 to −0.9 would indicate a strong negative correlation.
78. Answer: **C**. The symbol shown in this fault tree is that of an "OR" logic gate. This means that failure of any components in the tree will cause the overall system to fail; that is, component 1 can fail, or component 2 can fail, or component 3 can fail, etc. This arrangement is often called series construction. The + shown in the gate represents the engineering symbol for the "OR" function. The rare event approximation cannot be used in this problem. See the next question.

$$P_{Total} = P_1 + P_2 + P_3 - (P_1 \times P_2 \times P_3)$$
$$P_{Total} = 0.02 + 0.04 + 0.06 - (0.02 \times 0.04 \times 0.06) = 0.1199 \text{ or } 11.99\%$$

79. Answer: **A**. The symbol shown in the fault tree is that of the "AND" logic gate. The * shown in the gate represents the engineering symbol for the "AND" function. This means that failure of all the devices in the system must occur before the entire system will fail. This arrangement is often called parallel construction. To determine the total probability of failure for this representation, the bottom event probabilities would be multiplied.

Note: If any of the minimal cut set event probabilities were higher than about 1×10^{-2}, using the rare event approximation would be inappropriate. See the preceding question.

$P_{Total} = P_1 \times P_2 \times P_3$

$P_{Total} = 0.002 \times 0.004 \times 0.006 = 0.000000048$ or 4.8×10^{-8}

80. Answer: **C**. In product safety work, *private* is defined as "a direct relationship between the injured party and the party whose negligence caused an accident." Early English law held that there could be no negligence without *privity*. However, this rule was broken in the United States in the early 1900s when Judge Benjamin Cardozo ruled that an automobile manufacturer was liable for an injury accident involving a failed wheel. The automobile manufacturer based its defense on the *privity rule*.

    The company had sold the car to a dealer, had no contract with the injured party, and was therefore not liable to the plaintiff. The dealer was not liable since he had not built the car. The ruling, however, indicated that the car manufacturer had a duty to inspect the product sold for defects and to fail to do so was negligence.

81. Answer: **B**. A manufacturer or distributor would not have to label a large-bladed hunting knife because the product involves an **obvious peril**, sometimes called an obvious hazard, that is well known to the public.

    The term **res ipsa loquitur** (the thing speaks for itself) is involved in accidents where the damage-producing agent was under the sole control of the defendant and the accident would not have happened if the defendant had exercised proper control.

    Foreseeability involves liability for actions that a normal person would have known to exist and would have taken precautions to prevent.

    Tort is a wrongful act or failure to exercise due care that results in damage or injury in the broadest sense.

    Strict liability is the concept that a manufacturer of a product is liable for injury due to a defect, without necessity for a plaintiff to show fault or negligence.

82. Answer: **A**. An express warranty is a written or oral statement by a manufacturer or dealer that a product will perform in a specific manner, be suitable for a specific purpose, or contain specific safeguards.

83. Answer: **C**. The three basic legal principles that can be used in most states are:
    - Negligence, which tests the conduct of the defendant
    - Strict liability and implied warranty, which test the quality of the product
    - Express warranty and misrepresentation, which test the performance of the product against the manufacturer's/seller's representations.
    - Where legal liability is established, typical product liability insurance covers damage awards.

84. Answer: **A**. The five categories of violations are willful, serious, repeat, other than serious, and de minimis. De minimis includes areas where there is no immediate threat to safety and health.

85. Answer: **D**. According to the NSC Injury Facts booklet, although highway traffic incidents are the leading cause of all work-related fatal injuries, assaults and violent acts by persons (homicide) is the leading cause in the wholesale and retail trade industry. An example would be an armed robbery.

86. Answer: **D**. During production "go-ahead" evaluation, distributors, dealers, and field representatives should be asked to review the prototype for familiarization and comment. Personnel who may have to maintain or repair the product must be instructed about any potential hazards, safeguards, and precautionary measures. Service manuals and test equipment must be made available.

87. Answer: **A**. The static pressure is always measured perpendicular to the direction of flow.

88. Answer: **A**. Explanation: Various types of conjunctivitis, or inflammation of the mucous membrane, can develop beneath the eyelids. The eye becomes scratchy and red and has a discharge. Most often the cause is viral, bacterial, or allergic. All causes produce varying degrees of redness, which is often referred to as "pink eye." Viral infections usually produce tearing.

    Glaucoma is a leading cause of blindness in America. The most common form, primary open-angle glaucoma (POAG), was originally thought to develop when the fluid that normally fills the eyeball, the aqueous humor, fails to drain properly. Ordinarily, the fluid is continuously produced in the eye and excess drains off through a small duct near the iris. Aging, infection, injuries, congenital defects, and other causes can constrict or block the duct. Fluid pressure then builds up and the pressure, if great and of long duration, can damage the optic nerve.

Cataracts are opacities that form on the lens and impair the vision of many elderly and some younger people. Many cases are associated with metabolic disease or aging, but there are also traumatic cases associated with industrial exposures to ionizing radiation, ultraviolet radiation, infrared radiation, foreign bodies, and certain chemicals. Cataracts can also be caused by certain medications, particularly prolonged treatment with corticosteroids. There is also evidence that cigarette smoking increases cataract development. If the vision impairment is severe, the diseased lens can be removed, and is generally replaced with a plastic implant.

Nystagmus, involuntary movement of the eyeballs, may occur among workers who, for extended periods, subject their eyes to abnormal and unaccustomed movements. Complaints of objects dancing before the eyes, headaches, dizziness, and general fatigue are associated symptoms; all can clear up quickly if a change of work is made. The involuntary movements of the eyeball characteristic of nystagmus can sometimes be induced by occupational causes affecting the eyes through the central nervous system or by some extraneous cause. The most prevalent form of occupational nystagmus is seen in miners.

89. Answer: **D**. ANSI Z89.1-1997 establishes specifications for helmets (hard hats) to protect the heads of industrial workers from impact and penetration by falling objects and from high-voltage electrical shock.

Helmet Types

Class E (Electrical) helmets are intended to reduce the danger of exposure to high-voltage electrical conductors, and are proof tested at 20,000 volts. Class E is tested for force transmission first, then tested at 20,000 volts for 3 minutes, with 9 milliamps maximum current leakage; then tested at 30,000 volts, with no burn-through permitted (formerly Class B).

Class G (General) helmets are intended to reduce the danger of exposure to low-voltage electrical conductors, and are proof tested at 2200 volts. Class G is tested at 2,200 volts for 1 minute, with 3 milliamps maximum leakage (formerly Class A).

Class C (Conductive) helmets are not intended to provide protection from electrical conductors. Class C is not tested for electrical resistance (no change in class designation).

Definitions expanded: new test protocol section, including preparation, mounting, number, and sequence of test samples; summary of failure criteria

- The product was tested within a 3-inch circle on top of the helmet in "as worn" position.
- A 2.2-pound pointed steel penetrator, with 60° angle, was dropped from a simulated free-fall height of 8 feet.
- The penetrator can't make contact with the head form.
- Test apparatus includes an electronic contact indicator, a velocity indicator, and electronic recording equipment.
- No differentiation is made for helmet classes.

90. Answer: **C**. The limit for ionizing radiation in the United States is established by the Nuclear Regulatory Commission at 5 rem per year.
91. Answer: **C**. Two measurements are essential for radiation protection: the measurement of the dose of radiation absorbed by the body and assessment of risk associated with this absorbed dose. Two units were thus created: gray and sievert; an annual limit of 5 rem (0.05 Sv or 0.05 Gy) total effective dose equivalent (TEDE). Conversions are as follows:

1 Gy = 100 rad
1 mGy = 100 mrad
1 Sv = 100 rem
1 mSv = 100 mrem

Units of Measurement

Quantity measured	International system (SI)	Definition (SI)
Dose absorbed	Gray (Gy)	1 Gy: Energy released by joule per kilogram of matter
Equivalent dose and effective dose	Sievert (Sv)	Sv: Gy multiplied by a weighting factor specific to each type of radiation and organ

92. Answer: **D**. Since the components are in parallel, the configuration indicates an "AND" gate situation; that is, C_1 and C_2 and C_3 and C_4 must fail before the output fails. The symbol for an "AND" gate is "*" which indicates multiplication; this leads

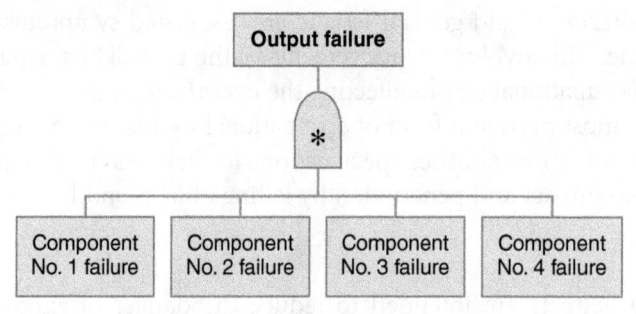

Figure 49 Output Failure "AND" Gate Example 1

to the correct answer. Multiply the failure rates of each component. $F_1 \times F_2 \times F_3 \times F_4$, or since the failure rates are all the same, F_4.

Note: When dealing in probability of failure, the general rules are:
- Parallel construction indicates "AND" = multiply
- Series construction indicates "OR" = addition

93. Answer: **D**. The safety culture is a group's attitude that everyone in the group will try to behave in a way that protects the safety of each other. Recognition will reinforce their trust in the culture. An important factor in developing a safety program is to incorporate concepts of job enrichment, participation, and employee-centered leadership. Management will most likely support a proactive safety effort when prevention of losses relates to achievement of company objectives.

94. Answer: **A**. People with normal cones and light-sensitive pigment (trichromasy) are able to see all colors and subtle mixtures of them by using cones sensitive to one of three wavelengths of light: red, green, and blue. A mild color deficiency is present when one or more of the three cones' light-sensitive pigments are not quite right and their peak sensitivity is shifted. Approximately 5% to 8% of all men and 0.5% of all women of the world are born color-blind. That total equals one out of twelve men and one out of two hundred women. People who are protans (red weak) and deutans (green weak) comprise 99% of this group.

95. Answer: **D**. The 1991 NIOSH lifting equation is expressed as:
RWL = LC × HM × VM × DM × AM × FM × CM

Where,
RWL = Recommended Weight Limit,
LC = load constant,
AM = asymmetric multiplier,
HM = horizontal multiplier,
FM = frequency multiplier,
VM = vertical multiplier,
CM = coupling multiplier, and
DM = distance multiplier.

Note: The load constant of 51 pounds is the maximum weight to be lifted under ideal conditions.

96. Answer: **D**.

$$\text{RWL} = 23\left(\frac{25}{H}\right)(1 - .003\,|\,V - 75\,|)\left(.82 + \frac{4.5}{D}\right)(1 - (.0032 \times A))(FM)(CM)$$

$$\text{RWL} = 23\left(\frac{25}{36}\right)(1 - .003\,|\,64 - 75\,|)\left(.82 + \frac{4.5}{44}\right)(1 - (.0032 \times 0))(.85)(1)$$

RWL = 23 × 0.694 × 0.967 × 0.922 × 1 × 0.85 × 1

RWL = 12.1 kg

97. Answer: **D**. Treatment of hazardous wastes to eliminate their toxicity and/or their hazardous characteristics can be achieved using a wide spectrum of technologies that revolve around two main pathways: namely, *chemical* and *mechanical (physical)*.
    Chemical treatment includes all forms of chemical reactions, such as reduction, oxidation, thermal oxidation, precipitation, neutralization, electrochemical, photolytic, biological degradation, etc.
    Mechanical or **physical treatment** includes those procedures that modify the physical properties of waste materials; for example, filtration, phase separation, filter pressing of suspended materials, centrifugation, agitation, adsorption, etc.

98. Answer: **C**. According to the NSC, the valuable attributes of interactive computer-assisted training, sometimes called distance learning, are:
    - Workers can work at their own pace.
    - Records of all training can be automatically kept.
    - Correct answers are required before the student can proceed.
    - Workers receive training as time is available.
    - Instructors can guide workers step by step through the lesson plan.
    - Organizations with a small workforce or those that cannot remove large groups from their jobs at any one time benefit greatly.
    - When students complete coursework away from an actual training facility, it is generally called distance learning. This is an umbrella term for many types of learning, including online training and training available through the mail.

99. Answer: **D**. According to Robert F. Mager in *Making Instruction Work*, answer D is correct. To build positive classroom discipline, instructors should model appropriate behavior, and use appropriate classroom management methods. Instructors must convey dignity and cooperation. If students feel they are respected as individuals, they will want to act with similar behaviors. Likewise, when instructors act maturely and competently, students will see them as role models after whom they will pattern their own behavior.

100. Answer: **D**. Communications consists of three basic elements: the sender, the message, and the receiver. When communicating, whether orally or in writing, people must always provide for feedback. This is the only way to ensure that the message was received.

Self-Assessment Exam 3 Questions

1. A solution contains 10^{-1} hydrogen ions per liter. This solution would be considered:

  A. a strong acid.
  B. a weak acid.
  C. a strong base.
  D. a weak base.

2. Under what conditions would the use of a 5000-fpm exhaust duct velocity be justified for extended periods in a ventilation system?

   A. To increase efficiency
   B. To reduce abrasion
   C. To reduce noise
   D. To reduce settling

3. Having an R number above 2100 implies what about flow characteristics in a ventilation system?

   A. 2000 is the breaking point for square ducts.
   B. Turbulent flow
   C. Laminar flow
   D. Too fast for round ducts

4. What do all organic materials contain?

   A. Carbon
   B. Hydrogen
   C. Oxygen
   D. Nitrogen

5. Critical pressure is defined as the:

   A. point where the temperature is 460°R.
   B. point where the temperature is 473°K.
   C. point where no liquid-vapor phase transition occurs.
   D. point of vapor pressure release.

6. Which of the following has the highest vapor pressure?

   A. Benzene
   B. Acetone
   C. Toluene
   D. Xylene

7. Btu is a traditional unit of energy equal to about 1055 joules. It is the amount of energy needed to cool or heat one pound of water by _____.

   A. 1 degree C
   B. 4 degrees K
   C. 1 degree F
   D. 4 degrees R

8. In the art and science of human factors, presentation of information is extremely important and follows certain rules. In which situation presented below would the presentation of an audio signal be *more appropriate* than a visual display?

   A. The message is long.
   B. The message is very complex.
   C. The message does not require a verbal response.
   D. The message requires immediate attention.

9. The inverse square law, as applied to illumination, states:

   A. The light source as perceived varies inversely as the square of the power.
   B. Light intensity on a surface varies inversely with the square of the distance between the source and surface.
   C. The light intensity of the source varies inversely as the distance in lumens.
   D. Surface illumination varies directly with the inverse square of the distance.

10. **Respirators are generally divided into which of the following categories?**
    A. Particulate and air-supplying
    B. Self-cleaning and non-self-cleaning
    C. Air-purifying and supplied air
    D. Gas masks and air hoods

11. **The inverse square law applies to all of the following *except*:**
    A. heat.
    B. illumination.
    C. noise.
    D. radiation.

12. **Unprotected eyes can be damaged by exposure to a welder's arc. This damage could be caused by exposure to:**
    A. infrared light.
    B. invisible radiation.
    C. sensible light.
    D. ultraviolet radiation.

13. **All of the following are characteristic of local exhaust ventilation when compared to dilution ventilation *except*:**
    A. it is less expensive than dilution ventilation.
    B. it is more suitable for highly toxic substances.
    C. it is good for ventilating point source emissions.
    D. it pushes less air than dilution ventilation.

14. **Which *best* describes the term *tidal volume* when used with reference to human lung volumes and capacities?**
    A. The maximum volume of air that can be forcibly inspired following a normal inspiration
    B. The volume of air inspired or expired during each normal respiratory cycle
    C. The maximum volume of air that can be forcibly expired following a normal expiration
    D. The sum of all four of the primary lung capacities

15. **The *most appropriate* response to a person suffering heatstroke is to:**
    A. immediately treat for shock.
    B. decrease the body temperature.
    C. place the victim in shade and provide liquids.
    D. fan the victim, place the victim in a cool area, and replenish body fluids.

16. **Chemical asphyxiants prevent the uptake of oxygen by the cells. For example, hydrogen sulfide, at high enough concentrations, paralyzes the respiratory center of the brain. Which of the following is considered a chemical asphyxiant?**
    A. Carbon monoxide
    B. Nitrogen
    C. Methane
    D. Hydrogen

17. **In a large percentage of industrial applications, round ducts are preferred to square ducts because round ducts:**
    A. can be sealed much more easily.
    B. use less material for the same size.
    C. are much stronger.
    D. offer less friction to airflow.

18. The National Electrical Code utilizes a Class, Division, and Group hazard identification system. Class II hazards involve which materials?

    A. Flammable liquids
    B. Powders
    C. Fibers
    D. Dusts

19. The major classifications of automatic sprinkler systems include wet pipe, dry pipe, deluge, foam water, special types, and:

    A. pre-action.
    B. AFFF.
    C. water cannon.
    D. combination.

20. A combustible gas indicator operates by sensing some characteristic of a sample drawn into the instrument and translating these characteristics into usable data. These instruments usually work on which principle?

    A. Thermal expansion in a confined chamber
    B. Rapid ionization of the sample gas
    C. Measurement of the weight of the sampled gas
    D. The Wheatstone bridge

21. When water damage is a major concern, the sprinkler system designed to offer the *best* protection is a:

    A. deluge system.
    B. pre-action system.
    C. dry pipe system.
    D. wet pipe system.

22. Which of the following *best* describes the system safety term "common cause failure"?

    A. Failure of common components from the same cause
    B. Failure of different components at the same time from a common cause
    C. Failure of components of similar design and specifications from the same cause
    D. Failure of any number of components in a system from a common cause

23. Which building has the *least* ability to resist structural damage from a fire?

    A. Fire resistive
    B. Noncombustible
    C. Ordinary
    D. Heavy timber

24. In states that have a Right to Know law, the federal OSHA Hazard Communication Standard 1910.1200:

    A. is preempted.
    B. preempts the state law in all cases.
    C. preempts the state law in occupational settings.
    D. preempts the state law in situations covered by OSHA.

25. You are conducting a training needs assessment on a newly acquired piece of equipment. When should learning objectives be completed?

    A. Prior to the construction phases
    B. While products are designed
    C. Before employees are trained
    D. Before a change is initiated

26. Which ANSI standard covers construction hard hats?
   A. ANSI Z 87.1
   B. ANSI B 16.4
   C. ANSI A 12.1
   D. ANSI Z 89.1

27. After reading the OSHA regulations, regarding occupational noise exposure, what should a CSP's first action be?
   A. Have the plant engineer determine noisy areas.
   B. Conduct a sound pressure survey.
   C. Conduct immediate audiometric testing of all employees.
   D. Contact a hearing protection supplier for advice.

28. The *most* common occupational disease that occurs in industry is:
   A. dermatitis.
   B. dysbarism.
   C. fibrosis.
   D. silicosis.

29. The reaction rate (rate of reaction) or speed of reaction for a reactant or product in a particular reaction is intuitively defined as how fast or slow a reaction takes place. This also equates to the quantity of material being used or produced per unit of time. If the total volume of the reacting system is doubled, and all other conditions being constant, the amount of matter produced per second is doubled. This means the "rate" is doubled. Which of the following *best* describes the effect heat has on rate of reaction?
   A. If heat is increased, the reaction rate will increase.
   B. If heat is increased, the reaction rate will decrease.
   C. If heat is increased, the reaction rate will decrease as the square of the energy added.
   D. If heat is decreased, or removed, the reaction rate will slow inversely proportional to the initial activation energy.

30. Self-contained breathing apparatus (SCBA) used as emergency or rescue equipment must be inspected:
   A. weekly.
   B. monthly.
   C. semiannually.
   D. annually.

31. A symptom a person would *not* experience when suffering a heatstroke is:
   A. a severe headache.
   B. loss of consciousness.
   C. profuse sweating and cool, moist skin.
   D. rapid temperature rise and hot, dry skin.

32. In an industrial environment, female workers perform many tasks that were designed for males. Which of the listed activities would provide the greatest compatibility between males and females in manual operations?
   A. Lowering
   B. Pushing
   C. Lifting
   D. Carrying

33. Which factor does *not* affect quality of light?

   A. Color
   B. Diffusion
   C. Direction
   D. Foot-candles

34. An endemic disease can be defined as:

   A. present in certain populations or regions.
   B. the rapid spread to a large number of persons in a given population within a short period of time.
   C. a propagated outbreak.
   D. affecting an entire population.

35. Certain occupations tend to contract tenosynovitis. Which of the following jobs would *most likely* induce this condition?

   A. Administrative assistant
   B. Assembly line worker
   C. Company CEO
   D. Crane operator

36. The damage a structure receives during an earthquake is dependent upon several factors, including composition. Ductility is an important quality in constructing earthquake-resistant structures. Which of the following would provide the greatest ductility?

   A. Wood
   B. Steel
   C. Masonry
   D. Brick veneer

37. Which of the following metals is generally considered to be *most* pyrophoric?

   A. Strontium
   B. Calcium
   C. Magnesium
   D. Sodium-potassium

38. Which of the following is *not* considered an acceptable method in controlling electrostatic discharge (ESD) in industrial operations?

   A. Dissipating wrist straps
   B. Static discharger
   C. Ion generator
   D. Dehumidification

39. What is the allowed volume of flammable and combustibles liquids to be kept in a flammable storage cabinet?

   A. 60 gallons of flammables or 120 gallons of combustibles
   B. 70 gallons of flammables or 40 gallons of combustibles
   C. 80 gallons of flammables or 80 gallons of combustibles
   D. 90 gallons of flammables or 140 gallons of combustibles

40. All of the following are alternatives to use of explosion-proof electrical equipment in Class I locations *except*:

   A. totally enclosing equipment in an inert atmosphere.
   B. using intrinsically safe equipment.
   C. using Class II, Division 1 equipment.
   D. providing equipment with supplied air to prevent explosive mixtures from entering the enclosure.

41. Which of the following firefighting agents could be effectively used on a Class A fire?

    A. Purple K
    B. Dry chemical (ammonium phosphate)
    C. Halon 1301
    D. Dry chemical (potassium chloride)

42. Destructive testing is carried out to determine structural performance or behavior under different loads. Which of the following could be considered an example of destructive testing?

    A. Pressure testing
    B. Dye injection
    C. Eddy current
    D. Radioscopic examination

43. Assured grounding programs require:

    A. installation of GFCI devices in construction areas.
    B. periodic testing of circuits and tools.
    C. an on-duty electrical worker at all times.
    D. specialized and very expensive equipment.

44. A generally accepted practice for use of a video display terminal is to locate the VDT slightly below the operator's horizontal line of sight (HLOS). The recommended angle is:

    A. 5° below horizontal line of sight.
    B. 5° to 35° below horizontal line of sight.
    C. 15° to 35° below horizontal line of sight.
    D. 15° to 25° below horizontal line of sight.

45. Neutron shielding is *best* accomplished by the use of:

    A. plastic.
    B. concrete.
    C. water.
    D. lead.

46. Safety in the design, fabrication, and inspection of boilers and pressure vessels is governed by the American Society of Mechanical Engineers' *Boiler and Pressure Vessel Code*, commonly referred to as the ASME boiler code. The ASME boiler code exempts several categories of unfired pressure vessels, including:

    A. underground or underwater pressure vessels.
    B. small vessels of less than 120 gallons of water under pressure.
    C. vessels with a pressure of less than 15 psig or greater than 3000 psig.
    D. hot water storage tanks.

47. Which of the following agencies publishes TLVs and PELs?

    A. ACGIH and OSHA
    B. OSHA and MSHA
    C. ACGIH and MSHA
    D. NIOSH and OSHA

48. Which of the following is *not* a known carcinogen?

    A. Benzene
    B. Vinyl chloride
    C. Formaldehyde
    D. Potassium permanganate

49. The principle of "time - distance - shielding" is *most* closely associated with which of the following disciplines?

   A. Ergonomics
   B. Health physics
   C. Fire protection engineering
   D. Industrial hygiene

50. **Of the following statements associated with heat stress measurement, which is incorrect?**

   A. t_{wb} is normally measured with a psychrometer.
   B. t_a is generally referred to as dry bulb, or DB.
   C. A t_g temperature globe is also called radiant temperature.
   D. The WGT index is not used in the United States because it has no correlation with the WBGT index.

51. **Which of the following incidents would *not* require reporting under the current DOT reporting guidelines?**

   A. Truck accident involving six fatalities
   B. Semi-tractor trailer incident resulting in a hazardous chemical release
   C. Driver provided with on-scene first aid
   D. Driver transported to a hospital for medical attention

52. **What color is used to identify workplace tripping hazards?**

   A. Red
   B. Blue
   C. Yellow
   D. Green

53. **Information is denoted by what color in an industrial setting?**

   A. Red
   B. Blue
   C. Yellow
   D. Orange

54. **The organization that is commonly responsible for compressed gas cylinder safety is:**

   A. CGA.
   B. OSHA.
   C. ANSI.
   D. ASTM.

55. **The acronym REM represents:**

   A. relevant equivalence man.
   B. radiation emendation man.
   C. rabelaisian equivalent man.
   D. roentgen equivalent man.

56. **Warning labels must contain all of the following *except*:**

   A. steps to be taken to avoid injury.
   B. avoidance actions to prevent damage.
   C. consequences of improper actions.
   D. additional safety precautions access concerning this class of product.

57. **The foremost cause of heat gain for a person is the body's internal heat. This is referred to as:**
    A. metabolic heat.
    B. internal heat.
    C. total work heat.
    D. work-produced heat.

58. **Identify the organization established and operated by the American Chemistry Council to provide emergency response information.**
    A. Chemical Center for Accident Response Information
    B. Chemical Transportation Emergency Center
    C. Chemical Manufacturers Association
    D. Chemical Emergency Center for Transportation

59. **During firefighting on a residential structure, what would be the likely cause of an adjacent building heating?**
    A. Convection
    B. Irradiance
    C. Radiation
    D. Conduction

60. **The purpose of epidemiological studies is to describe the symptoms of a disease and to uncover the relationship with the etiological (causative) agent. Which of the following statements *best* describes retrospective studies?**
    A. Retrospective studies are the most expensive.
    B. Retrospective studies look back in time on populations exposed to the agent under investigation.
    C. Retrospective studies are also called cohort or incident studies.
    D. Retrospective studies are considered the most scientifically useful.

61. **The type of system safety analysis used in the early stages of a project for determination of the gross hazards that may exist is:**
    A. PHA.
    B. FMEA.
    C. FTA.
    D. MORT.

62. **Which of the following concepts is *not* widely accepted in today's safety community?**
    A. Multiple accident causation
    B. Accident proneness
    C. Motivational training
    D. Behavior modification

63. **A conclusion from the Hawthorne study indicated that employees would respond to:**
    A. discipline first, education second.
    B. supervisors who had job knowledge.
    C. both positive and negative forms of attention.
    D. safety professionals before supervisors.

64. **An important function of management is to set goals and objectives. Which of the following methods is used as a tool to accomplish this task?**
    A. MBO system
    B. Zero-based budgeting
    C. Performance review
    D. All responses listed are correct.

65. The approach used to make a job safe, by identifying hazards and developing measures to prevent those hazards, is called:
   A. a fault tree.
   B. MORT analysis.
   C. job safety analysis.
   D. probabilistic risk assessment.

66. Senior management can *best* support health and safety training by:
   A. signing policy letters about H&S training importance.
   B. hiring professional educators.
   C. talking about S&H at staff meetings.
   D. showing active and sincere interest in the program.

67. Safety sampling measures the effectiveness of a line manager's safety actions. The four steps of safety sampling include all of the following *except*:
   A. developing corrective measures.
   B. preparing a code.
   C. validating the sample.
   D. taking the sample.

68. The technique of system safety analysis can be applied to which of the following processes/systems?
   A. Generally, only the most complex
   B. Any that have interacting components
   C. Very simple ones, with only a single component
   D. Any, but only after some loss has occurred

69. According to some safety experts, there are 10 basic principles of safety. These include all of the following *except*:
   A. Safety management should be treated separately and different from other company management.
   B. The key to effective line safety performance is management procedures that affix accountability.
   C. An unsafe act, an unsafe condition, and an accident are all symptoms of faulty management.
   D. A certain set of circumstances will prevent severe injuries.

70. The term *incident rate* is used quite often in the expanding field of safety and health. In industrial safety work, the term is most commonly associated with minor mishaps or the frequency of all mishaps. In epidemiology, the term *incidence rate* is often used to indicate (the number of) _____ that occurred in a given period of time.
   A. prevalent cases
   B. all cases
   C. specific cases
   D. new cases

71. Measuring injuries and illness resulting in days away, restricted, or transferred from normal duty is frequently used in industrial safety work. This indicator should be used as:
   A. an absolute rate to compare with other industries.
   B. an indicator of serious injury frequency.
   C. a yardstick after converting to a million hours worked.
   D. an accident severity rate to compare severity and frequency against other similar industry rates.

A. training objectives.
B. training staff.
C. training methods.
D. content of the training program.

76. Which is the *most* important feature of a maintenance department's energy isolation program?

    A. Safety training of workers and supervisors
    B. A written and enforced lock-out procedure
    C. Knowledge of job requirements
    D. Safe scheduling of maintenance tasks

77. Within a company's structure, the individual *most* responsible for implementing response actions required by the Emergency Action Plan is the:

    A. security director.
    B. operations manager.
    C. safety professional.
    D. supervisor.

78. Which of the following tests is associated with the *Otis-Lennon Mental Ability Test*?

    A. Personality Inventory Test
    B. Personnel Classification Test
    C. IQ Test
    D. Multiple Aptitude Test

79. Who must implement the actions identified in a facility's emergency response or action plan?

    A. Security
    B. Corporate manager
    C. Operations manager
    D. Supervisors

262 ASP Exam Study Workbook

80. According to the Factory Mutual Engineering Corporation, the three principal causes of fire in the United States are:

    A. electrical, smoking, and hot surfaces.
    B. static sparks, lightning, and cutting and welding.
    C. friction, cutting and welding, and smoking.
    D. smoking, hot surfaces, and spontaneous ignition.

81. Section 1910.1000 (Air Contaminants) in the General Industry Standards would be classified as what kind of standard?

    A. Optional
    B. Vertical
    C. Specification
    D. Performance

82. When two parties involved in a disagreement agree to accept the determination of a third party, this process is known as:

    A. negotiation.
    B. arbitration.
    C. obfuscation.
    D. concession.

83. In assessing the capabilities of a computer and humans, which of the following statements is *incorrect*?

    A. Humans are better at abstract judgment situations, such as emergency management.
    B. Computers are better at voluminous searches of data.
    C. Humans are better at exercising inductive reasoning, making judgments based on experience and reasoning.
    D. Computers are better at following a random and variable strategy.

84. In order for health and safety training to provide maximum effectiveness, enabling learning objectives should be developed. Which of the following requirements of enabling learning or training objectives is the *least* important?

    A. Enabling training objectives should be reasonable.
    B. Enabling training objectives should be measurable.
    C. Enabling training objectives should be obtainable.
    D. Enabling training objectives should be written.

85. Which of the following is of *least* importance when considering an instructor for a safety and health training project in an industrial setting?

    A. Appearance
    B. Desire to instruct
    C. Knowledge of subject
    D. Presentation style

86. Which of the following is the *best* indicator of training effectiveness?

    A. Favorable student critiques
    B. Correct student response to questions
    C. Increase in effectiveness of job performance
    D. Testing meets expected norms

87. In order to make verbal communication, which of the following is required?

    A. Directing
    B. Evaluating
    C. Listening
    D. Responding

88. What is the minimum number of people required for a group?

    A. 2
    B. 3
    C. 4
    D. 5

89. Which of the following is a disadvantage of the lecture method?

    A. There is a lack of audience participation
    B. Instructors have control of the information presented.
    C. It's the most effective way to teach knowledge-level objectives.
    D. Large amounts of information are presented in a short period of time.

90. Calculate the incidence rate for a company if recordable accidents are 20 and the total man-hours are 1,750,000.

    A. 8.3
    B. 6.3
    C. 3.3
    D. 2.3

91. An industrial facility has experienced 36 recordable mishaps involving days away from work. The facility has 850 full-time employees. Calculate the lost workday rate for this facility.

    A. 42.3
    B. 4.23
    C. 32.45
    D. 3.45

92. An assembly line worker burned the tip of his finger with a soldering iron while installing a circuit board component. He went to see the on-site Registered Nurse (RN) who treated the burn and applied a dressing. The RN said he would not need additional treatment; however, she requested he return the next day for observation. Which of the following is the *best* OSHA classification for the incident?

    A. Recordable first-aid injury
    B. Recordable lost time injury
    C. Recordable medical treatment, greater than first-aid
    D. Not recordable, less than medical treatment

93. The American Industrial Hygiene Association (AIHA) publishes a set of Emergency Response Guidelines (ERGs®) that provides values intended as estimates of concentration ranges. The primary focus of the ERGs® is to provide guideline levels for once-in-a-lifetime, short-term (typically 1-hour) exposures to airborne concentrations of acutely toxic, high-priority chemicals. The number of levels of ERGs is:

    A. 2.
    B. 3.
    C. 4.
    D. 5.

94. During a training presentation, an instructor uses both verbal and nonverbal communications. Nonverbal refers to voice inflection, body movements, and even dress for the presentation. Which of the following indicates a power image?

    A. Open-collared shirt, many hand motions
    B. Light-colored suit, high rate of speech, rigid posture
    C. Dark suit, relaxed body motions, closed-arm stance
    D. Memorized presentation, rigorous time schedule

95. Which of the following is the common language of client/server database management?

    A. SQL
    B. URL
    C. HTML
    D. HTTP

96. The presentation of a safety training session is *least* effective when:

    A. training occurs after an accident.
    B. training occurs after a plant explosion.
    C. training occurs after the monthly accident data shows an increase in the incident rate.
    D. training occurs after the company announces it is downsizing.

97. Which of the following is *not* an expected outcome of group training?

    A. Becoming actively involved in planning and implementation of company policy
    B. Gaining skills
    C. Evaluating information
    D. Sharing ideas

98. Communication is defined as:

    A. sharing information and/or ideas with others and gaining approval.
    B. sharing opinions and/or ideas with others and being understood.
    C. sharing information and/or ideas with others and being understood.
    D. sharing opinions and/or ideas with others and gaining approval.

99. The minimum pressure for a standard hydrostatic test of a compressed air bottle, according to the ASME Code, must be 150% of which of the following pressures?

    A. Burst pressure
    B. Normal operating pressure
    C. Required pressure relief valve setting
    D. Maximum operating pressure

100. When fixed guards are not possible or practical, safeguarding devices may be used to protect workers from point-of-operation hazards where moving parts actually perform work on stock. Which type of safeguarding device requires adjustment for each individual operator?

    A. Movable-barrier device
    B. Two-hand control device
    C. Pullback device
    D. Presence-sensing device

Self-Assessment Exam 3 Answers

1. Answer: **A**. 10^{-1} H$^+$ ions is equal to a pH of 1. This is a strong acid solution.
2. Answer: **D**. This high velocity would normally only be used if dust or heavy contaminants were involved, such as lead dust with small chips, moist cement dust, asbestos chunks from transite pipe cutting machines, quick lime dust, etc. High velocities do not always increase efficiency but they do always increase abrasion and noise.
3. Answer: **B**. The Reynolds number is a dimensionless ratio used to predict if flow is turbulent or laminar. If the Reynolds number is less than 2000, the flow is laminar; if greater than 2100, the flow is turbulent.
4. Answer: **A**. Organic is defined as compounds that contain carbon.
5. Answer: **C**. The critical pressure of a substance is that pressure at which no liquid-vapor phase transition occurs at any temperature.
6. Answer: **B**. Acetone has the highest vapor pressure. This is easily recognized by its rapid evaporation rate.

MATERIAL	V. P.
Benzene	75 mm
Toluene	22 mm
Xylene	10 mm
Acetone	227 mm

7. Answer: **C**. The British Thermal Unit (Btu) is the amount of heat required to raise the temperature of 1 pound of water 1 degree Fahrenheit.
8. Answer: **D**. Use visual presentation methods when:
   - Operator is in one position
   - Immediate attention is not required
   - Information is complex
   - Environment is noisy

   Use audio presentation methods when:
   - Message is simple and short
   - Immediate attention or action is required
   - Illumination limits vision
   - Message deals with a time-critical sequence

   The above listing is definitely incomplete.
9. Answer: **B**. Light intensity on a surface does vary inversely with the square of the distance between the source and the surface. A way to show this relationship as an equation is:

   $$RI = \frac{I_0}{X^2}$$

   Where RI = radiation intensity, I_0 = initial intensity, and X = distance.
10. Answer: **C**. All respirators can be placed in two categories:
    - Air-purifying
    - Supplied air
11. Answer: **A**. Utilizing the inverse square law for measurements concerning noise, illumination, and radiation is acceptable, but not for heat.
12. Answer: **D**. Damage to eyes from ultraviolet radiation is much more violent than visible or infrared. A severe burn can be produced with little or no warning and significant damage to the eye lens can occur.

266 ASP Exam Study Workbook

13. Answer: **A**. Local exhaust ventilation almost always costs more than dilution ventilation. Dilution ventilation is defined as the removal or addition of air to keep the concentration of a contaminant below hazardous levels. The process can use natural or forced air movement through open doors, windows, etc., or exhaust fans can be mounted on roofs, walls, or windows. Local exhaust systems trap an air contaminant near its source, which usually makes this method much more effective, but more expensive than dilution.

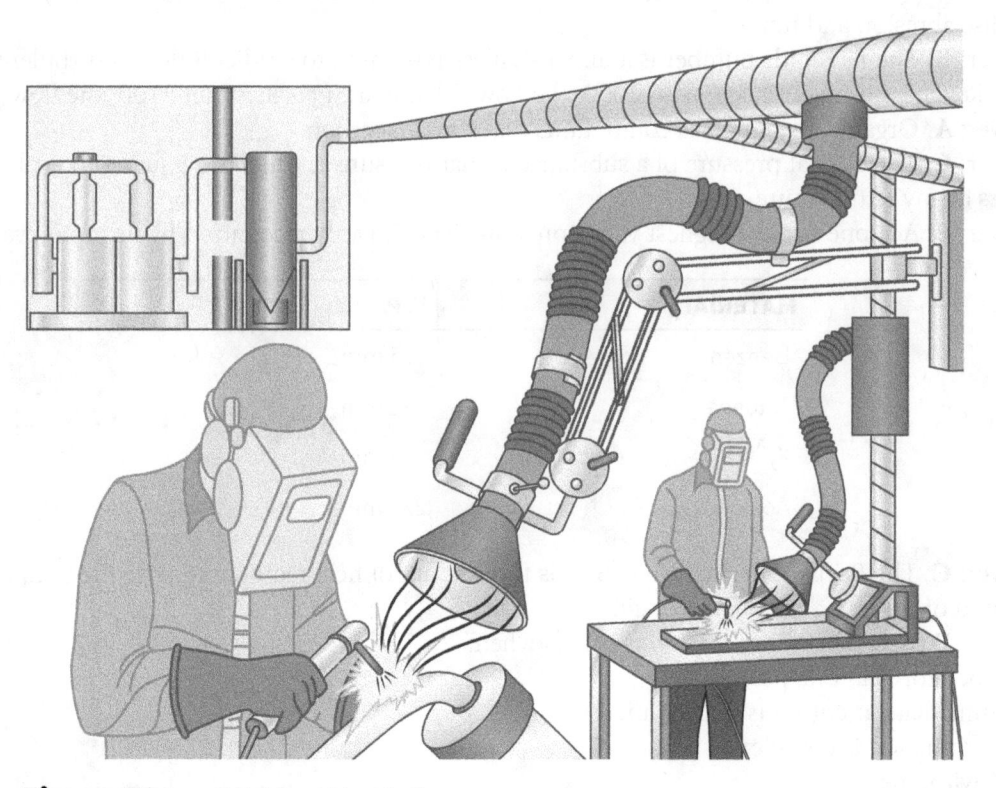

Figure 50 Local Exhaust Ventilation

14. Answer: **B**. Tidal volume (TV) is normally considered to be the volume of air or gases inspired or expired during each respiratory cycle. Selection A is the definition of inspiratory reserve volume (IRV). Selection C is the definition of expiratory reserve volume (ERV). Selection D is the definition of total lung capacity (TLC).
15. Answer: **B**. Heatstroke is the most serious heat illness. It occurs when the body temperature is so high that sweating stops, allowing the temperature to rise to levels where tissue damage and even death can occur. Proper emergency measures are all-important and involve reducing body temperature by whatever means available. Wet sheets, ice baths, water spray, and fans have all been used to successfully lower body temperature.
16. Answer: **A**. Asphyxiants cause harm by reducing the amount of oxygen in the blood. Simple asphyxiants displace oxygen, while chemical asphyxiants (through direct chemical action) prevent oxygen from reaching the blood. Carbon monoxide is a chemical asphyxiant.
17. Answer: **C**. In industrial applications, high velocities and therefore high SPs are normally used. This condition results in duct collapses. Circular ducts are better able to withstand this stress.

18. Answer: **D**. The NEC Class II hazard classification includes combustible dusts. Refer to NFPA 70 Article 500.

CLASS	DIVISION 1	DIVISION 2
I Gases, Vapors, and Liquids (ART. 501)	Normally explosive and hazardous	Not normally present in an explosive concentration (but may accidentally exist)
II Dusts (ART. 502)	Ignitable quantities of dust normally are or may be in suspension or conductive dust may be present	Dust not normally suspended in an ignitable concentration (but may accidentally exist). Dust layers are present.
III Fibers and Flyings (ART. 503)	Textiles, woodworking, etc. (easily ignitable but not likely to be explosive)	Stored or handled in storage (exclusive of manufacturing)

Electrical standards reference manual, U.S. Department of Labor, Occupational Safety and Health Administration, Office of Training and Education, 1988.

19. Answer: **A**. The NFPA lists six major classification of automatic sprinkler systems:
    - Wet pipe
    - Dry pipe
    - Pre-action
    - Deluge
    - Foam water
    - Special types
20. Answer: **D**. Most combustible gas analyzers use a Wheatstone bridge circuit, which includes an active element of platinum. Catalytic combustion takes place when the atmosphere tested comes in contact with this active element and the change in resistance is indicated on an electric meter.
21. Answer: **B**. Pre-action systems are dry pipe. When a fire occurs, a supplementary fire-detecting device in the protected area is actuated. This opens a valve, which permits water to flow into the piping system before a sprinkler is activated, thus allowing redundant protection from inadvertent activation and water damage.
22. Answer: **D**. The search for common causes of component failure, sometimes called *common killers*, is a prime system safety responsibility. Often, a common environmental cause can cripple otherwise redundant subsystems to the point where the entire system is adversely affected. A short list of common causes might include:
    - Moisture
    - Metal fatigue
    - Vibration
    - Test voltage/current
    - Temperature
    - Common vendor errors
    - Pressure
    - Substandard fasteners
    - Corrosion
    - Mud daubers

    An often-cited common cause in system safety texts concerns a mishap involving a four-engine aircraft that suffered complete engine failure due to moisture in a large electrical connector. The connector (a multi-pin cannon plug) provided a single point at which all electrical control for certain fuel feed valves could be affected by a combination of moisture and cold. When the fuel panel was configured for cruise and the aircraft encountered the cold of altitude after flying through a rain shower, all engines quit. The engines were able to be restarted only because the emergency checklist selected a different fuel feed arrangement. After returning the fuel panel to the cruise configuration, the engines again failed, causing the flight crew great consternation.

23. Answer: **C**. Ordinary construction has all the inherent hazards attributed to construction where wood or other combustible material is used and is the least protected of answer choices.
    NFPA 220 provides the following classifications:
    Type I – Fire Restive
    Type II – Non Combustible
    Type III – Ordinary
    Type IV – Heavy Timber
    Type V – Frame
24. Answer: **D**. The Federal Hazard Communication Standard preempts state law where the two laws conflict.
25. Answer: **C**. If hazard identification, evaluation, and controls have been determined, learning objectives should be identified before employees are trained, to reinforce desired safe performance.
26. Answer: **D**. **ANSI Z 87.1** deals with Occupational and Educational Eye and Face Protection. **ANSI Z 1 6.4** concerns Uniform Recordkeeping for Occupational Injuries and Illnesses. **ANSI A 12.1** is the standard for Floor and Wall Openings, Railing, and Toeboards. **ANSI Z 89.1** is the authority on Protective Headgear for Industrial Workers.
27. Answer: **B**. The OSHA occupational noise exposure standard 1910.95 requires employers to determine workplace noise exposure and establish a hearing conservation program *if noise exposure exceeds an 8-hour time weighted average of 85 dBA*. Audiograms may be required if a hearing conservation program is required.
28. Answer: **A**. Dermatitis is by far the most frequently reported disease occurring in industry and accounts for almost 50% of occupational diseases reported to OSHA.
29. Answer: **A**. In general, it is found that a small increase in temperature will increase rates of simple reactions by a large amount. The magnitude of this effect on increasing temperature depends on the reaction activation energy. Those reactions, having large activation energy, will be more sensitive to temperature changes than reactions having low activation energy. This principle is explained via Arrhenius' equation in most advanced chemistry texts.
30. Answer: **B**. OSHA requires monthly inspections for self-contained breathing apparatus (SCBA). Nondisposable respirators should be cleaned and inspected before and after each use.
31. Answer: **C**. During heatstroke (sunstroke), the body temperature rises and reaches a point where the heat-regulating mechanism breaks down completely. The body temperature then rises rapidly. The symptoms are hot and dry skin, severe headache, visual disturbances, rapid temperature rise, and loss of consciousness.
32. Answer: **B**. Females generally have the capacity to perform 80% of those jobs designed for male workers when tasks require pushing. They can perform only 50% of those jobs involving carrying, 65% for lifting, and 65% for lowering tasks.
33. Answer: **D**. Quality of illumination refers to distribution of brightness in the visual environment. It includes glare, diffusion, direction, uniformity, color, and brightness. It does not include quantity.
34. Answer: **A**. Endemic simply means that the problem is localized to a particular population, e.g., in the Southwest, on islands, in the desert.
35. Answer: **B**. Tenosynovitis is an inflammation of the connective tissue sheath of a tendon. It is a repetitive motion affliction common to assembly line workers or others who perform repetitive actions without adequate rest periods.
36. Answer: **B**. Ductility is the ability to undergo distortion or deformation—bending, for example—without resulting in complete breakage or failure. A rigid cement block is an example of a structure with extremely low ductility.
37. Answer: **C**. A pyrophoric substance (from Greek, *pyrophoros*, "fire-bearing") ignites spontaneously in air at or below 55°C (130°F). Pyrophoric metals are those, usually in fine powder form, that ignite spontaneously when exposed to air! All metals listed burn and require special firefighting tactics. Water

used on all of these materials except for magnesium can lead to explosion, even at room temperatures. Magnesium is considered the most pyrophoric.

38. Answer: **D**. Please note that humidity has a significant effect on the induced charge. It is not recommended to have relative humidity (RH) that is too low, say, below 30%. ESD control becomes especially challenging at low RH levels. A relative humidity between 40% and 60% is recommended for the typical assembly area. Detailed information on ESD grounding can be found in the ESD Association standard ANSI/ESD S6.1, Grounding, and the ESD Handbook ESD TR20.20, and/or the CLC/TR 61340-5-2 User Guide.

    Six basic principles in the development and implementation of effective ESD control programs are:
    a) **Design in protection** by designing products and assemblies to be as robust as reasonable against the effects of ESD.
    b) **Define the level of control** needed in your environment.
    c) **Identify and define** the electrostatic protected areas (EPAs), the areas in which you will be handling ESD-sensitive parts (ESDS).
    d) **Reduce electrostatic charge generation** by reducing and eliminating static-generating processes, keeping processes and materials at the same electrostatic potential, and by providing appropriate ground paths to reduce charge generation and accumulation.
    e) **Dissipate and neutralize** by grounding, ionization, and the use of conductive and dissipative static control materials.
    f) **Protect products from ESD** with proper grounding or shunting and the use of static-control packaging and material-handling products. Reproduced from "ESD fundamentals"

39. Answer: **A**. OSHA 1926.152 requires that a flammable storage cabinet hold no more than 60 gallons of flammable or 120 gallons of combustible liquids in any one cabinet. Additionally, no more than three storage cabinets may be located in a single fire area.

40. Answer: **C**. As an alternative to "explosion-proof" equipment and wiring it is permissible to totally enclose equipment and provide supplied air to create positive-pressure ventilation, or totally enclosed inert gas–filled equipment may be used. Lastly, intrinsically safe equipment may be used. The use of equipment approved for use in Class II or III locations is not permitted because this equipment was designed for a different purpose. Equipment for use in Class II and III locations is designed to be dust ignition–proof and will not resist internal explosions.

41. Answer: **B**. The only agent listed that is rated for Class A firefighting is selection B, ammonium phosphate, which is rated as an A:B:C extinguisher. Purple K, potassium bicarbonate, is well known as an effective agent for flammable liquid fires and is often used in combination with AFFF. Halon 1301, a halogenated agent, and the dry chemical potassium chloride are rated only B, C. Of the multipurpose dry chemicals, monoammonium-phosphate-base is by far the most common and although considered nontoxic, will cause irritation if breathed for extended periods. Another problem with ammonium phosphate is corrosion. The agent is acidic and, when mixed with even minuscule amounts of water, will corrode most metals, so immediate cleanup is very important.

42. Answer: **A**. Pressure testing can result in violent failure and adequate safeguards must be established.

43. Answer: **B**. An assured grounding program is sometimes used in lieu of ground fault circuit interrupters on construction sites. The program requires extensive testing of all equipment and circuits to insure integrity of equipment grounding conductors.

44. Answer: **D**. Although there is not complete agreement on this design principle, most references, including the NSC Accident Prevention Manual, suggest that 15° to 25° below horizontal line of sight is the proper placement for video display terminals. This allows the operator to assume a normal head position that develops a slightly lowered sight or viewing angle. This means the video monitor top is placed at eye level to allow proper head and neck position.

45. Answer: **C**. Shielding for neutrons is best accomplished by materials with light nuclei such as hydrogen atoms. Accordingly, water or other media rich in hydrogen content is frequently used. Graphite (carbon atoms) can also be used effectively.

46. Answer: **B**. The American Society of Mechanical Engineers' *Boiler and Pressure Vessel Code*, commonly referred to as the ASME boiler code, covers the safety of design, fabrication, and inspection of boilers and pressure vessels in the United States. The current code contains 11 sections and occupies 2.5 feet of shelf space. The ASME boiler code exempts several categories of unfired pressure vessels, including:
    - Any vessel that is covered by a U.S. governmental entity
    - Small pressure vessels with a capacity of 120 gallons of water under pressure
    - Hot water storage tanks heated by steam or indirect means with a water temperature of 200°F
    - Vessels with an inside diameter not exceeding 6 inches (pipes)
    - Vessels having an operating pressure of 15 psig or less

    Because of the extra hazards involved in pressures over 3000 psi, the ASME code requires the design of these pressure vessels to be based on an extremely detailed stress design that is certified by a registered professional engineer (PE) competent in pressure vessel design.

    Note: An extremely valuable reference for pressure vessels operating at less than 15 psig is the American Petroleum Institute (API) standard 620, *Recommended Rules for Design and Construction of Large, Welded, Low-Pressure Storage Tanks*.

47. Answer: **A**. The American Conference of Governmental Industrial Hygienists publishes the Threshold Limit Values (TLVs) in wide use in industry. OSHA publishes the Permissible Exposure Limits (PELs).

48. Answer: **D**. Vinyl chloride has been associated with tumors of the liver, brain, lung, and hematolymphopoietic system. There is also sufficient evidence for the carcinogenicity of benzene in humans. Many case reports and case studies have described the association of leukemia with exposure to benzene, either alone or in combination with other chemicals. Methyl iodide has been re-evaluated and is now considered "equivocal." Formaldehyde is a potential carcinogen. Almost all applications of potassium permanganate exploit its oxidizing properties. As a strong oxidant that does not generate toxic by-products, $KMnO_4$ has many uses, such as in water treatment.

49. Answer: **B**. The principles of "time - distance - shielding" are basic principles of protection closely associated with the discipline of health physics:
    - Dose or exposure is directly related to time, so if time is reduced, exposure will be reduced as well.
    - Distance is a function of the inverse square law (assuming free field conditions), so doubling the distance from a point source will result in a fourfold reduction in exposure.
    - Providing a barrier or shield between energy and employees is widely used for protection, for example lead aprons for dental X-rays.

50. Answer: **D**. The Wet Globe Temperature (WGT) index has been accepted and does have a high correlation with the WBGT; however, the correlation is not constant for all environmental conditions. The accepted relationship is WGT + 3.6°F = WBGT. Selection A is correct as t_{wb} is usually obtained with a psychrometer either motor driven or manually with a sling psychrometer. Selection B is also correct. In most industrial hygiene texts, t_a and DB are synonymous. Answer C is true, as t_g is radiant temperature. One such globe thermometer is a thin-wall black, 6-inch sphere with thermometer attached. This device depends on transfer of radiant heat to the indicating thermometer and one must wait at least 20 minutes for the transfer to take place before accurate readings can be obtained. See the ACGIH Industrial Ventilation Manual for a short but excellent review on heat stress.

51. Answer: **C**. Under current DOT reporting guidelines, only the mishap involving on-scene medical attention is not reportable. This assumes that the operator does not later seek medical attention for the same injuries.

52. Answer: **C**. Yellow is normally used to identify physical tripping hazards.

53. Answer: **B**. Blue is the color utilized to denote information.

54. Answer: **A**. The CGA (Compressed Gas Association), as the name indicates, is the primary organization dealing with compressed gas safety in the United States.

55. Answer: **D**. Rem is the expression used to indicate Roentgen equivalent man, which is the quantity of radiation that produces a physiological effect equivalent to that produced by absorption of one roentgen of gamma or X-radiation.
56. Answer: **D**. According to ANSI Z535.4-1991, in addition to the signal word DANGER, WARNING, or CAUTION, warning labels should be understandable to all potential users. This means they may have to be multilingual. They must include instruction about action to be taken to avoid damage or injury and severity of consequence that might result if the indicated action is not taken. And depending on the product and user, additional information might be required. For example, if the product is designed for the blind, Braille symbols might be needed; if the product may be ingested, an antidote might be included; specific colors or symbols may be required by international standards, etc.
57. Answer: **A**. The main source of heat gain is the body's own internal heat. Called metabolic heat, it is generated within the body by biochemical processes that sustain life and by energy used in physical activity. The body exchanges heat with its surroundings mainly through radiation, convection, and evaporation of sweat.
58. Answer: **B**. CHEMTREC, the acronym for Chemical Transportation Emergency Center, is a 24-hour telephone center operated by the American Chemistry Council that provides assistance in response to hazmat incidents in transportation.
59. Answer: **C**. Since there is no connection between the two structures, heating is probably caused by radiant heat transfer. Conduction occurs when there is a direct contact between two materials (e.g., coffee heats the outside of a cup). Convection heat transfer depends on mixing (e.g., warm air currents in a convection oven). Radiant heat transfer is transmission of thermal energy between objects, as between the sun and Earth; no physical contact needs to take place.
60. Answer: **B**. Epidemiological studies are divided into three separate types:
    - Cross-sectional or prevalence studies
    - Retrospective or case control studies
    - Prospective studies or cohort or incident studies

    Retrospective studies look back in time on populations exposed to the agent under investigation. They are the most inexpensive. However, these studies suffer from lack of data such as what dose was received, for how long, what other agents were present, etc. These questions cannot be answered since exposure occurred in the distant past. They rely heavily on estimated data and experimental statistical methods that affect validity.

    It is generally accepted that the most scientifically useful study is the *prospective* study, which is initiated before commencement of exposure to the agent under study and is continued until appearance of disease. Recently some more progressive major companies have initiated prospective epidemiological studies for all new chemicals introduced into the workplace. The process, however, is quite expensive. Plans must be established well in advance for methods of gathering exposure data, establishing the history of workers, other agent exposure, etc.

    Cross-sectional studies deal with real-time relationships between an agent and infection or disease. They are based on existing relationships and investigate only present-time cases.
61. Answer: **A**. PHA (Preliminary Hazard Analysis) is used to identify apparent hazards very early in pre-design stages. It is a gross hazard search to identify potential problems that may determine the depth of future hazard analysis techniques.
62. Answer: **B**. The concept of accident proneness is rejected today by most progressive safety professionals.
63. Answer: **C**. The Hawthorne studies proved only that people, including workers, respond to attention.
64. Answer: **A**. The Management by Objective (MBO) system is an excellent method for employees and supervision to set goals and rate performance. A key component of an objective is that it must be obtainable.
65. Answer: **C**. The process of job safety analysis examines job hazards during each step of the job and results in improved procedures that almost always increase accident prevention.

66. Answer: **D**. Management can best support any health and safety effort by showing active and sincere interest in the program. This support can take many forms, but it is vitally important that the message that reaches the company floor be consistent and sincere. If the boss really values safety, so, most likely, will the workers. Management is inclined to give support to safety efforts when prevention of losses related to achievement of company objectives is thoroughly understood.

67. Answer: **A**. The four steps in safety sampling are:
    - Prepare a code.
    - Take the sample.
    - Validate the sample.
    - Prepare the report.

    Safety sampling can be a successful method to verify effectiveness of a safety strategy, provided the technique is adapted to the operation, a sound basic incident prevention program is in place, and management is familiar with the technique.

68. Answer: **B**. The discipline of system safety can be applied to almost any system that has interacting components. It is an application of systematic and forward-looking techniques to identify and control hazards. The discipline is most effective if it begins at the conceptual phases of project development and should continue throughout the entire life of the project or product.

69. Answer: **A**. According to Dan Peterson in *Techniques of Safety Management*, there are 10 basic principles of safety. These are:
    - An unsafe act, an unsafe condition, and an accident are all symptoms of something wrong in the management system.
    - We can predict that certain sets of circumstances will prevent severe injuries. The circumstances can be identified and controlled.
    - Safety should be managed like any other company function. Management should direct the safety effort by setting achievable goals and by planning, organizing, and controlling to achieve them.
    - The key to effective line safety performance is management procedures that affix accountability.
    - The function of safety is to locate and define the operational errors that allow accidents to occur.
    - The causes of unsafe behavior can be identified and classified.
    - In most cases, unsafe behavior is normal human behavior, a result of people reacting to their environment.
    - There are three major subsystems that must be dealt with in building an effective safety system: (1) physical, (2) managerial, and (3) behavioral.
    - The safety system should fit the culture of the organization.
    - There is no one right way to achieve safety in an organization; however, for a safety system to be effective, it must meet certain criteria.

    Reproduced from Petersen, D. (1998). Safety Management: A Human Approach. (2nd ed.). Des Plaines, Illinois: American Society of Safety Professionals

70. Answer: **D**. Incidence rate is the rate of development of *new cases* of a specific disease over a given time period.

71. Answer: **D**. The OSHA DART is useful in industrial safety work as an indicator of an accident frequency rate to compare an organization's accident severity and frequency against other similar industry rates. The least reliable method is to use lost workday cases.

72. Answer: **C**.

    $$\text{RATE} = \frac{\text{recordables} \times 200{,}000}{\text{total hours worked}}$$

    $$\text{RATE} = \frac{33 \times 200{,}000}{1{,}909{,}910}$$

    $$\text{RATE} = 3.46 \text{ cases}$$

73. Answer: **B**. The OSHA 300 form must be maintained in the workplace for 5 years. Records of investigation must be maintained for 30 years.

74. Answer: **B**. Workers only have the right to contest an abatement date of an OSHA citation; they cannot change an abatement date nor negotiate corrective actions. There are many other "rights" of workers under the OSH Act including, but not limited to, the right to request an inspection and have inspections made by a compliance officer: Section 8 (f). Employees have the right to have the employer maintain an accurate record of exposures to toxic or harmful materials: Section 8 (c)(3). Employees have the right to examine records of their exposure to harmful agents: Section 8 (c)(3). Employees have the right to be notified if he or she has been exposed to harmful agents at or above the PEL: Section 8 (c)(3).
75. Answer: **A**. The training objective must be firmly established before a training program is undertaken. The primary purpose of the objectives is to describe the intended training outcome.
76. Answer: **B**. Although all of the functions listed are very important, the best answer is a written and enforced lock-out procedure.
77. Answer: **D**. The person responsible for performing most of the actions required by the emergency action plan is the line supervisor.
78. Answer: **C**. The Otis-Lennon Mental Ability Test, often referred to as the *Otis test*, is used extensively in IQ testing. There is, and has been, huge controversy within the educational community concerning the use of this type of testing. The controversy is multifaceted and involves test content, methods used in test administration, methods used in test scoring, etc. The generally accepted premise in industrial safety work is that cognitive ability tests such as the Otis test are **not** reliable indicators of an employee's ability to do well in industrial or safety training efforts.
79. Answer: **D**. The supervisor controls most immediate and many amelioration actions.
80. Answer: **A**. The leading cause of fires in the United States is electrical (22%), generally related to wiring and motors. Smoking accounts for 9% of all industrial fires and hot surfaces are responsible for 9%. Some sources also list fires maliciously set by intruders, juveniles, unhappy employees, etc. These fires account for 10% of all industrial fires in the United States. The CSP examinations have historically not included this category.
81. Answer: **D**. OSHA Standard 1910.1000 is a performance standard that deals with more than one industry, which also makes it a horizontal standard.
82. Answer: **B**. The definition of arbitration is "the settlement of a dispute by a person or persons chosen to hear both sides and come to a decision."

Webster's New World College Dictionary, Fifth Edition Copyright © 2014 by Houghton Mifflin Harcourt Publishing Company.

83. Answer: **D**. Computers must follow programmed instructions. They have no inductive capability and cannot perform complex tasks that require subjective decision-making. They are very good at routine, repetitive tasks and mathematical calculations.
84. Answer: **D**. Training objectives should above all be reasonable, measurable, and obtainable. It is very desirable, but not imperative, that objectives and goals for any program be written so as not to be misplaced or relegated to a low priority.
85. Answer: **A**. There are many attributes that complement a successful trainer or educator. Some of these attributes are more important than others. The motivation of students and their level of sophistication will determine to a great extent which attribute is the most important. In an industrial setting, appearance is generally considered of less importance than the desire to instruct, knowledge of subject, and presentation style. This is not to imply that appearance is unimportant, just that it has less impact on the learning process.
86. Answer: **C**. Job performance is the most effective and final measure of any training program.
87. Answer: **C**. No oral communications take place unless someone listens. To be effective leaders and make valid decisions, professionals must be skillful listeners.
88. Answer: **B**. The interaction between two people is different than what takes place between three or more. The larger the group, the more relationships there are to maintain.
89. Answer: **A**. One of the major disadvantages of the lecture is that there is limited audience participation. The major advantage is that it is the most efficient way to teach knowledge-level objectives to train a large group in one setting.

90. Answer: **D**. The formula to calculate incident rate is recordable accidents times 200,000 divided by total man-hours worked. This formula yields the rate of injuries per hundred full-time workers.

$$\frac{20 \times 200,000}{1,750,000} = 2.29$$

91. Answer: **B**. Select formula and solve

$$\text{Accident Rate} = \frac{\text{Cases} \times 200,000}{\text{Total hours worked}}$$

$$AR = \frac{36 \times 200,000}{850 \times 2000}$$

$$AR = \frac{7,200,000}{1,700,000} = 4.23$$

92. Answer: **D**. First-aid treatment is defined by OSHA (1974) as "any one-time treatment, and any follow-up visit for the purpose of observation of minor scratches, cuts, burns, splinters, and so forth, which do not ordinarily require medical care. Such one-time treatment, and follow-up visit for the purpose of observation, is considered first-aid even though provided by a physician or registered professional personnel."

93. Answer: **B**. The ERPG-3 is the maximum airborne concentration below which it is believed nearly all individuals could be exposed for up to one hour without experiencing or developing life-threatening health effects.

    The ERPG-2 is the maximum airborne concentration below which it is believed nearly all individuals could be exposed for up to one hour without experiencing or developing irreversible or other serious health effects or symptoms that could impair their abilities to take protective action.

    The ERPG-1 is the maximum airborne concentration below which it is believed nearly all individuals could be exposed up to one hour without experiencing other than mild transient adverse health effects or perceiving a clearly defined objectionable odor. Because human responses do not occur at precise exposure levels, they can extend over a wide range of concentrations.

94. Answer: **C**. Making quality presentations requires an attitude and appearance of being in control of the situation and having a high level of knowledge of all the material being presented. A dark conservative business dress style is accepted as the highest and most powerful dress code for a presentation. Being nervous and having excess hand and body motions show lack of control. Generally, memorized material is perceived as boring or unimportant and a high-pitched voice indicates that the instructor may be stressed.

95. Answer: **A**. SQL is the abbreviation for Structured Query Language. It is a standardized application language for relational databases that is used to enter data into a database, modify data, delete data, and retrieve data.
    URL is the abbreviation of Uniform Resource Locator, the global address of documents and other resources on the World Wide Web.
    HTML stands for Hyper Text Markup Language and is used for web publishing.
    HTTP stands for Hyper Text Transfer Protocol and is a file transfer protocol.

96. Answer: **D**. There are three things that will hinder a person from active listening: word barriers such as *death, liar, layoff, IRS*, etc.; emotional barriers such as bias, boredom, envy, fatigue, etc.; and distractions.

97. Answer: **B**. Group techniques encourage participation from a selected audience. These methods allow trainees to share ideas, evaluate information, and become actively involved in planning and implementation of company policy.

98. Answer: **C**. According to the NSC, communications is defined as "sharing information and/or ideas with others and being understood."

99. Answer: **D**. The ASME Code calls for 150% of the *maximum operating pressure*.

100. Answer: **C**.
   - *Movable-barrier* devices protect the operator by enclosing the point of operation before a press stroke begins.
   - *Two-hand tripping* devices or *two-hand control* devices require concurrent application of both operator control buttons to activate the machine, thus keeping the operator's hands a safe distance from the danger area while the machine completes its closing cycle.
   - *Presence-sensing* devices create a sensing field or area that deactivates the press when an operator's hand or any other body part is within the field or area. These devices can be photoelectric (optical), radio frequency (capacitance), or electromechanical.
   - *Pullback* devices utilize a series of cables attached to the operator's hands, wrists, and/or arms. When the slide/ram is up between cycles, the operator can access the point of operation. When the slide/ram begins to cycle by starting its descent, a mechanical linkage automatically withdraws the operator's hands from the point of operation. Because of the variations in the sizes of operators' hands and varying characteristics of different dies, the pullback device must be adjusted for each operator and after each change of die.
   - *Restraints* (wrist straps and fully anchored cords or cables) can also be used to prevent the operator from reaching into the point of operation at any time and must also be adjusted for each operator.

Self-Assessment Exam 4 Questions

1. **The term *anhydrous* in anhydrous ammonia means:**

   A. 100% pure.
   B. without impurities.
   C. without water.
   D. hospital grade.

2. **The specific gravity of water is:**

   A. equal to 1.
   B. 5.
   C. 1.
   D. 5 to 1.

3. **A load is to be suspended by a three-point sling. The weight to be lifted is 10,000 pounds. The slings have a 30,000-pound breaking strength (your company requires a safety factor of 5). Sling angle to load is 50 degrees. Can the load be lifted?**

   A. No, it is out of limits by more than 20%.
   B. No, it is out of limits by 10%.
   C. Yes, it is within limits by 20%.
   D. Yes, it is within limits by 40%.

4. **Which of the following laws specify that gases behave consistently with temperature changes?**

   A. Charles's Law
   B. Boyle's Law
   C. Newton's Law
   D. Dalton's Law

5. A maintenance worker is using a torch to cut the end from a small steel tank. Assume the pressure in the sealed tank is increased four times as a result of heating. If the original temperature was 45 degrees Celsius, what is the new temperature?

   A. 45°K
   B. 1272°K
   C. 555°R
   D. 1450°K

6. Given a velocity pressure reading of 0.50 in a circular duct, determine the velocity in feet per minute.

   A. 2832 fpm
   B. 27 fpm
   C. 2800 fpm
   D. 1234 fpm

7. The evaluation of tasks involving steps, hazards, and solutions is *best* described by:

   A. System Safety Analysis (SSA).
   B. Fault Tree Analysis (FTA).
   C. Management Oversight and Risk Tree (MORT).
   D. Job Safety Analysis (JSA).

8. A 10-foot beam is supported on each end and loaded at 30 pounds per foot (300 pounds, total weight). Determine the moment.

   A. 900 foot-lbs
   B. 1200 foot-lbs
   C. 1500 foot-lbs
   D. 3000 foot-lbs

9. An empty handcart weighs 200 pounds; coefficient of friction is 0.045. Determine the weight the cart can transport with a 20-pound pushing force. $F = \mu N$

   A. 340 lbs
   B. 244 lbs
   C. 348 lbs
   D. 20 lbs

10. Which of the following is *not* a halogen?

    A. Astatine
    B. Bromine
    C. Chlorine
    D. Neon

11. The vertical grouping of elements in the periodic table is called a _____.

    A. transition
    B. family
    C. period
    D. metaloid

12. In ventilation work, TP, or total pressure, is:

    A. the difference between SP and VP.
    B. normally positive on the suction side.
    C. measured parallel to the axis of flow.
    D. the product of SP and VP.

13. The Poisson distribution is used when the occurrences of an event are small, but the number of cases is large enough to assure a few occurrences.

    A. True
    B. False
    C. Need standard deviation to calculate
    D. Not enough information

14. What is the audible range for an average young person with unimpaired hearing?

    A. Below 20 Hz
    B. Above 20,000 Hz
    C. Between 20 and 20,000 Hz
    D. Between 50 and 30,000 Hz

15. The three layers of skin are:

    A. hair follicles, capillary, and muscle.
    B. epidermis, dermis, and subcutaneous.
    C. id, ego, and superego.
    D. cuticle, blood vessel, and muscle.

16. The basis for operation of *most* hydraulic and pneumatic systems is related to which law?

    A. Boyle's Law
    B. Newton's Law
    C. Charles's Law
    D. Pascal's Law

17. On December 6, 1991, the Occupational Safety and Health Administration (OSHA) originally promulgated the Occupational Exposure to Bloodborne Pathogens Standard (29 CFR 1910.1030). Which of the following *best* describes the term "universal precautions" as defined in the OSHA standard?

    A. Precautions taken for spilled blood
    B. Treat all blood as if it were infectious
    C. Define rules for cleanup
    D. Define all body fluids and substances as infectious

18. What is the force required at point A?

    A. 100 lbs
    B. 133 lbs
    C. 660 lbs
    D. 800 lbs

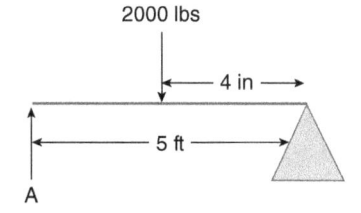

    Figure 51 Mechanical Advantage

19. What physical characteristic allows a lead oxide particle to settle more rapidly than a silica particle?

    A. Shape
    B. Size
    C. Density
    D. Electrostatic charge

20. A white light entering a triangular prism would be refracted downward and separated into the colors of the spectrum. Which color would be refracted *most*?

   A. Red
   B. Orange
   C. Blue
   D. Violet

21. Using the illustrated chart below, determine the length of time per hour a worker could consistently produce work requiring effort at a 400 kcal/hr level with a WBGT heat load of 25°C.

   A. 15 min/hr
   B. 30 min/hr
   C. 45 min/hr
   D. 60 min/hr

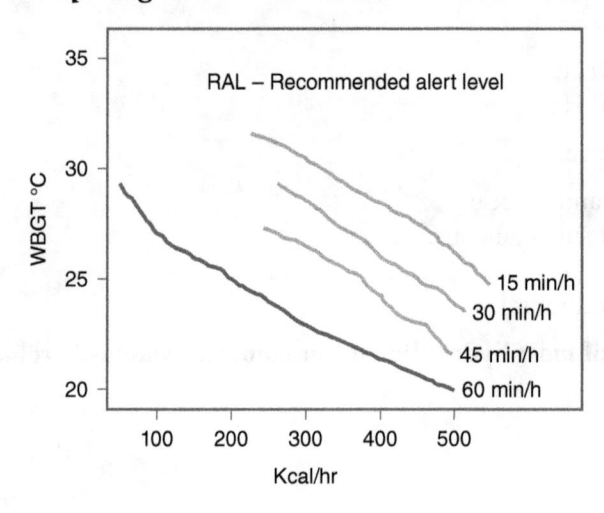

Figure 52 Metabolic Heat Load

22. A calorie is defined as the amount of heat required to raise the temperature of one kilogram of water by _____.

   A. 1 degree F
   B. 1 degree K
   C. 1 degree C
   D. 1 degree R

23. Tensile strength is defined as:

   A. the capacity of a material or structure to withstand loads tending to reduce size.
   B. the maximum stress that a material can withstand while being stretched or pulled before failing or breaking.
   C. behavior of solid objects subject to stresses and strains.
   D. the stress at which a material begins to deform plastically.

24. Given the following atomic weights: O = 16, H = 1, C = 12, how many ft³ of oxygen are necessary to burn 10 ft³ of C_2H_6 gas using the reaction:

$$2C_6H_6 + 14O_2 \rightarrow 4CO_2 + 6H_2O$$

   A. 25
   B. 50
   C. 70
   D. 100

25. **A curie is defined as:**
    A. one curie weighs 3.7×10^{10} grams.
    B. one curie is the radioactivity of one gram of polonium.
    C. one curie is the radioactivity of one gram of radium.
    D. one curie is the amount of radiation that can be absorbed by a normal healthy person without long-lasting adverse effects.

26. **The responsibility for promulgation of OSHA standards falls to:**
    A. the Secretary of Labor.
    B. OSHRC.
    C. NIOSH.
    D. OSHA.

27. **The governmental agency with jurisdiction over the shipment of materials between states and that sets rules and regulations concerning those shipments is the:**
    A. Interstate Commerce Commission.
    B. Department of Transportation.
    C. National Highway Safety Commission.
    D. Highway Safety Administration.

28. **To determine the cause or causes of any mishap or series of mishaps in order to prevent further incidents of a similar kind is:**
    A. performance analysis.
    B. to use the OSHA 300 log.
    C. baseline analysis.
    D. accident analysis.

29. **Accident costs are generally divided into two areas, which are:**
    A. budgeted and nonbudgeted.
    B. insured and uninsured.
    C. direct and indirect.
    D. direct and uninsured.

30. **Often in safety work, certain supervisors are called "Key Persons." This reference would *best* apply to which of the following?**
    A. Company president
    B. Mid-level supervision
    C. Chief Executive Officer
    D. Line manager

31. **Sources of information that might be used for injury accident analysis include all of the following *except*:**
    A. first-aid reports.
    B. an insurance rate table.
    C. a first report of injury form.
    D. a supervisor accident investigation.

32. **Accidents are usually the result of:**
    A. personality factors.
    B. environmental factors.
    C. physical limitations.
    D. a combination of all the factors listed.

33. Project management is the process and activity of planning, organizing, motivating, and controlling resources, procedures, and protocols. The work that must be performed is called:

    A. the project schedule.
    B. the project scope.
    C. program evaluation.
    D. the project evaluation management plan.

34. Prior to the passage of worker's compensation laws, workers were often provided limited injury benefits due to the doctrine of contributory negligence. This doctrine stated that the:

    A. company would pay for all mistakes.
    B. worker was always wrong.
    C. worker assumed responsibility for accidents.
    D. responsibility for negligence was shared.

35. An OSHA compliance officer has issued a citation to a company for not having a guard in place on a power saw while performing custom work. How much time does the company have to contest the citation?

    A. 1 day
    B. 7 working days
    C. 15 working days
    D. 30 calendar days

36. Many NIOSH employees are commissioned officers in which of the following organizations?

    A. American Federal Health Officers Association
    B. United States Coast Guard
    C. Public Health Service
    D. American Medical Association

37. A Root Cause Analysis report contains all the following *except* information on:

    A. negligent individuals.
    B. identification of problem areas.
    C. underlying causes.
    D. recommended corrective actions.

38. Which of the following statements is *correct* according to McGregor's Theory X and Theory Y?

    A. Theory X assumes the worker is essentially uninterested and unmotivated to work.
    B. Theory Y assumes the worker is essentially uninterested and unmotivated to work.
    C. Theory X assumes the worker is basically interested but unmotivated to work.
    D. Theory Y assumes the worker is basically uninterested but motivated to work.

39. The agency responsible for the reduction of injuries, deaths, and economic losses resulting from traffic accidents is:

    A. UNLV.
    B. ICC.
    C. NHTSA.
    D. DOT.

40. All of the following actions are required of a company that receives an OSHA citation *except*:

    A. paying the fine.
    B. paying the fine and posting notice of violation.
    C. correcting the violation.
    D. retraining all employees.

41. The Federal Motor Vehicle Safety Standards developed and issued by the U.S. Department of Transportation are designed to accomplish all of the following *except*:

   A. to provide a safe, fuel-efficient vehicle.
   B. to prevent crashes.
   C. to reduce injury severity.
   D. to minimize damage following crashes.

42. The recommended way to deal with minor infractions of operational safety rules is to:

   A. provide an oral reprimand.
   B. issue a written reprimand.
   C. ignore the infractions or violations.
   D. suspend guilty workers.

43. Routes of entry for exposure to a toxic are:

   A. inhalation, skin absorption, and ingestion.
   B. inhalation, capillary absorption, and intravenous.
   C. inhalation, respiration, and breathing.
   D. inhalation, skin absorption, and eating.

44. Which of the following *best* describes the term *TLV-STEL*?

   A. A concentration that should never be exceeded
   B. A dose permitted for a 30-minute exposure
   C. A level generally below the TLV-TWA
   D. A level for rescue workers

45. The A-weighted sound-level measurement is used as the "standard" scale in occupational noise measurement because:

   A. it weights intermittent and impact noise.
   B. weighing is related to effects of noise on the ears.
   C. it filters out "white" noise.
   D. it has a built-in dose-response curve.

46. Boiling point is *best* described by which of the following?

   A. Transition of a substance directly from the solid to the gas phase
   B. Lowest temperature at which a substance can vaporize to form an ignitable mixture
   C. When vapor pressure of a liquid is greater than the atmospheric pressure
   D. The phase change from liquid to a solid

47. The testing and approval of any respiratory protection devices is done by:

   A. ANSI.
   B. OSHA.
   C. DOT.
   D. NIOSH.

48. The purpose of local exhaust ventilation in industrial settings is to:

   A. prevent any entrance of air contaminants.
   B. remove contaminants at their source.
   C. provide dilution ventilation.
   D. provide spot ventilation for comfort.

49. A company has purchased a used vehicle with a very high noise level. This vehicle is operated over the road for extended periods of time. Which device should be selected for monitoring the noise exposure of vehicle operators?

   A. Sound-level meter
   B. Octave-band analyzer
   C. Noise dosimeter
   D. Annual audiogram

50. Given equal thickness, which of the following matter would be the *most* effective shield for gamma radiation?

   A. Concrete
   B. Water
   C. Red iron
   D. Lead

51. Which of the following diseases have, in the past, been known as "potter's rot" and "stonemason's disease"?

   A. Silicosis
   B. Fibrous mitosis
   C. Eczema
   D. Asbestosis

52. For which of the following applications is the use of a pitot tube measuring device suggested?

   A. Checking airflow in a vent hood
   B. Flow testing a fire hydrant
   C. Checking the particulate count on an electrostatic precipitator
   D. Determining flow through a cyclone scrubber

53. Which of the following chemicals is *not* being used as a solvent in the operation described?

   A. Alcohols in paint cleanup
   B. Ketones in spray painting
   C. Hydrocarbons in metal cleaning
   D. Epoxies in core making in foundries

54. The eye contains all of the following *except*:

   A. rods and cones.
   B. a cochlea.
   C. a cornea.
   D. a retina.

55. The *most* economical method of treating acidic industrial waste with a pH of 2 or less is:

   A. dilution to raise the pH.
   B. use of a stabilization pond.
   C. neutralization.
   D. oxygenation.

56. To be classified as a fiber, the aspect ratio (length to diameter) must be greater than:

   A. 1 to 1.
   B. 2 to 1.
   C. 3 to 1.
   D. 4 to 1.

57. In electroplating processes using chromium, the *most* prevalent danger is:

    A. mists of chromic acid.
    B. splashes of acid.
    C. high-voltage electrical currents.
    D. extremely slippery floors.

58. Which of the following sound frequency ranges is generally considered to be the *most* harmful to hearing, especially in the speech range?

    A. 37.5–500 Hz
    B. 1000–4000 Hz
    C. 8000–16,000 Hz
    D. 16,000–32,000 Hz

59. The leading causative agent for fish kills in streams is:

    A. depletion of oxygen.
    B. lack of a food supply.
    C. the toxic effects of pollutants.
    D. increased temperature of the water.

60. Air sampling is frequently performed to determine effectiveness of dust control measures. Not all dust created poses a health hazard and generally measurements of dust deal with that fraction of dust that causes pneumoconiosis. Which of the following correctly indicates the size of dust particles that are deposited and retained by the lungs?

    A. 1 to 10 μm
    B. 5 to 10 μm
    C. 1 to 5 μm
    D. 1 to 15 mm

61. The *best* description of the medical condition of *emphysema* is:

    A. fluid in the lungs.
    B. an abscess in the lungs.
    C. scarring in the lungs.
    D. expanded or ruptured alveoli.

62. Which of the following rules involving parking of a commercial vehicle transporting hazardous materials (Explosives "A" or Explosives "B") is *not* true?

    A. The vehicle may not normally be parked within 300 feet of a bridge.
    B. The vehicle can be left unattended in a safe haven.
    C. The driver can have someone watch the vehicle when parked on a public street.
    D. The vehicle must not be parked within 5 feet of the traveled section of a roadway.

63. Which of the following is an unacceptable method of protecting an employee from a radiant heat source?

    A. Reducing the temperature of an infrared source
    B. Providing infrared shadows
    C. Using reflecting protective equipment
    D. Increasing ventilation

64. Which of the following is a term used to describe the condition *epicondylitis*?

    A. Trigger finger
    B. Rotator cuff
    C. Roofer's wrist
    D. Carpenter's elbow

65. If an ionizing radiation shield consists of three half-value layers, how much radiation will pass through the shielding from a 1800-mR source?

    A. 900 mR
    B. 450 mR
    C. 225 mR
    D. 125 mR

66. Which of the following statements is *most* correct concerning the National Institute for Occupational Safety and Health (NIOSH)?

    A. NIOSH is assigned under OSHA.
    B. OSHA is assigned under NIOSH.
    C. NIOSH reports to HHS.
    D. PHS reports to NIOSH.

67. In reference to electrical equipment, the term *explosion proof* means capable of:

    A. containing internal arcs.
    B. venting hot gases.
    C. use in gasoline fume areas.
    D. containing internal explosions.

68. Which of the following NFPA standards deals with fire extinguishers?

    A. NFPA 10
    B. NFPA 70
    C. NFPA 13
    D. NFPA 30

69. In general, there are three classifications or varieties of safeguards: fixed guards, interlocking guards, and _____.

    A. adjustable
    B. electrical
    C. mechanical
    D. automatic

70. The main reason for enclosing a grinding wheel is to:

    A. maintain the collection system.
    B. contain parts should the wheel shatter.
    C. support the tool rest.
    D. prevent the wheel from breaking.

71. What is the standards organization for boilers and pressure vessels?

    A. ANSI
    B. ASME
    C. UL
    D. ASSP

72. The proper angle for a portable straight ladder is _____ feet vertical to _____ feet horizontal.

    A. 12; 6
    B. 12; 5
    C. 12; 4
    D. 12; t3

73. A room designed for recharging lead-acid batteries requires all of the following *except*:

  A. an eyewash/safety shower.
  B. ventilation.
  C. facilities to neutralize acid.
  D. pressure-relief panels.

74. Forklift operators should keep the tines of the forks approximately what distance above the traveling surface?

  A. 2 inches
  B. 4 inches
  C. 6 inches
  D. 8 inches

75. Which ANSI standard deals with accident reporting?

  A. ANSI Z16.1
  B. ANSI Z87.1
  C. ANSI Z12.1
  D. ANSI Z358.1

76. There are *no* established safety specifications for which of the following?

  A. Bump caps
  B. Safety spectacles
  C. Respiratory protection
  D. Boilers

77. Which color identifies major moving machine parts?

  A. Red
  B. Magenta
  C. Green
  D. Orange

78. What is the distance above the ground when guardrails and toeboards are required for any construction scaffolding platform?

  A. 5 feet
  B. 8 feet
  C. 10 feet
  D. 12 feet

79. Power presses are normally equipped with _____.

  A. barrier guards
  B. remote controls
  C. sensing circuits
  D. location guards

80. Which of the following organizations regulates PITs?

  A. OSHA
  B. DOT
  C. ASME
  D. ASTM

81. Which of the following elements determine the safety factor for natural fiber rope?

    A. Size of rope, material, and tensile strength
    B. Type of fiber and strength
    C. Environmental factors and size
    D. Use and exposure data

82. When inspecting a hoisting and lifting chain hook, the measurement between the shank and the narrowest point of the hook opening (throat) should *not* exceed what percent of the original dimension?

    A. 20%
    B. 10%
    C. 15%
    D. 5%

83. Safeguarding of power transmission parts involves the principle of covering all moving parts in such a manner that no part of the body can come in contact with any moving part. Within the industrial safety community it is widely accepted that moving parts _____ or less from the floor must be guarded.

    A. 9 feet
    B. 7 feet
    C. 8 feet
    D. 10 feet

84. A gantry crane equipped with a hoist and hook block is reeved with six parts of cable. The crane is lifting a load of 16 tons. What is the load on the haul line (discount friction)?

    A. 2225 lbs
    B. 5333 lbs
    C. 9370 lbs
    D. 24,000 lbs

85. A paint spray booth has a 5-foot by 5-foot flanged exhaust duct opening that is fed by a 16-inch circular duct. If the velocity of airflow measured at the face of the flanged opening is 120 fpm, what is the approximate velocity of air flowing in the duct?

    A. 2150 fpm
    B. 3000 fpm
    C. 1230 fpm
    D. 1843 fpm

86. Which of the following situations has the greatest chance of igniting?

    A. Wood chips stored alone
    B. Wood stored against a heating duct
    C. Saw dust stored with wood chips
    D. Pressure-treated lumber

87. Which of following metals is flammable?

    A. Aluminum
    B. Magnesium
    C. Molybdenum
    D. Iron

88. The reason acetylene cylinders are stored in an upright position is:
   A. to prevent liquid acetone from escaping.
   B. to allow the bottle to be properly secured.
   C. to prevent liquid acetylene from escaping.
   D. None of the responses listed is correct.

89. To determine the correct fire-suppression agent for a fire involving a combustible metal used in the plant, which agent should be chosen?
   A. Green triangle with an A in the center
   B. Red square with a B in the center
   C. Blue circle with a C in the center
   D. Yellow star with a D in the center

90. A deserted chemical dump site is discovered on company property where leaking containers of perchloric acid, ether, and other unidentified chemicals are observed. What is the appropriate action to be taken?
   A. Segregate chemicals by hand.
   B. Call an experienced Hazmat team.
   C. Call the EOD team.
   D. Remove the chemicals to safe storage.

91. Without proper storage, which one of the following chemicals would be considered to have significant dangerous properties?
   A. Nitric acid
   B. Trichloroethylene
   C. Perchloric acid
   D. Orthodichlorobenzene

92. A paint spray booth is classified as a Class I, Div 1 Hazardous Location. What is the proper classification for the paint storage area where paint is dispensed to a spray gun reservoir?
   A. Class I, Div. 1
   B. Class I, Div. 2
   C. Class II, Div. 1
   D. Class II, Div. 2

93. The *most* economical method of preventing corrosion of an elevated fire water tank is to:
   A. install a fiberglass tank.
   B. circulate the water.
   C. double-insulate the tank and ground it.
   D. install cathodic protection.

94. Which article of the National Electrical Code deals with hazardous locations?
   A. Article 407
   B. Article 101
   C. Article 20
   D. Article 500

95. The specific heat of a material is determined by measuring:
   A. heat flow and caloric transfer.
   B. the heat capacity per unit mass of a material.
   C. thermal conductivity.
   D. thermal expansion, time, and distance.

288 ASP Exam Study Workbook

96. **Which of the following is the ideal flash point for an industrial cleaning solvent?**
    A. 73 degrees F
    B. 90 degrees F
    C. 140 degrees F
    D. 120 degrees F

97. **All of the following compressed cylinders require safety relief devices *except*:**
    A. oxygen.
    B. nitrogen.
    C. poison-A.
    D. argon.

98. **How frequently does a water fire extinguisher require hydrostatic testing? Every:**
    A. year.
    B. 3 years.
    C. 5 years.
    D. 7 years.

99. **Which of the following refers to the process of bonding a flammable liquid dispensing can?**
    A. Connecting the can to a grounding rod
    B. Connecting the can to a grounding strap
    C. Connecting the can to the equipment ground
    D. Connecting the can to other conductive objects

100. **When experiencing a natural disaster, ERPs usually call for which of the following as the first consideration?**
    A. Turn the responsibility over to authorities for protection of resources.
    B. Safeguard people and abandon systems.
    C. Shut down processes involving hazardous/toxic materials.
    D. Safeguard both personnel and equipment/processes.

Self-Assessment Exam 4 Answers

1. Answer: **C**. Anhydrous means without water.
2. Answer: **C**. Specific gravity (sp. gr.) is the weight ratio of a certain volume of liquid or solid as compared to the weight of an equal volume of water.
3. Answer: **B**. Double divided slings are SIN full. Divide the load by two and then divide by the SIN of the angle.

$$10,000 \div 2 \div \sin 50 = 6527 \text{ lbs}$$

    The third leg on the sling is not considered because if the load should shift (which it certainly must, with only three legs) the entire weight of the load will be carried by the remaining two sling legs.
4. Answer: **A**. Gases behave consistently with temperature changes. This is stated in Charles's Law: At a constant pressure, the volume of a confined gas varies directly as the absolute temperature; and at a constant volume, the pressure varies directly as the absolute temperature.
   Note the use of absolute temperature!
5. Answer: **B**.

$$t_{°C} = \frac{(t_{°F} - 32)}{1.8}$$

$$t_{°K} = t_{°C} + 273$$

$$t_{°R} = t_{°F} + 460$$

$$\frac{P_1}{T_1} = \frac{P_2}{T_2}$$

$$\frac{1}{318} = \frac{4}{T_2}$$

$$T_2 = 1272$$

6. Answer: **A**.

   $V = 4005 \sqrt{VP}$

   $V = 4005 \times \sqrt{.50}$

   $V = 4005 \times 0.7071$

   $V = 2832$ ft per min

7. Answer: **D**. Job safety analysis is a systematic analysis of job elements. It results in an in-depth evaluation by workers and first-line supervisors of individual steps and hazards. SAs also offer protective measures or solutions to identified hazards. Option A (System Safety Analysis) is a broad term covering all of the various system safety tools used in the analysis of system risk. Option B, Fault Tree Analysis, is the process of using deductive logic to determine the combination of events that caused a hazardous event to occur. It normally is accompanied by a companion report that evaluates the overall likelihood of failure and provides solutions to findings discovered in FTA. Option C, MORT, Management Oversight and Risk Tree, is a formal decision tree used in the evaluation of safety programs or as an accident investigation tool. The tool is exhaustive, offering about 1500 events to be evaluated. For this reason it is often considered overkill for all but the largest evaluations or mishaps. However, the system logic is sound and recently several practitioners have produced "mini-MORT" charts that have proven to be useful tools for smaller applications.

8. Answer: **C**. An equally loaded beam represents the same loading as a single load located in the middle of the beam. The moment must be measured from one of the support points.

   $M =$ Weight $\times$ Distance

   $M = 300 \times 5$ ft $= 1500$ ft-lbs

9. Answer: **B**. Force to move the cart = the force of friction times the weight of the cart plus the load (n). This is the weight that can be moved with a 20-pound pushing force. This weight includes the load and the cart. To determine load, subtract out the cart:

   $W = N -$ cart $\qquad\qquad F = \mu N$

   $W = 444 - 200 = 244$ lbs $\qquad 20 = 0.045 \times N$

   $\qquad\qquad\qquad\qquad\qquad\qquad 20 = \frac{20}{0.045} = 444$ lbs

10. Answer: **D**. Neon is the obvious and correct choice.
11. Answer: **B**. Vertical groupings are families and horizontal groupings are periods.
12. Answer: **C**. Total pressure is measured parallel to the direction of flow.
13. Answer: **A**. A Poisson distribution is useful when dealing with repeated or multiple accident events. For example, it may be used over a period of time where a worker may have more than one accident in a year or where the same type of accident may reoccur.
14. Answer: **C**. Below 20 Hz is subaudible; above 20,000 is ultrasonic. The average measured hearing range of an unimpaired person is 20–20,000 Hz.
15. Answer: **B**. The three layers of skin are the epidermis (outer layer), the dermis (true skin), and the subcutaneous tissue.
16. Answer: **D**. Pascal's Law is the basis of operation of most hydraulic and pneumatic systems. This law is stated as follows: Pressure applied upon a confined fluid is transmitted equally in all directions.

17. Answer: **B**. "Universal Precautions" is OSHA's required method of control to protect employees from exposure to all human blood and OPIM (defined below). The term *Universal Precautions* refers to a concept of blood-borne disease control, which requires that all human blood and certain human body fluids be treated as if known to be infectious for HIV, HBV, and other blood-borne pathogens. Universal Precautions are not limited to PPE, but also include sharps management and contaminated equipment management procedures. Selection D, *defines all body fluids and substances as infectious*, is more descriptive of the concept of Body Substance Isolation (BSI), which is an allowed control method and defines all body fluids and substances as infectious.

    OPIM is defined as the following human body fluids: saliva in dental procedures, semen, vaginal secretions, cerebrospinal, synovial, pleural, pericardial, peritoneal, and amniotic fluids; body fluids visibly contaminated with blood, along with all body fluid in situations where it is difficult or impossible to differentiate between body fluids; unfixed human tissues or organs (other than intact skin); HIV-containing cell or tissue cultures, organ cultures, and HIV- or HBV-containing culture media or other solutions; and blood, organs, or other tissues from experimental animals infected with HIV or HBV.

18. Answer: **B**.
    Step 1 Draw a diagram.

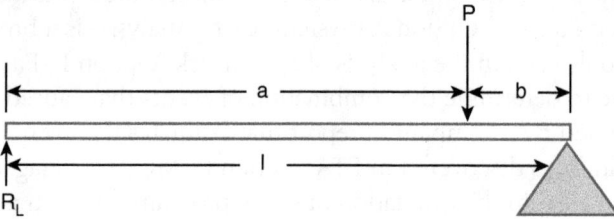

    Figure 53 Mechanical advantage 2

    Step 2 Select a formula and solve.

    Alternate Solution
    Use the mechanical advantage of 15 offered by the difference of 5 feet to 0.33 feet to calculate force needed.

    $$R_L = \frac{Pb}{l}$$

    $$R_L = \frac{2000 \times 0.33}{5} = \frac{660}{5} = 132 \text{ lbs}$$

    $$A = \frac{\text{force}}{\text{MA}}$$

    $$A = \frac{2000}{15} = 133 \text{ lbs}$$

19. Answer: **C**. Settling velocity is directly proportional to particle density. Which is more dense: lead or silica?

20. Answer: **D**. A beam of white light entering a triangular prism results in separation of colors. Light is dispersed into colors by a prism because the different frequencies travel at different speeds in the glass. Red refracts least and violet refracts most. The range can be remembered by "ROY G BIV," red, orange, yellow, green, blue, indigo, and violet.
    Note: The heat produced by different colors of light is directly proportional to frequency (i.e., the higher the frequency, the more heat produced). Thus, if the light from a prism falls on an absorbing material, violet light would produce the most heat and red light would produce the least.

21. Answer: **C**.

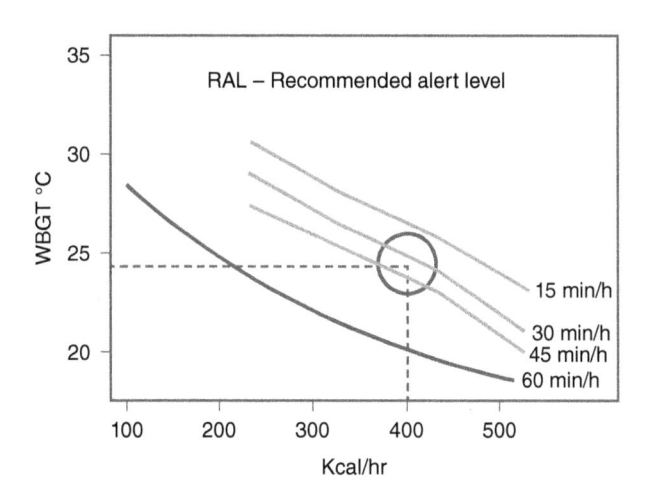

Figure 54 Metabolic heat load 2

22. Answer: **C**. The calorie is the amount of heat required to raise the temperature of one gram of water one degree Celsius.
23. Answer: **B**. The tensile strength is the same as the breaking strength of a material when exposed to a stretching force.
24. Answer: **C**. The balanced formula indicates that the ratio of oxygen to ethane is 7:1 because in the formula there are 14 moles of oxygen and only 2 moles of ethane. Therefore, it would take 70 cubic feet of oxygen to burn 10 cubic feet of ethane.
25. Answer: **C**. A curie is defined as the measure at which a radioactive material emits particles. The curie was named for Pierre and Marie Curie, who discovered several elements, including radium, radon, and polonium. The radioactivity of one gram of radium is a curie.
26. Answer: **A**. The Secretary of Labor promulgates OSHA standards.
27. Answer: **B**. The Department of Transportation (DOT) is concerned with the shipment of materials between states. The Interstate Commerce Commission regulates the buying and selling of goods, especially when done on a large scale between cities or states. The key words are *shipment of materials*.
28. Answer: **D**. The goal of accident analysis is to uncover problem areas.
29. Answer: **C**. Accident costs have for many years been divided into direct and indirect costs. Direct costs are those costs directly and often immediately associated with accidents, such as transportation of the injured, medical services, days lost from work, etc. Indirect costs include lost production, replacement of injured workers, replacement worker training cost, etc.
30. Answer: **B**. Mid-level supervisors are often referred to as key persons in safety terminology.
31. Answer: **B**. The insurance rate table provides little or no useful information for analysis of accidents because it is most often based on past experience.
32. Answer: **D**. Accidents are usually multicausal in nature and cannot be attributed entirely to any single factor.
33. Answer: **B**. This is the definition of a project scope. A program evaluation is similar to an audit and is defined as a measurement of results against accepted criteria.
34. Answer: **C**. Prior to enactment of workers' compensation laws, only one means existed by which a worker could receive compensation for an injury resulting from employment. This was to prove that the employer's negligence had been the entire cause of the employee's injury. If there had been contributory negligence, no employee benefits were granted. Workers could expect no damages if they had been negligent to any extent, no matter how minor.
35. Answer: **C**. The citation must be contested within the 15-working-day period. If not, the citation becomes final and can no longer be appealed.

36. Answer: **C**. Some NIOSH employees are also commissioned officers in the Public Health Service.
37. Answer: **A**. The report summarizes the underlying causes and their relative contributions, begins to identify administrative and systems problems that might be candidates for redesign, and recommends corrective actions.
38. Answer: **A**. McGregor's Theory X assumes all workers are uninterested and unmotivated toward work. His Theory Y assumes all workers are basically interested and motivated to work.
39. Answer: **C**. The basic goal of the National Highway Traffic Safety Administration (NHTSA), a branch of the Department of Transportation, is reduction of injuries, deaths, and economic losses resulting from traffic accidents.
40. Answer: **D**. Training of employees may not be required by every citation issued by OSHA.
41. Answer: **A**. The Federal Motor Vehicle Safety Standards are designed to:
    - Prevent crashes by providing safe brake systems and components, rearview mirrors, etc.
    - Reduce injury severity in crashes by use of improved occupant restraint systems, glazing materials, seating systems, door locks, etc.
    - Minimize damage and injury following crashes by insuring the integrity of fuel systems, flammability resistance of vehicle materials, etc.
42. Answer: **A**. Progressive companies believe the proper way to deal with minor rule infractions is to issue an oral reprimand for the first offense. Progressively more severe discipline is then administered for additional violations.
43. Answer: **A**. The most common ways for toxic materials to enter the body are through the skin by absorption, by inhalation, and through ingestion.
44. Answer: **A**. The Threshold Limit Values and Biological Exposure Indices Booklet (2015) (TLV booklet) states: "STEL is defined as a 15-minute TWA exposure which should not be exceeded at any time during a workday even if the 8-hour TWA is within the TLV-TWA. Exposures above the TLV-TWA up to the STEL should not be longer than 15 minutes and should not occur more than four times per day. There should be at least 60 minutes between successive exposures in this range. An averaging period other than 15 minutes may be recommended when this is warranted by observed biological effects."
45. Answer: **B**. The A-weighting most closely weights the sound to the injurious effects of noise on the ears.
46. Answer: **C**. When the vapor pressure of a liquid is greater than the atmospheric pressure, the material has reached its boiling point.
47. Answer: **D**. Within the United States, both NIOSH and MSHA test and approve respiratory protection.
48. Answer: **B**. The purpose of local exhaust ventilation is to remove air contaminants at the source, not to dilute them.
49. Answer: **C**. Sound-level meters require constant readings and a technician to note the readings. The same holds true for octave-band analysis. Annual audiograms are an after-the-fact measure. Noise dosimeters are easy to use and provide the measurement desired in this case.
50. Answer: **D**. The following comparison is offered:
    Lead thickness required 0.3 inch
    Sheet steel thickness required   1.3 inches
    Concrete thickness required   2.7 inches
    Water thickness required   8.3 inches
51. Answer: **A**. Silicosis is a lung disease caused by inhalation of free silica particulates and has in the past been known as:
    - Potter's rot
    - Stonemason's disease
    - Miner's asthma
    - Grinder's consumption
    - Miner's phthisis
    - Miner's lung
    - Rockman's rot

52. Answer: **B**. The only measurement possible with a pitot tube is flow from a fire hydrant.
53. Answer: **D**. To be a solvent, the chemical must be used as a cleaner or used to dissolve something. The use of epoxies is generally to establish a resin matrix to bind material together.
54. Answer: **B**. The cochlea is a cone-shaped winding structure in the inner ear containing the organ of Corti, which is the receptor for hearing.
55. Answer: **C**. Neutralization probably would be the most economical method of treating very low pH acid waste. However, the other methods might provide satisfactory results, depending on the particular situation.
56. Answer: **C**. Fibers are particles that have a length at least three times their width.
57. Answer: **A**. The most common and most damaging hazard in chrome electroplating is inhalation of chromic acid mists.
58. Answer: **B**. The ear is most susceptible to noise in the 1000–4000-Hz range.
59. Answer: **A**. The main reason many fish die in streams polluted by industrial waste is because the waste depletes the available oxygen. Although the other factors do cause grave ecological damage, lack of oxygen is the best answer.
60. Answer: **C**. It has been widely accepted that only dust particles smaller than approximately 5 microns (micrometers) in aerodynamic diameter are deposited and retained in the lungs. A large percentage of particles larger than 3 microns are deposited in the upper respiratory system (i.e., the nasal cavity, trachea, bronchial tubes, etc). Approximately half the smaller particles find their way into alveolar or pulmonary air spaces. Almost all really small particles (less than 1 micron) collect in alveolar spaces. The portion of dust that is small enough to penetrate into pulmonary spaces is known as "respirable dust" and varies as a part of the total dust cloud from 5% to 50%. Thus, several methods of measuring only harmful dust have been developed. A thorough review of principles of dust-collection methods prior to taking the Safety Fundamentals examination is highly recommended. The fourth edition of the National Safety Council's *Fundamentals of Industrial Hygiene* provides several excellent chapters covering this topic.

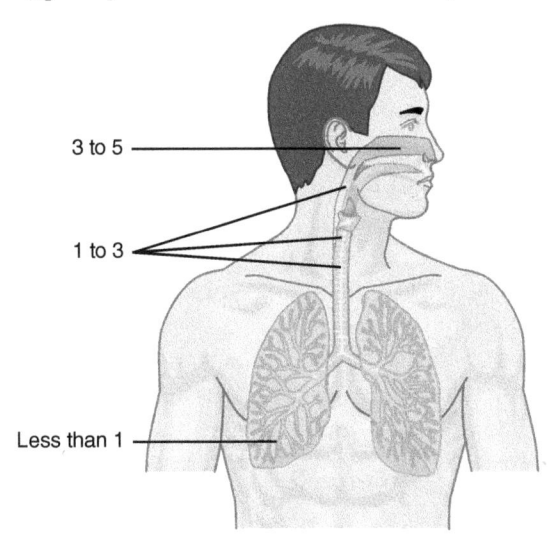

Figure 55 Dust particles in the respiratory system

61. Answer: **D**. Emphysema is a condition in which the walls of the individual alveoli rupture or dilate. The wall of the resulting larger sac has lost its naturally elastic recoil, and so does not exhaust air as efficiently, and does not offer the large area for gas transfer afforded by several smaller sacs.
62. Answer: **C**. Never park with EXPLOSIVES A or EXPLOSIVES B within 5 feet of the traveled part of the road. Unless work requires it, parking is forbidden within 300 feet of:
    - A bridge, tunnel, or building
    - A place where people gather
    - An open fire

294 ASP Exam Study Workbook

If parking is imperative for safety work, it should be done briefly. Avoid parking on private property (including fueling and eating facilities) unless the owner is aware of the danger. In all cases, someone must watch the parked vehicle, but **only** if the vehicle is:
- On a shipper's property
- On a carrier's property
- On a consignee's property

A vehicle may be left unattended in a "safe haven." A safe haven is a government-approved place for parking unattended vehicles loaded with explosives.

Note: Reference - 49 CFR part 397.5.

63. Answer: **D**. Ventilation does not control radiant heat.
64. Answer: **D**. The disorder "epicondylitis" is often called tennis elbow or sometimes carpenter's elbow. The disorder is a result of combined motion causing pronation of the hand and ulnar deviation. For a carpenter, this involves swinging heavy hammers and in tennis, swinging a racket. The affliction causes considerable pain in the hand, forearm, and elbow. The term *rotator cuff* is associated with the tearing of a ligament in the shoulder. Roofer's wrist is a common name for carpal tunnel syndrome, a disorder caused by compression of the median nerve. Trigger finger is an affliction caused by repeated use of the finger pulling levers or triggers (e.g., paint spray operators).
65. Answer: **C**. Three half-value layers would reduce the radiation to 225 mR. The easiest way to solve these problems is by building a table.

	AFTER		
Source	1st Half Value	2nd Half Value	3rd Half Value
1800	900	450	225

66. Answer: **C**. The National Institute for Occupational Safety and Health (NIOSH) is administratively located within the Centers for Disease Control (CDC), which functions as a member of the Public Health Service (PHS) and reports to the Department of Health and Human Services (HHS). NIOSH was originally founded within the Department of Health, Education and Welfare, which is now HHS, under the provisions of the OSH Act. It has prime responsibility for research to eliminate occupational health and safety hazards. NIOSH has the responsibility to identify hazards and recommend changes in the regulations. It performs testing and certification of workers' personal protective equipment, mainly respirators. NIOSH has a very active training grant program that supports university training throughout the country and conducts excellent courses at regional centers. NIOSH also does workplace investigations under 42 CFR Part 85, largely to conduct epidemiological methods research and studies.
67. Answer: **D**. Generally, equipment installed in NEC Class 1 locations must be approved as *explosion-proof*. This is because it is impractical to keep flammable gases outside of the enclosure. So, arcing equipment must be installed in enclosures that are designed to withstand an explosion. This minimizes the risk of having an external explosion occur when a flammable gas enters the enclosure and is ignited by the arcs. Not only must the equipment be strong enough to withstand an internal explosion, but the enclosures must be designed to vent resulting explosive gases. The venting must ensure that gases are cooled to a temperature below that of the ignition temperature of hazardous material involved before being released into the hazardous atmosphere.
68. Answer: **A**. NFPA 10 is the Standard for Portable Fire Extinguishers.
69. Answer: **D**. The generally recognized types of machine guards are fixed, interlocking, and automatic. Adjustable, electrical, and mechanical are subdivisions of these general classifications.
70. Answer: **B**. The primary reason for installing full enclosure guards on grinding wheels is to contain pieces of the wheel should it break during operation.
71. Answer: **B**. The American Society of Mechanical Engineers (ASME) is the primary agency providing oversight for boilers and pressure vessels in the United States and also develops the *Boiler and Pressure Vessel Code*, plus code for all components associated with boilers and pressure vessels.

72. Answer: **D**. The safe procedure for setting up a ladder requires the base to be one-fourth the ladder length; 3/12 = 1/4.
73. Answer: **D**. Pressure-relief panels are not required in battery-charging locations.
74. Answer: **C**. Operators of lift trucks should keep the tines as close to the ground as possible. The generally accepted rule is 6 inches.
75. Answer: **A**. *ANSI Z16.1* deals with classification of injuries. *ANSI Z87.1* is concerned with Occupation and Educational Eye and Face Protection. *ANSI/NFPA Z12.1* addresses Floor and Wall Openings, Railings and Toeboards. *ANSI Z358.1* is the standard for Emergency Eyewash and Shower Equipment.
76. Answer: **A**. There are no standards for bump caps.
77. Answer: **D**. Orange is the color used to indicate moving machine parts.
78. Answer: **C**. With few exceptions, guardrails and toeboards are required on platforms over 10 feet above ground. OSHA (1926.451)

    CAUTION: The general industry standards at 1910.23 generally require a standard guardrail anytime a drop of more than 4 feet is encountered.

    Modified from OSHA 29 CFR 1910.23(e)(4).

    A standard toeboard shall be four inches nominal in vertical height from its top edge to the level of the floor, platform, runway, or ramp. It shall be securely fastened in place and with not more than ¼ inch clearance above floor level. It may be made of any substantial material either solid or with openings not over 1 inch in greatest dimension.
79. Answer: **B**. Most power presses are equipped with remote control types of guards. An excellent source of information on this subject is the Accident Prevention Manual for Business & Industry (National Safety Council).

    Where point-of-operation protection is necessary for a shear point, an opening of ¼ inch must be made for operational purposes, and the minimum distance that must be maintained between the point of the hazard and the guard is ½ inch.
80. Answer: **A**. OSHA regulates fork trucks for industry in the United States.
81. Answer: **A**. The generally accepted factors used in determining the safety factor for the use of natural fiber rope, such as manila, cotton, flax, asbestos, jute, silk, etc., are the size of rope, construction material (type of fiber), and the tensile or breaking strength (based on new, unused rope). For example, a new ⅜ inch diameter manila rope has a tensile strength of 1200 pounds and a recommended safety factor of 10, which makes the working load 120 pounds. A new 1 inch diameter manila rope has a tensile strength of 8000 pounds and a recommended safety factor of 7, which makes the working load 1150 pounds. Generally, manila rope from 3/16 inch to ⅜ inch requires a safety factor of 10, above ⅜ inch but less than 9/16 inch requires a 9 safety factor, above 9/16 inch but less than ¾ inch has a safety factor of 8, and so on. These factors are guides, and judgment based on professional risk analysis must be used in many cases.
82. Answer: **C**. The opening on a lifting chain hook, if not overloaded, should remain constant. Any change in dimension indicates excessive loading and the hook should be taken out of service. The generally accepted tolerance for throat openings is 15%; however, it varies a small amount from manufacturer to manufacturer. One reference might be OSHA 1910.184.
83. Answer: **B**. Moving parts 7 feet or less from the floor must be provided with safeguarding to prevent inadvertent contact by individuals working in the area.
84. Answer: **B**. The mechanical advantage is roughly equal to the parts of the line when hoisting with a two-block system. Because of this relationship, it is very easy to compute tension on the haul line by using the simple formula:

$$\text{Lead} - \text{line pull} = \frac{\text{load to be lifted}}{\text{parts of line}} \times F$$

$$F = \text{Multiplication Factor}$$

The multiplication factor is required because each time a rope passes over a sheave, friction is produced, which reduces the block's efficiency. In practice, losses are discounted for *rough* calculations. However, you must be aware that this produces a calculated load that is significantly lower than the actual lead-line stress. The final calculations should divide the load by the ratio of line parts or use a multiplication factor for each block (as shown below). Both depend on bearings used, type of sheave, etc. The following chart illustrates the concept.

Parts of Line	Ratio	Multiplication Factor	Parts of Line	Ratio	Multiplication Factor
1	0.96	1.04	5	4.39	1.14
2	1.87	1.07	6	5.16	1.16
3	2.75	1.09	7	5.90	1.19
4	3.59	1.12	8	6.60	1.21

85. Answer: **A**.
    Step 1   Determine the area of the hood.
    A = Length × Height
    A = 5 ft × 5 ft = 25 ft^2

    Step 2   Determine the volume of air flowing through the hood.
    Q = V × A
    Q = 120 × 25 = 3000 cfm

    Step 3   Compute the duct area.
    A = π × r^2
    A = 3.14 (8/12)^2
    A = 1.395 ft^2

    Step 4   Determine the rate of airflow in the duct.
    Q = V × A
    V = Q / A
    V = 3000 / 1.395 = 2150 fpm

86. Answer: **B**. Wood stored against a heating duct may undergo pyrolysis (chemical decomposition of a substance by heat) and become easily ignitable.
87. Answer: **B**. Examples of metals considered combustible other than magnesium include titanium, zirconium, sodium, and potassium. Fires involving these metals are Class D fires.
88. Answer: **A**. Acetylene cylinders must always be stored in an upright position to allow proper securing and to prevent liquid acetone from escaping. If cylinders used for gas welding are stored lying down or upside down, liquid acetone will enter valve passages. When the torch is used, highly flammable liquid acetone will flow from the torch, instead of desired acetylene gas.
89. Answer: **D**. The green triangle with an "A" is for ordinary combustible fires. "B" is for flammable liquids. "C" is for electrical equipment. "D" is for fires involving certain combustible metals.
90. Answer: **B**. When dealing with some potentially unstable chemicals, experts should be consulted.
91. Answer: **C**. Perchloric acid with age can become unstable. One indication is crystal growth around the lid.
92. Answer: **A**. Following the requirement of the National Electrical Code, a Class I, Div. 1 rating is required. This high level of protection is required because flammable solvents are used, vapors can travel, and, if no protection was provided, a source of ignition may be found. Refer to NFPA 70 ART. 500.
93. Answer: **D**. The use of a sacrificial anode to protect from corrosion is an accepted and economical method widely used in industry.
94. Answer: **D**. Article 500 of the NEC deals with classifications of hazardous locations.
95. Answer: **B**. B is the correct choice because it describes the proper method of computing the specific heat of any material.
96. Answer: **C**. Every attempt should be made to obtain and use industrial solvents that are nonflammable. When this is not possible, solvents having a flash point of 140 degrees or higher are considered to pose an acceptable risk.

97. Answer: **C**. Very toxic or poisonous gases do not require a safety relief device because of the hazard that release of these materials could cause. Most other bottled or compressed gases are required to be equipped with frangible disks, fusible disks, bursting disks, etc.
98. Answer: **C**. NFPA requires hydrostatic testing of water extinguishers every five years. The *Fire Protection Handbook* has an excellent discussion of fire extinguishers.
99. Answer: **D**. *Bonding* is the process of connecting two or more conductive objects together by means of a conductor to minimize a potential electrical difference between them. *Grounding* is the process of connecting the conductive object to the ground, and is a specific type of bonding. A conductive object may also be grounded by bonding it to another conductive object that is already connected to the ground. *Bonding* minimizes potential differences between conductive objects. *Grounding* minimizes potential differences between conductive objects and the ground. In dealing with flammable liquids, both *bonding and grounding* are very important. When flammable liquids are being transferred between containers, static electricity is the hazard workers protect against.
100. Answer: **D**. When planning for an emergency, one must consider the protection of all resources. Naturally, the saving of life must come first; however, protection of processes and equipment is also of utmost concern. Should the decision be made to abandon hazardous processes, an additional disaster could be created.

Self-Assessment Exam 5 Questions

1. The atomic mass of an element is a combination of:

A. neutrons and electrons.
B. protons and neutrons.
C. protons and electrons.
D. protons.

2. Determine the pH of a solution in which [H+] = 2.5 × 10⁻⁵ moles per liter.

A. 4.6, a weak acid
B. 2.6, a strong acid
C. 13.3, a strong base
D. 7.4, a weak base

3. The type of friction relative to solid surfaces is called:

A. dry.
B. fluid.
C. lubricated.
D. kinetic.

4. Sensorineural hearing loss in an industrial setting is typically caused by:

A. prolonged exposure to loud noise.
B. abnormalities in the hair cells of the organ of Corti in the cochlea.
C. lack of development (aplasia) of the cochlea.
D. the continued use of hearing protection.

5. The difference between pounds per square inch absolute and pounds per square inch gage is:

A. 14.7 psi.
B. 15 psi.
C. 29.92 psi.
D. There is no difference.

6. The correct formula to determine the percent slope of a ramp is:
   A. rise over run.
   B. run over rise.
   C. rise times run.
   D. run times rise.

7. A 20,000-pound semi-tractor is traveling at 70 mph. Nearly how much kinetic energy is being developed?
   A. 120,000 ft-lbs
   B. 1,270,000 ft-lbs
   C. 3,320,000 ft-lbs
   D. 880,563 ft-lbs

8. A solid material weighs 1800 ounces. When placed in water, it weighs 1200 oz. What is the material's specific gravity?
   A. 1.5
   B. 0.15
   C. 3.0
   D. 0.3

9. Matter that has a definite volume, but no definite shape, is a:
   A. liquid.
   B. solid.
   C. gas.
   D. vapor.

10. According to OSHA regulations regarding cadmium exposure, all of the following are true *except*:
    A. all contaminated debris, waste, scrap, PPE, and clothing must be bagged with impermeable material prior to disposal.
    B. cleanup of dust should be done with HEPA-filtered vacuum cleaners.
    C. exposure over the PEL requires clothing change rooms, showers, and a lunchroom facility.
    D. exposure over the PEL requires biological monitoring, such as a urine test for hippuric acid at the work shift end.

11. **Strong oxidizing agents:**
    A. always react violently with bases.
    B. can cause serious burns.
    C. can be safely stored in steel containers.
    D. are always shipped with a Class 2 label.

12. Which of the following statements is *incorrect* regarding the OSHA standard on benzene?
    A. Employees requiring medical examination will be afforded an examination within 30 days of initial assignment.
    B. A medical surveillance program is required for exposure to benzene at or above the action level.
    C. A medical surveillance program is required for exposure above the PEL for 10 or more days per year.
    D. A medical surveillance program is required for tire-building machine operators who use solvents.

13. What is the specific gravity of dry air?
    A. 1.1 to 1
    B. 1 to 5
    C. 1
    D. 5

14. In the study of human behavior, the term *population stereotype* concerns the human expectation that results from the movement of controls and fixtures. Which of the following violates the principle of this stereotype?

    A. Movement of the control lever of an air-boat forward to turn right
    B. A switch that moves up to shut off a pump
    C. In electronics, a knob turns clockwise to increase gain.
    D. A key switch that turns right to start a car

15. Using the t-distribution table, compute the range of values that will include 95% of means recorded in a sample test. Assume 9 degrees of freedom for this calculation due to estimated data.

    A. −1.833 to +1.833 standard deviation
    B. −1.476 to +1.476 standard deviation
    C. −2.833 to +2.333 standard deviation
    D. −08.13 to +08.13 standard deviation

Table of Percentage Points of the t-Distribution

df \ p	0.25	0.1	0.05	0.01
1	1.000	3.078	6.314	31.821
2	0.816	1.886	2.920	6.965
3	0.765	1.638	2.353	4.541
4	0.741	1.533	2.132	3.747
5	0.727	1.476	2.015	3.365
6	0.718	1.440	1.943	3.143
7	0.711	1.415	1.895	2.998
8	0.706	1.397	1.860	2.896
9	0.703	1.383	1.833	2.821
10	0.700	1.372	1.812	2.764
15	0.691	1.341	1.753	2.602
20	0.687	1.325	1.725	2.528
25	0.684	1.316	1.708	2.485
30	0.683	1.310	1.697	2.457
∞	0.674	1.282	1.645	2.326

16. A mixture is prepared by diluting 150 mL of sulfur dioxide with clean air. The final volume is 2 cubic meters. What is the concentration of sulfur dioxide in the mixture?

    A. 150 ppm
    B. 75 ppm
    C. 750 ppm
    D. 1500 ppm

17. A 200-pound metal bar with a specific gravity of 9 is submerged in quenching oil (SG = 0.7) for heat treatment. What is the bar's weight when submerged in the oil?
    A. 100 lbs
    B. 127.8 lbs
    C. 184 lbs
    D. 200 lbs

18. Calcium carbide (CaC$_2$) has a melting point of 2300°C, a specific gravity of 2.22 g/cm, a molecular weight of 54.2 grams, a vapor density of 2.2, and is a grayish-black solid with a garlic-like odor. Which of the following would be a safety issue concerning the use and handling of calcium carbide?
    A. It reacts with water, producing acetylene.
    B. It combusts spontaneously with air.
    C. It is a flammable solid.
    D. It cannot be extinguished if involved in combustion.

19. An entire class of safety professionals received the following scores on the ASP examination: 59, 67, 80, 75, 54. Compute the standard deviation:
    A. 9.6
    B. 5.8
    C. 10.8
    D. 6.7

20. A direct current rotary generator has a commutator ring, whereas an AC generator has _____.
    A. slip rings
    B. brushes
    C. armature
    D. field coils

21. Epidemiological studies compare two groups of people who are alike except for one factor, such as exposure to a chemical or the presence of a health effect; the investigators try to determine if any factor is associated with the health effect. These studies use biostatistical methods to evaluate cause-and-effect relationships. Which of the following statements concerning epidemiological studies is *most* correct?
    A. Cross-sectional studies are the most expensive.
    B. Retrospective studies are considered the most scientifically useful.
    C. Epidemiological studies have been severely restricted by the courts and must prove cost/benefit before proceeding.
    D. Prospective studies are also called cohort or incident studies.

22. What is the center mass for a 2-meter beam loaded with 20 kg on one end and 10 kg on the opposite end?
    A. 66.7 cm from 20 kg
    B. 61.5 cm from 10 kg
    C. 61.5 cm from 20 kg
    D. 66.7 cm from 10 kg

23. An accident at your plant has caused the piping from a large H_2SO_4 (sulfuric acid) tank to leak acid into a nearby stream. The acid is leaking at a rate of 25 gallons a minute. Due to the toxicity of the material and several other factors, you are unable to stop the leak until equipment arrives from another location. Assuming that the level of acid was 18 inches from the top of the tank when the leak started, how long before this leak empties the 9-foot-tall, 6-foot-diameter tank? Sulfuric acid has a specific gravity of 1.9.

    A. 64 minutes
    B. 25 minutes
    C. 76 minutes
    D. 85 minutes

24. **What are workers' rights with respect to OSHA citations?**

    A. Workers have limited rights under OSHA.
    B. Workers have the right to appeal the abatement date of OSHA citations.
    C. Workers have the right to appeal a citation penalty.
    D. Workers have the right to bargain remedial actions suggested by the CoSHO.

25. **Which state had the first Workers' Compensation Act to become law and remain in effect?**

    A. California
    B. Colorado
    C. Nevada
    D. Wisconsin

26. **Workers *not* likely covered by workers' compensation would include:**

    A. domestic workers.
    B. maritime employees.
    C. farm workers.
    D. all of those listed above.

27. **Responsibility for safety in operations belongs to:**

    A. operations management.
    B. the safety manager.
    C. line supervisors.
    D. top management.

28. **Program audits are intended to achieve which of the following?**

    A. Ensure compliance with codes and standards
    B. Assess cost effectiveness of safety program
    C. Check on recordkeeping and code violations
    D. Ascertain if programs are following the designated plan

29. **In the United States, the *primary* cause of on-the-job injuries is:**

    A. falls.
    B. motor vehicle accidents.
    C. fires.
    D. workers not using appropriate PPE correctly.

30. **The *most* frequent errors run into during the preparation and use of computer-generated statistical analysis of accident and injury data are:**

    A. syntax errors.
    B. computer downtimes.
    C. data entry errors.
    D. fourth-generation language incongruences.

31. Which of the following is *least* important in a maintenance department's accident prevention effort?

   A. Performing a job safety analysis
   B. Having knowledge of job hazards
   C. Having knowledge of preventive maintenance items
   D. Reviewing the written work order procedure

32. All of the following would be reportable accidents under DOT regulations *except*:

   A. an injury not requiring a medical response.
   B. death of operator at the scene.
   C. property damage in excess of $1500.
   D. an injury requiring a medical response.

33. Retrospective rating of workers' compensation insurance premiums is based on how many years' loss record?

   A. Previous year
   B. Projected one year beyond the current year
   C. Last three years
   D. Last five years

34. When using the formula $S \cong 6\,CE$ for gamma emitters, one must be careful to determine the correct radiation energy. Some materials, such as cobalt-60, emit more than one gamma. In this case, energies must be totaled. The Mev for cobalt-60 is 1.1 and 1.3. Given this information, what radiation reading would result from an unshielded 75-millicurie source of cobalt-60, at a distance of 1 foot?

   A. 2.3 R/hr/1ft
   B. 1080 mR/hr/1ft
   C. 1100 R/hr/1ft
   D. 1800 mR/hr/1ft

35. The critical first step in the development of an accident data collection system is to:

   A. differentiate between human error and design error.
   B. define ensuing use of the data.
   C. create accident-reporting responsibilities.
   D. codify statistics to conform to presented data sources.

36. Safety programs should give priority attention to all of the following *except*:

   A. inspections and surveys.
   B. the physical demands of the workplace.
   C. the accident predisposition among workers.
   D. the production pressure in the work environment.

37. The *best* method for safety professionals to ensure that safety considerations are well thought out in the project design phase is to:

   A. inspect facilities prior to acceptance.
   B. examine the project design with engineers.
   C. instruct the design engineers in safety codes.
   D. make subcontractors correct mistakes.

38. Supervisors are often in the *best* situation to provide SH&E training and information to employees because:

   A. they always have plenty of spare time.
   B. they are responsible for production.
   C. they know production schedules.
   D. they provide better training than the training department.

39. During design, which of the following is the *best* method of visualizing plant layout prior to actual construction?

   A. Study the plot plan blueprints
   B. Study a three-dimensional model
   C. A computer-generated CAD printout
   D. Calculations on square feet per occupant

40. Which of the following *best* describes the assessment of tasks involving steps, hazards, and solutions?

   A. System Safety Analysis (SSA)
   B. Fault Tree Analysis (FTA)
   C. Job Safety Analysis (JSA)
   D. Management Oversight and Risk Tree (MORT)

41. The *primary* reason safety professionals perform accident investigation is to:

   A. discipline rule violators.
   B. provide regulatory agencies and other safety professionals with valid information.
   C. satisfy insurer requirements.
   D. ascertain causal circumstances.

42. Which of the following reflects the *best* use of the management tool, Failure Modes and Effects Analysis (FMEA)?

   A. Survey instrument
   B. Inspection checklist
   C. Preventive maintenance indicator
   D. Alternate for fault tree

43. In an 8-hour workday, what is the allowable time limit for exposure to a 101.8-dBA noise, according to 29 CFR 1910.95?

   A. 30 minutes
   B. 2 hours
   C. 1 hour and 30 minutes
   D. 15 minutes

44. A company makes it publicly known that it has a 3.5 accident rate. With 1800 employees, this generates approximately _____ recordable accidents.

   A. 91
   B. 63
   C. 105
   D. 88

45. After completing a review course, your college had 35 recent graduates sit for the 200-question ASP examination. The mean of the students was 140, with a range of 155 to 70. If the $\Sigma(x - \bar{x})^2 = 4900$, then what is the sample standard deviation?

   A. 12
   B. 11.8
   C. 9
   D. 18.8

46. Abraham Maslow is often cited on his theory of human needs in the basic study of behavioral science. In Maslow's theory, a need is a deficiency a person feels the compulsion to satisfy. Central to this theory is the progressive principle, meaning that needs are arranged in a hierarchy. Only after a lower-level need is satisfied can the next highest level become active. Which of the following needs are at the lowest level in Maslow's hierarchy?

   A. Esteem
   B. Social
   C. Safety
   D. Physiological

47. Which of the following is *not* responsible for ensuring that each container of a hazardous chemical leaving the workplace is labeled?

   A. Chemical manufacturer
   B. Distributor
   C. Importer
   D. Advertising representative

48. 1,1,1-trichloroethane (methyl chloroform) is sometimes substituted for trichloroethylene because it has a:

   A. higher boiling point.
   B. greater TLV.
   C. lower flash point.
   D. lower volatility.

49. Carbon tetrachloride (CCl_4) is *most* likely to cause physiologic damage to which organ or body system?

   A. Heart
   B. Lungs
   C. Liver
   D. Skeletal

50. Employees becoming accustomed to heat is generally achieved by requiring the employee to work:

   A. at 50% of the desired work rate.
   B. at 75% of the desired work rate.
   C. for 2 hours per day for 2 weeks.
   D. for 6 hours per day for 2 months.

51. Should a radioactive powder be spilled in a lab, the first required action is to:

   A. report the incident to OSHA.
   B. clean up as quickly as possible.
   C. evacuate personnel and reroute traffic.
   D. notify NRC immediately.

52. A single short exposure to a chemical above the established TLV is permissible as long as the TWA is not exceeded.

   A. Yes, unless the TLV-C is exceeded.
   B. No, the TLV may not be exceeded without an OSHA waiver.
   C. TLVs are meaningless.
   D. TLVs should only be used as guidelines and are not enforceable.

53. **Which of the following *best* describes a zero-mechanical state, also known as a ZESP (zero energy state procedure) being assured?**
    A. All electrical energy is off.
    B. The equipment is nonfunctional (i.e., locked out)
    C. All energy sources are rendered safe and all potential energy is dissipated.
    D. Guards are in a zero or down position.

54. **The *most* common health hazard found in a brass foundry is:**
    A. dust, toxic gases, fumes, and acid vapors.
    B. lead.
    C. noise.
    D. copper, zinc, lead fumes, and dust.

55. **Employees working in slaughterhouses have an increased potential of contracting the disease known as:**
    A. norovirus.
    B. MRSA.
    C. Q fever.
    D. byssinosis.

56. **Which disease is associated with animal products?**
    A. Anthracosis
    B. Pneumoconiosis
    C. Anthrax
    D. Presbycusis

57. **An infection that is connected with milk is:**
    A. brucellosis.
    B. bursitis.
    C. laryngitis.
    D. pleurisy.

58. **When confirming the electrical ground in a duplex receptacle, which of the following provides the *best* method? Check continuity between the _____.**
    A. black wire and the white wire.
    B. green wire and the outlet box.
    C. white wire and the outlet box.
    D. green wire and the building ground.

59. **All of the following elements of a respirator maintenance program are required *except*:**
    A. inspection.
    B. cleaning.
    C. selection and purchase.
    D. repair.

60. **If 2 gallons of gasoline are consumed in a fire, what is the total heat produced?**
    A. 224,000 Btu
    B. 112,000 Btu
    C. 144,000 Btu
    D. 448,000 Btu

306 ASP Exam Study Workbook

61. **The safety director of a textile plant had an OSHA inspection and the plant was cited for several violations. Which of the following actions is *most* accurate?**

   A. The management has 15 working days to pay any fines on cited violations.
   B. The workers must be allowed to see the citations.
   C. The safety director must correct the cited violations within 30 days.
   D. The employer must post citations for at least three days.

62. **Which of the following *best* describes an audiogram?**

   A. A hearing-loss device
   B. A written record of audible range level measured at different frequencies
   C. An indicator of hearing loss
   D. An instrument used to measure and record sound frequencies and pressure levels in dB

63. **Managing noise exposure through use of engineering controls is extremely complicated. Often reduction in noise level is possible through use of material with high absorption coefficients (α). The α is defined as the ratio of sound energy absorbed to the sound energy incident upon the surface of a material exposed to a sound field. Which of the following factors would *not* contribute to the α of a material used for noise attenuation?**

   A. Frequency of the noise
   B. Density of the material
   C. Color
   D. Surface condition and porosity

64. **Which of the following would provide the lowest emissivity while engineering a shield for a high radiant heat source (industrial furnace)? Assume the shield will be constructed from flat plate materials.**

   A. A painted flat black surface
   B. A polished black surface
   C. A white surface
   D. A polished light-colored surface

65. **Carpal tunnel syndrome is a repetitive motion disease that affects many production workers. Recently efforts to prevent injuries in the slaughter industry have met with great success. The symptoms of carpal tunnel syndrome include all of the following *except*:**

   A. numbness in the little finger.
   B. pain in the wrist upon exertion.
   C. pain in the second and third fingers.
   D. inflammation and swelling of the wrist.

66. **All of the following are true concerning the affliction metal fume fever (MFF) *except*:**

   A. MFF is an acute condition of short duration.
   B. MFF is a permanent condition, which is compensable through the workers' compensation system in all states.
   C. daily exposure will produce an immunity to MFF.
   D. recovery from MFF is very quick (usually one or two days).

67. **Due to company downsizing, an entire plant, including several metal-working shops, is being relocated to a place with an elevation of 5000 feet. The welding hood exhaust systems for these shops were all originally designed to operate at sea level. Which of the following correctly describes the results of this relocation?**

   A. Fan static pressure will not be affected.
   B. CFM will not change.
   C. Horsepower will not change.
   D. RPM will change per density calculations.

68. **Which of the methods listed below is *not* allowed in supplying air for SCBA, airline respirators, or combination units?**
    A. Filtered breathing air grade "d" or higher
    B. Manifold cylinders of high-pressure air
    C. Oil-pumped compressed air with filtering
    D. Medical grade oxygen

69. **Which of the following statements is incorrect regarding carbon monoxide (CO)?**
    A. The current TLV for CO is 1500 ppm.
    B. CO mixtures in air are flammable.
    C. CO poisoning does not cause injury to red blood cells.
    D. CO reduces the oxygen-carrying capacity of red blood cells.

70. **Any agent that can disturb the development of an embryo or fetus is termed a:**
    A. mutagen.
    B. carcinogen.
    C. teratogen.
    D. halogen.

71. **In order to reduce emissions of fork trucks using gasoline in a warehouse, a safety professional's *best* option in lieu of electrical truck usage is to:**
    A. convert to diesel.
    B. convert to LP.
    C. provide respirators.
    D. None of the responses listed is correct.

72. **When using Crosby clamps to secure a ½-inch wire rope, workers should use:**
    A. two clamps with a saddle on the dead end.
    B. two clamps with a U-bolt on the live end.
    C. three clamps with a U-bolt on the live end.
    D. three clamps with a saddle on the live end.

73. **In which case could a double-insulated, two-wire portable drill produce a shock hazard?**
    A. All cases require a third ground wire.
    B. If a short exists between the neutral and the load wire
    C. If a short exists between the case and a hot wire
    D. If an energized drill was dropped in water

74. **Which of the following constitutes the majority of accidents and injuries in an office environment?**
    A. Electrical shocks
    B. Falls
    C. Lack of PPE
    D. Being struck by falling objects

75. **When a high-pressure fitting begins leaking, the correct repair course of action is to:**
    A. depressurize to gage zero immediately.
    B. tighten all fittings with a brass wrench.
    C. install a saddle repair device and tighten securely.
    D. evacuate and post the area.

76. **Preparation of a diluted solution of an acid is accomplished by pouring water into the acid.**
    A. True
    B. False
    C. Except for hydrochloric acid
    D. Only true for sulfuric acid

77. **Performing background checks on driving records is permissible under the DOT regulations of new hires for transport hazardous materials.**
    A. This is a DOT requirement and therefore permissible.
    B. This violates civil rights and is not allowed.
    C. It is permissible only if the new hire is suspected of having a prior felony conviction.
    D. It is allowable if the employee has given prior consent.

78. **The load boom indicator on a mobile crane:**
    A. is a load indication device.
    B. is the data plate identifying critical information for operation.
    C. monitors crane capacity.
    D. is optional.

79. **What is the angle of a flight of stairs that rises 10 feet vertical for every 12 feet horizontal?**
    A. Almost 90 degrees
    B. Almost 50 degrees
    C. 40 degrees
    D. 30 degrees

80. **The type of guard frequently used with an automatic guillotine paper cutter is:**
    A. an enclosed guard.
    B. a remotely activated control.
    C. a two-hand pull-away.
    D. a swing-away (adjustable) enclosure guard.

81. **Which of the following is *most* correct concerning the use of structural reinforcing steel in concrete structures?**
    A. Steel is used to prevent cracking.
    B. Steel should not be used in floor slabs.
    C. Plastic is commonly used as a reinforcing medium.
    D. Steel reinforcement is often placed on metal chairs to prevent displacement while pouring.

82. **A 50,000-pound housing is being lifted by a 250-ton mobile crane. The pick requires a long boom (250 feet) and a blind lift due to the configuration of adjacent structures. A safety factor of 5 is assigned to the rigging, which consists of a single shackle connecting the load block hook to a two-leg sling shackled to a strongback (spreader bar). It is equipped with two parallel 40-foot pendants that are shackled to the housing at engineered pick points. The total weight of the rigging is 2400 pounds. Although the shackles are the weakest link in the rigging chain, what strength must they be able to support?**
    A. 9900 lbs
    B. 52,400 lbs
    C. 100,000 lbs
    D. 131,000 lbs

83. **Which of the following factors determine the safety factor for natural fiber rope?**

    A. Size of rope, material, and tensile strength
    B. Type of fiber and strength
    C. Environmental factors and size
    D. Use and exposure data

84. **Which of the following devices is *most* commonly used to change electrical direct current (DC) to alternating current (AC)?**

    A. Inverter
    B. Rectifier
    C. Transformer
    D. Capacitor

85. **When designing point-of-operation protection on machinery having running nip points, some guard designers have used the formula shown below to good advantage. Using this formula, what is the distance for a guard opening located 6 inches from the danger zone?**

    A. ½ inch
    B. ⅝ inch
    C. ¾ inch
    D. 1 inch

    $$O_{Max} = 0.25 + (0.125D)$$

    Where O_{Max} = Maximum Safe Opening

    D = Distance from danger zone in inches

86. **Why is a canopy hood an unacceptable ventilation system for a large solvent dip tank containing methylene chloride? Methylene chloride has a vapor pressure of 359 mm Hg and a vapor density of 1.326 g/cm³.**

    A. The hood would be unacceptably large.
    B. Larger fans are needed.
    C. Methylene chloride would be drawn through the breathing zone.
    D. The hood would get in the way of the lifting device.

87. **What is the *primary* consideration in storing chemicals?**

    A. Appropriate ventilation
    B. Proper segregation
    C. Adequate fire-suppression systems
    D. Bonding and grounding

88. **Photoelectric smoke detectors are particularly effective in what setting/situation?**

    A. In covered areas
    B. For smoldering fires or low-temperature pyrolysis of PVC
    C. In fuel loading platforms
    D. In areas where a flame flicker is seen

89. **The Life Safety Code includes the term exit in an overall definition of means of egress. A means of egress includes three parts, which are: the exit, the access, and the _____.**

    A. width of isles
    B. number of doors
    C. height of the tread riser
    D. exit discharge with unhindered lanes from the building

90. **NFPA classifies six types of fire-protective signaling systems. Which of those listed below are included in this classification?**

    A. Supervisory, local, remote
    B. Smoke, fire, supervisory
    C. Local, central station, proprietary
    D. Household, auxiliary, pull-station

91. Which type of building construction material has the greatest ability to resist structural damage from a fire?

    A. Wood veneer
    B. Fire resistive
    C. Heavy timber
    D. Common

92. Which of the following is done to minimize the potential differences between conductive objects?

    A. Bonding
    B. Electrical neutralization
    C. Grounding
    D. Earthing

93. What is the recommended spacing for fire-detection systems?

    A. Every 15 feet
    B. 15 to 20 feet
    C. Every 20 feet
    D. According to the manufacturer's specifications

94. Which of the following fire-detection systems experiences thermal lag?

    A. Photoelectric
    B. Fixed temperature
    C. Infrared
    D. Ultraviolet

95. How is static accumulation, associated with aircraft fueling operations, minimized?

    A. Grounding the aircraft
    B. Grounding the aircraft and bonding to the fueler
    C. Bonding to the fueler unless in an electrical storm
    D. Grounding the aircraft, grounding the fueler, and bonding both

96. When a fire-detection system is electrically supervised, it means that a single outage in the power supply system, such as an open ground circuit, will signal the presence of a fault.

    A. True
    B. False; it means the system has a watchman.
    C. False; the electronic supervision circuit will be affected by the power outage.
    D. False; the supervision circuit only monitors the detection system. It will not sense a problem with input power.

97. Which of the following is the *best* inside stairwell design in the event of fire?

    A. Straight stairwell with 1-hour walls
    B. Doors at each level
    C. Smoke-proof tower with pressurized stair tower
    D. Smoke-free stairs with horizontal exits

98. How high should a fire-resistive wall separating oxygen and fuel gases be?

    A. Must extend 6 inches beyond tallest cylinder
    B. Approximately 5 feet
    C. 4 feet
    D. 6 feet

99. In fire-protection engineering, some problems involving piped water supplies and fire-protection systems require substitution of one pipe for another. What length of 8-inch pipe (friction loss of 1.28 psi per 100 feet) is equivalent to 700 feet of 6-inch pipe (friction loss of 4.40 psi per 100 feet)?
   A. 3000 feet
   B. 2100 feet
   C. 1800 feet
   D. 2400 feet

100. Which of the following is considered the *primary* purpose of fire sprinkler systems?
   A. They provide life safety and protect property.
   B. They provide proper dispersion of water droplets.
   C. They provide both power cone and full fog water sprays.
   D. They automatically deliver water to a fire.

Self-Assessment Exam 5 Answers

1. Answer: **B**. The mass number of an element refers to the total number of protons and neutrons in the nucleus.
2. Answer: **A**. pH = –log [H⁺]. pH equals minus the logarithm of the hydrogen ion concentration in moles per liter. The pH scale extends from 0 to 14, with values less than 7 acids and greater than 7 bases.
3. Answer: **A**. Friction is the force resisting the relative motion of solid surfaces, fluid layers, and material elements sliding against each other. There are several types of friction:
   - Dry friction resists relative lateral motion of two solid surfaces in contact. Dry friction is subdivided into *static friction* between nonmoving surfaces and *kinetic friction* between moving surfaces.
   - Fluid friction describes the friction between layers of a viscous fluid that are moving relative to each other.
   - Lubricated friction is a case of fluid friction where a fluid separates two solid surfaces.
   - Skin friction is a component of drag, the force resisting the motion of a fluid across the surface of a body.
   - Internal friction is the force resisting motion between the elements making up a solid material while it undergoes deformation.

   Friction is a function of weight, surface, and contact. The maximum frictional force on a body resting on another body is proportional to the resultant of all forces perpendicular to the surfaces in contact and the coefficient of static friction.
4. Answer: **A**. Most industrial exposure is sensorineural or noise induced.
5. Answer: **A**. Pounds per square inch gage (Psig) is equivalent to Pounds per square inch absolute (Psia) minus one standard atmosphere or 14.7 psi.
6. Answer: **A**. The correct formula is rise over run. To determine the percent slope of a ramp with an elevation of 4 feet and a length of 10 feet = 4/10 or 0.4 = 40%.
7. Answer: **C**.

$$K.\,E. = \frac{m\,v^2}{2} = \frac{W\,v^2}{2g}$$

$$70 \text{ mph} \times 1.47 = 103 \text{ ft per sec}$$

$$\frac{20{,}000 \text{ lbs} \times (103 \text{ f/s})^2}{2 \times 32 \text{ f/s}^2} = 3{,}315{,}000 \text{ ft-lbs}$$

8. Answer: **C**. Specific gravity is the ratio of the weight of substance (in this case a metal weight) to an equal volume of water. SG = ds/dw; d = w/v. Since the difference in weight on land and in water is 600 ounces,

then an amount of water the same density as the lead weight must weigh 600 ounces, but the weight weighs 1800 ounces, so 1800/600 = 3 times heavier than water. SG = 3.

9. Answer: **A**. A liquid has no definite shape but a definite volume. Gases and vapors have volume, but shape is determined by the container.
10. Answer: **D**. OSHA 1910.1027 requires that if biological monitoring is required for cadmium exposure, it will search for the following markers:
    - CdU – urinary cadmium (chronic damage)
    - CdB – blood cadmium (acute damage)
    - β2-M – urinary β2 microglobulin (β2-M damage/kidney disease)

    A review of 1910.1027 is in order prior to the Safety Fundamental Examination. Selection D references the biological determinant hippuric acid in urine at the end of each shift, which might be used for toluene exposure.
11. Answer: **B**. Oxidizers do not always react violently with bases nor can they be stored safely in steel containers. Shipping labeling and placards are Class 5.1 and 5.2 for oxidizers.
12. Answer: **A**. OSHA 1910.1028 requires the employer to make available a medical surveillance program for employees who are or may be:
    - Exposed to benzene at or above the action level 30 or more days per year
    - Exposed to benzene at or above the PEL 10 or more days per year
    - Exposed to 10 ppm of benzene for 30 days or more in a year prior to current employment
    - An employee involved in tire-building operations called tire-building machine operators who use solvents containing greater than 0.1 percent benzene

    The initial medical examination shall be conducted at or before the time of initial assignment. A review of OSHA 1910.1028 is suggested prior to sitting for the Safety Fundamentals Examination. Modified from OSHA 1910.1028
13. Answer: **C**. The specific gravity of gases is defined as the ratio of the weight of a certain volume of a gas to the weight of an equal volume of dry air.
14. Answer: **B**. The term "population stereotype" or "operational stereotype" in the field of human engineering refers to the expectation of humans in response to the movement of controls. In other words, when operating a control, workers expect a certain response. Research and experience have proven that some standardized movements are expected by a large segment of the population. For example, in North America it is expected to turn on house lights by flipping the switch to the up position. A lever is pushed forward to increase speed and when a wheel turns to the right generally the movement is to the right. These compatibilities are learned tendencies, not universal behaviors, and violations of these principles have been documented in accident reports since the beginning of time. Any text dealing with ergonomics will discuss the subject in greater detail.
15. Answer: **A**. From the table included on the exam: f = 9, P = 0.95. Solution = 1.833.

Table of Percentage Points of the t-Distribution

df \ p	0.25	0.1	0.05	0.01
1	1.000	3.078	6.314	31.821
2	0.816	1.886	2.920	6.965
3	0.765	1.638	2.353	4.541
4	0.741	1.533	2.132	3.747
5	0.727	1.476	2.015	3.365
6	0.718	1.440	1.943	3.143

Table of Percentage Points of the t-Distribution				
7	0.711	1.415	1.895	2.998
8	0.706	1.397	1.860	2.896
(9)	0.703	1.383	(1.833)	2.821
10	0.700	1.372	1.812	2.764
15	0.691	1.341	1.753	2.602
20	0.687	1.325	1.725	2.528
25	0.684	1.316	1.708	2.485
30	0.683	1.310	1.697	2.457
∞	0.674	1.282	1.645	2.326

16. Answer: **B**.
    Step 1 Determine the concentration.
    $$\frac{150 \text{ mliter}}{2 \text{ M}^3} = \frac{150 \times 10^{-3} \text{ liter}}{2 \times 10^3 \text{ liter}} = 75 \times 10^{-6}$$

    Step 2 Multiply by 1,000,000.
    $(75 \times 10^{-6}) \times (1 \times 10^6) = 75$ ppm

17. Answer: **C**. Concept: Specific gravity is the ratio of the steel bar's weight to an equal volume of water. When an object is immersed in a fluid, the force of buoyancy on it is equal to the weight of the displaced fluid.
    Step 1 Determine the weight of the bar if it were water.
    $$D = \frac{m}{V}$$
    $$9 = \frac{200}{x}$$
    x = 22.2 lbs

    Step 2 Correct for the lesser weight of the oil; SG = 0.7.
    x = 22.2 × 0.7
    x = 15.44 lbs

    Step 3 Subtract from the land-based weight.
    200 lbs − 15.54 = 184 lbs

18. Answer: **A**. Alkali and alkaline earth carbides are not compatible with water. Calcium carbide combines with water [$CaC_2 + 2H_2O \rightarrow Ca(OH)_2 + C_2H_2$] to form acetylene. The heat of reaction is hot enough to ignite acetylene. Additionally, calcium carbide is a major source of acetylene and is also used to make the fertilizer, calcium cyanamide ($CaCN_2$), which is also very water reactive.

19. Answer: **A**. The population standard deviation is 9.6.

20. Answer: **A**. A DC generator needs a commutator to change the frequency or direction of current in the armature windings. The commutator is a cylindrical ring or disk assembly of conducting members, each insulated in a supporting structure with an exposed surface for contact with current-collecting brushes and mounted on the armature shaft. In an AC generator, two slip rings or collector rings enable the rotating loop to be connected to stationary wire leads for the external circuit.

21. Answer: **D**. Epidemiological studies are divided into three separate types:
    - Cross-sectional or prevalence studies
    - Retrospective or case control studies
    - Prospective studies or cohort or incident studies

    It is generally accepted that the most scientifically useful study is the *prospective* study, which is initiated before commencement of exposure to the agent under study and is continued until the appearance of disease. Recently some of the more progressive major companies have initiated prospective epidemiological studies for all new chemicals introduced into the workplace. As most people would expect, the process is quite expensive. Plans must be established well in advance for the methods of gathering exposure data, establishing history of the workers, other agent exposure, etc. *Retrospective* studies look back in time on populations exposed to the agent under investigation. These are the most inexpensive, but often suffer from lack of data. What dose was received, for how long, what other agents were present, etc.? These questions cannot be answered because the exposure occurred in the distant past. They rely heavily on estimated data and experimental statistical methods, which affect the validity. *Cross-sectional* studies deal with real-time relationships between an agent and infection or disease. They are based on existing relationships and investigate only present-time cases. Great effort is made to ensure that all persons affected will become part of these studies.

22. Answer: **A**.

    Step 1 Draw and label a free body diagram of the beam.

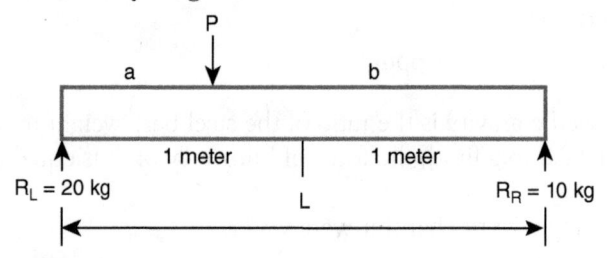

    Figure 56 Diagram of 2-meter beam

    Step 2 Select a formula and solve.

    $$R_R = \frac{Pa}{L}$$

    $$a = \frac{L \times R_R}{P}$$

    $$a = \frac{2 \times 10}{30} = \frac{20}{30} = 0.667 \text{ m or } 66.7 \text{ cm}$$

23. Answer: **A**.

    Step 1 Calculate the volume of the tank with a starting height of 7.5 feet (9 − 1.5).

    $$V = \frac{\pi d^2 \times h}{4}$$

    $$V = \frac{3.14 \times (6)^2 \times 7.5}{4}$$

    $$V = 212 \text{ cu ft}$$

    $$212 \text{ ft}^3 \times 7.48 \text{ gal/ft}^3 = 1586 \text{ gallons}$$

Step 2 Convert to gallons.
Step 3 Calculate time to drain at 25 gallons per minute.

$$\frac{1586 \text{ gallons}}{25 \text{ gal/min}} = 63.45 \text{ minutes}$$

24. Answer: **B**. Workers only have the right to contest the abatement date of OSHA citations. They have no say in the working of the compliance officer's citation and cannot negotiate corrective actions. Complaints can be made if corrective actions do not correct the violation.
    When a violation is issued and a penalty is assessed, the employer is not relieved from his or her responsibility to fix the violation by payment of the fine.
25. Answer: **D**. Wisconsin was the first state to establish an *effective* workers' compensation program.
26. Answer: **D**. Most likely none of these workers would be covered by a state program and are either not covered or receive federal benefits.
27. Answer: **A**. According to current thinking, Operations Management, which includes all levels of supervision, is responsible for safety. Actually, **everyone in the entire organization is responsible for safety**.
28. Answer: **D**. The primary purpose of a program audit is to determine if the program is following the plan. Performance measurement in well-performing companies includes the basic procedures of determining compliance, performing scheduled safety audits, and benchmarking.
29. Answer: **B**. Motor vehicle accidents are the largest cause of industrial injuries in the United States.
30. Answer: **C**. Operator entry mistakes are a common computer problem.
31. Answer: **D**. Although all factors listed are important to the safety effort, the least important is to review written work order procedures. There should be a process for submitting, prioritizing, and completing maintenance work orders.
32. Answer: **A**. Accidents involving injuries that do not require medical response are not recordable in accordance with DOT regulations.
33. Answer: **C**. Retrospective rating plans use the last three years' experience in order to determine the current charges.
34. Answer: **B**.

    $S \cong 6 \text{ CE}$

    $S \cong 6 \times 0.075 \times (1.1 + 1.3)$

    $S \cong 1.08 \text{ roentgen}$

    $S \cong 1080 \text{ milliroentgen}$

35. Answer: **B**. The first step in establishing any data collection system is to determine subsequent use of the data.
36. Answer: **C**. The concept of Accident Proneness is shunned by the current progressive safety community.
37. Answer: **B**. Involvement in the early stages of any project by safety professionals is the best way to insure that safety receives proper consideration.
38. Answer: **B**. The supervisor is responsible for production and this puts him/her in the best position to be an educator and trainer. He/she realizes what is critical to the operation and understands the workplace tempo.
39. Answer: **B**. A three-dimensional model is very helpful in visualizing plant layout prior to actual construction.
40. Answer: **C**. Job safety analysis is a systematic analysis of job elements. It results in an in-depth evaluation by workers and first-line supervisors of the individual steps and hazards. JSAs also offer protective measures or solutions to identified hazards. Option A (System Safety Analysis) is a broad term covering all various system safety tools used in the analysis of system risk. Option B, Fault Tree Analysis, is the process of using deductive logic to determine the combination of events that caused a hazardous event

316 ASP Exam Study Workbook

to occur. It is normally accompanied by a companion report that evaluates the overall likelihood of failure and provides solutions to findings discovered in FTA. Management Oversight and Risk Tree is a formal decision tree used in the evaluation of safety programs or as an accident investigation tool. The tool is exhaustive, offering about 1500 events to be evaluated. For this reason, it is often considered overkill for all but the largest evaluations or mishaps. However, system logic is sound and recently several practitioners have produced "mini-MORT" charts that have proven to be useful tools for smaller applications.

41. Answer: **D**. Accident investigations are conducted to determine cause factors so that mishaps can be prevented.

42. Answer: **C**. Preventive maintenance schedules can be developed from detailed analysis of a system or process that a Failure Mode and Effects Analysis (FMEA) provides. The analysis provides an indication of which component failure is maintenance dependent, as well as how the overall system will benefit from extended life of critical parts.

43. Answer: **C**.

$$T = \frac{8}{2^{\left(\frac{L-90}{5}\right)}} = \frac{8}{2^{\left(\frac{101.8-90}{5}\right)}} = \frac{8}{2^{\left(\frac{11.8}{5}\right)}} = \frac{8}{2^{2.36}} = \frac{8}{5.13}$$

$$T = 1.56 \text{ hours}$$

44. Answer: **B**. Select the formula, rearrange, and solve.

$$\text{Accident Rate} = \frac{\text{Cases} \times 200{,}000}{\text{Total hours worked}}$$

$$\text{Cases} = \frac{\text{AR} \times \text{Total hours worked}}{200{,}000}$$

$$\text{Cases} = \frac{3.5 \times (1800 \times 2000)}{200{,}000}$$

$$\text{Cases} = \frac{3.5 \times 3{,}600{,}000}{200{,}000}$$

$$\text{Cases} = \frac{12{,}600{,}000}{200{,}000}$$

$$\text{Cases} = 63$$

Note: Since the accident rate is per 100 workers, the same result can be obtained by $3.5 \times 18 = 63$.

45. Answer: **A**. Select the formula for a sample standard deviation and solve.

$$s = \sqrt{\frac{\Sigma(X - \bar{X})^2}{N - 1}}$$

$$s = \sqrt{\frac{4900}{35 - 1}}$$

$$s = \sqrt{144.12}$$

$$s = 12$$

46. Answer: **D**. At the bottom of Maslow's "hierarchy of human needs" are the physiological or survival needs of food, water, and physical well-being. According to the *progression principle,* as soon as these

survival needs are met, one attempts to satisfy the next level of needs; those of security, protection, and stability in day-to-day life activities. If these are met, one moves on to social needs, etc. The first three needs in the model are called lower order needs and are concerns for a person's desire for social and physical well-being. The top two needs in the pyramid are the high-order needs that satisfy psychological development and growth. Maslow's needs hierarchy is often used as the most elementary model in the complex study of man's needs and desires. **Figure 37** shows how needs are satisfied in life and in business.

47. Answer: **D**. The chemical manufacturer, importer, or distributor must ensure that hazardous chemical containers are labeled.
48. Answer: **B**. The TLV is higher for 1,1,1-trichloroethane than trichloroethylene and trichloroethylene is suspected of having carcinogenic activity. This is a recent, almost classic, example of the principle of "substitution of materials."
49. Answer: **C**. Carbon tetrachloride ("carbon tet") is an outlawed solvent that causes damage to the liver.
50. Answer: **C**. Acclimatization to heat is generally achieved by having the employee exposed to the hot environment for two hours per day for one or two weeks.
51. Answer: **C**. If radioactive materials that emit alpha particles such as radium are spilled, leak out of their container, or are involved in a fire, it is easy to spread them over a large area and thus create major problems.
52. Answer: **A**. A short excursion above the TLV but below the STEL is generally permissible. Many individuals refer to a published TLV or AC as a go or no-go value—that is, something to be used in a specific situation. This use of data overlooks the important qualification of these values set forth by the organizations establishing them.
53. Answer: **B**. *Zero mechanical state* (ZMS) is a common term used in ANSI, OSHA, and other well-recognized safety literature. It may also be called a zero energy state procedure, or ZESP. However, the term "locked-out" makes B the best selection, since by the standard definition, the lock-out procedure consists of four major steps: preparation, lock-out, release of stored energy, and verification.
54. Answer: **D**. Copper, zinc, and lead fumes and dust are all common hazards found in brass foundries.
55. Answer: **C**. Q fever is a rickettsial organism that infects meat and livestock handlers. Similar to tick fever, byssinosis is contracted by those exposed to large concentrations of cotton or flax dust. Noroviruses are a group of related viruses that causes gastroenteritis, which is inflammation of the stomach and intestines. This leads to stomach cramping, nausea, vomiting, and diarrhea. MRSA is methicillin-resistant *Staphylococcus aureus*, a bacterium responsible for several difficult-to-treat infections in humans.
56. Answer: **C**. Anthrax is a highly virulent bacterial infection contracted from animals and animal products. Pneumoconiosis is "dusty lung." Presbycusis is hearing loss due to age. Anthracosis is a disease of the lungs caused by prolonged inhalation of dust that contain particles of carbon and coal.
57. Answer: **A**. Brucellosis is an infection caused by drinking unpasteurized milk from cows with Bang's disease. Pleurisy is the pain caused by lack of lubrication of the outer lung lining. Laryngitis is an inflammation of the larynx. Bursitis is an inflammation of the connective tissue around bone joints.
58. Answer: **D**. In discussions on electrical wiring, the terms *ground*, *grounded*, and *grounding* will always be encountered. They all refer to deliberately connecting parts of a wiring installation to a grounding electrode or electrode system. Grounding falls into two categories:
    - System grounding: Grounding one of the current-carrying wires of the installation
    - Equipment grounding: Grounding noncurrent-carrying parts of the installation, such as the service equipment cabinet, frames of motors or equipment, duplex outlets connected to a metal conduit, or the metal armor of armored cable

    The only possible answer here is selection D, *check the continuity between the green wire and the building ground*. However, in many cases when metal armor or conduit is used, it provides the path and serves as the conductor for the equipment ground, so attaching the green wire to the metal duplex outlet that is connected to the conduit is sufficient. If the neutral (white) wire is properly grounded both at the transformer and at the building service equipment, there will be no resistance between the white and green wires. NFPA 70, *National Electric Code* provides the following definitions in Part 100-A:

Ground: A conducting connection, whether intentional or accidental, between an electrical circuit or equipment and the earth, or to some conducting body that serves in place of the earth.

Grounded: Connected to earth or to some conducting body that serves in place of the earth.

Grounded, Effectively: Intentionally connected to earth through a ground connection or connections of sufficiently low impedance and having sufficient current-carrying capacity to prevent the buildup of voltages that may result in undue hazards to connected equipment or to persons.

Grounded Conductor: A system or circuit conductor that is intentionally grounded.

Grounding Conductor: A conductor used to connect equipment or the grounded circuit of a wiring system to a grounding electrode or electrodes.

Grounding Conductor, Equipment: The conductor used to connect the noncurrent-carrying metal parts of equipment, raceways, and other enclosures to the system grounded conductor, the grounding electrode conductor, or both, at the service equipment or at the source of a separately derived system.

Grounding Electrode Conductor: The conductor used to connect the grounding electrode to the equipment grounding conductor, to the grounded conductor, or to both of the circuits at the service equipment or at the source of a separately derived system.

Ground-Fault Circuit-Interrupter: A device intended for the protection of personnel that functions to de-energize a circuit or portion thereof within an established period of time when a current to ground exceeds some predetermined value that is less than that required to operate the overcurrent protective device of the supply circuit.

Ground-Fault Protection of Equipment: A system providing protection of equipment from damaging line-to-ground fault currents by causing a disconnecting means to open all ungrounded conductors of the circuit. This protection is provided at current levels less than required to protect conductors from damage by a supply circuit overcurrent device." Reproduced from Article 500 of the National Electrical Code (NEC), NFPA 70, 2017 edition, National Fire Protection Association.

59. Answer: **C**: The respirator maintenance program should include inspection for defects, cleaning, disinfecting, and provisions for storage and repair. Selection and purchase by definition do not belong to the "maintenance" program.

60. Answer: **A**: Each kind of fuel has an energy or heat value per unit weight that is called the heat of combustion. Gasoline's is about 20,000 Btu/lb. The total heat produced during a fire is the product of the weight of fuel consumed and the heat of combustion for the fuel. The average density of gasoline is 5.6 lb/gal at 68°F. If 2 gallons of gasoline are consumed in a fire, the total heat produced would be calculated as follows:

$$20,000 \text{ Btu/lb} \times (2)(5.6 \text{ lb/gal}) = 224,000 \text{ Btu}$$

61. Answer: **D**. Employers are required by OSHA to post the citation at or near the location of the violation for three days or until corrected, whichever is longer.

62. Answer: **B**. The audiogram is a written record of the hearing threshold at certain specified frequencies and is normally presented in graph form. An audiometer produces tones that vary in frequency, usually from 125 or 250 to 8000 Hz, in octave or half-octave intervals. The amplitude or intensity from the audiometer can vary from zero dB to 110 or 115 dB and is plotted against frequency to provide a graphic record of hearing ability. Zero on the audiometer is slightly different from the 0.0002-microbar standard used in sound pressure level surveys. If a person experiences a 30-dB loss at 3000 Hz, it means that person cannot hear the tone unless it is raised 30 dB above the standard.

The illustration shown above depicts sensorineural hearing loss. The two measurements shown for the right ear show both air and bone conduction and show a sensorineural hearing loss in which the air conduction threshold and the bone conduction threshold have risen almost equally (no gap between them). These cases usually indicate a defect in the cochlea or possibly in central pathways.

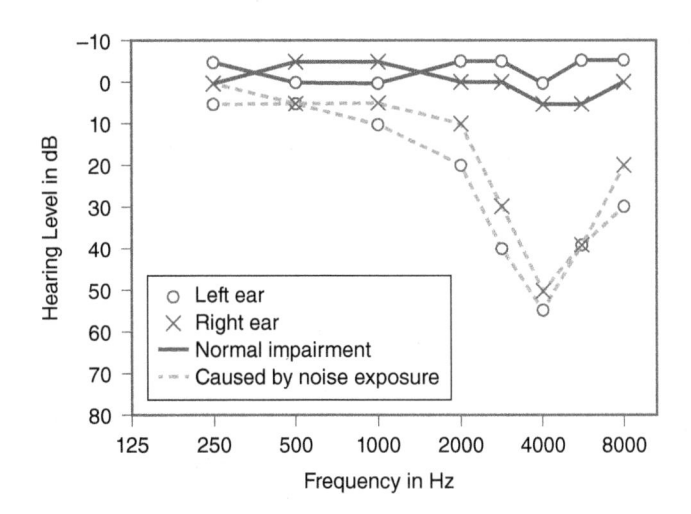

Figure 57 Sensorineural hearing loss

63. Answer: **C**. The absorption coefficient (α) of a material depends on many factors, among which are:
    - Angle relative to the noise source
    - Frequency of the noise source
    - Density
    - Condition/cleanliness
    - Type of mounting
    - Shape of surface

    Color is generally not considered a factor. The general rule is that a porous material (one through which air may be forced) will make a good sound absorbent. For example, fabric, felt, foam rubber, cheesecloth, carpet, Styrofoam, etc. Generally, materials that are thicker are better, with as many air gaps as possible. Many absorption materials are available and listings of the absorption coefficient of acoustical materials can be found in various advertising literature.

64. Answer: **D**. Emissivity is the capacity to radiate relative to a black body, which has a capacity of 1.0. Bright metal surfaces are poor emitters (good reflectors), having an emissivity of less than 0.1. When dealing with radiant heat sources in the infrared spectrum, emissivity of unpolished surfaces approaches that of a black body. Therefore, even light colors will not reflect well. The near side of a polished metal shield will reflect back 90% of the radiant heat from a furnace and the far side of that shield will emit only 10% of absorbed energy.

65. Answer: **A**. Carpal tunnel syndrome (CTS) is a median nerve entrapment neuropathy that causes paresthesia, pain, numbness, and other symptoms in the distribution of the median nerve due to its compression at the wrist in the carpal tunnel. The main symptom of CTS is intermittent numbness of the thumb, index, long, and radial half of the ring finger. The numbness often occurs at night.

66. Answer: **B**. Metal fume fever (MFF) is an acute affliction that produces flu-like symptoms (fever and chills). Recovery is normally complete within one to two days. Daily exposure will cause an immunity; however, any disruption such as a weekend off will result in reoccurrence of the symptoms, usually with greater severity. The cause of MFF is almost always inhalation of high concentrations of zinc oxide fumes. But there have been instances arising from exposure to magnesium oxide and copper oxides.

67. Answer: **B**. Assuming that the original system design was done using standard air with a density of 0.075 lb/ft^3, corrections will need to be made to meet actual operating conditions. Generally, no corrections are needed if temperatures range from 40°F to 100°F or for altitude changes of ±1000 feet. However, this large altitude increase will mean less dense air, which means the fan is moving less mass and will not need to develop as much static pressure. Additionally, the horsepower requirement is lower

since less air mass is being moved. *Changes in altitude do not affect the volume output of the fan (CFM),* which makes selection B the only correct answer. Additional reading includes the ACGIH Industrial Ventilation Manual.

68. Answer: **D**. It is very dangerous to provide breathing air with more than 23.5% oxygen and the practice is not permitted without equipment certified for oxygen service. Breathing air grade D or better will have 19.5% to 23.5% oxygen, less than 5 mg/m³ oil, 10 ppm or less CO, and less than 1000 ppm CO_2. Compressed oxygen can cause a fire to burn more intensely and therefore increases the fire risk in a hospital room.

69. Answer: **A**. OSHA's PEL for carbon monoxide is 35 ppm with a transitional limit of 50 ppm as an 8-hour TWA. OSHA's ceiling is 200 ppm for a 5-minute sample and 1500 ppm for an instantaneous sample. The ACGIH has a TLV-TWA of 50 ppm with a TLV-STEL of 400 ppm. NIOSH (1973d/Ex. 1-237) recommends an 8-hour TWA limit of 35 ppm with a 200-ppm ceiling. The current NIOSH pocket guide to chemical hazards lists the IDLH for CO at 1500 ppm. Carbon monoxide (CO) is a highly poisonous gas, and its mixtures with air are flammable and in some cases explosive. However, the greatest danger, in most cases, is the poisonous property of CO. Carbon monoxide exerts its harmful effect by reducing the oxygen-carrying capacity of the blood. CO entering the body through the lungs combines with hemoglobin in the blood to form carboxyhemoglobin. Hemoglobin has a greater affinity for CO than for oxygen and therefore at equilibrium the blood's carboxyhemoglobin-to-oxyhemoglobin ratio is 200 to 300 times higher than the CO-to-oxygen ratio in the inspired air. If CO is inhaled in small amounts, the formation of carboxyhemoglobin is a reversible reaction and red blood cells are apparently uninjured by the process. When exposure to CO ceases, oxygen replaces CO in the blood and oxyhemoglobin is formed once again.

70. Answer: **C**. Teratogens are chemicals that cause damage to a developing fetus, but the damage does not propagate across generational lines.

71. Answer: **B**. The best option would be to substitute LP trucks for gasoline trucks.

72. Answer: **D**. As the saying goes, "Never saddle a dead horse." Three clips are required with the saddles on the live end of the rope.

73. Answer: **D**. Double insulation cannot prevent conductive paths in extremely wet locations.

74. Answer: **B**. Falls are by far the most common cause of office mishaps.

75. Answer: **A**. At the first indication of a high-pressure leak, employees should immediately reduce pressure.

76. Answer: **B**. Pouring water into acid creates a violent reaction that often results in acid splashing and should be avoided. AAA = Always Add Acid.

77. Answer: **A**. The ability to check driving records of employees is required by the DOT and has stood up in court.

78. Answer: **C**. The term *load moment* is an engineering term that refers to the product of a force and its moment arm. The moment arm is defined as a perpendicular distance between the force vector and a reference point. The load boom indicator is a moment device that indicates the boom angle relative to horizontal.

79. Answer: **C**.

$$\text{Tan } A = \frac{a}{b} \quad a = 10 \quad b = 12$$

$$\text{Tan } A = \frac{10}{12}$$

$$A = \text{Tan}^{-1}\left[\frac{10}{12}\right] = 39.81°$$

80. Answer: **D**. Generally, shears of this type are remotely operated and require both hands to engage the clutch to ensure the safety of the operator.

81. Answer: **D**. Reinforced concrete is a composite material in which concrete's relatively low tensile strength and ductility are counteracted by the inclusion of reinforcement having higher tensile strength and/or ductility. Concrete structures must resist two kinds of forces: those of *compression* and *tension*. Design of

concrete slabs, beams, and girders involves computation of how much steel is required for strength in *tension* and how much concrete is required for strength in *compression*. The placement of reinforcement is a critical function if the structure is to resist the forces placed on it. All metal reinforcement should be accurately placed, and supported at the proper height by concrete or *metal chairs* to prevent movement during pouring. The actual placement in the slab or beam is dependent on forces the slab will experience. When a beam is supported at two or more points, it will tend to break by pulling apart at the bottom. To add strength, place steel near the bottom surface where it is needed most. When a beam is supported at one point, it is likely to fail by pulling apart at its upper surface first. So, we need to place reinforcing as high as possible (but not generally closer to the surface than one inch). The weakness of concrete in tension is illustrated in the failure of a cantilevered slab, which fails at the top of the slab. This requires the steel to be placed at the top of the slab.

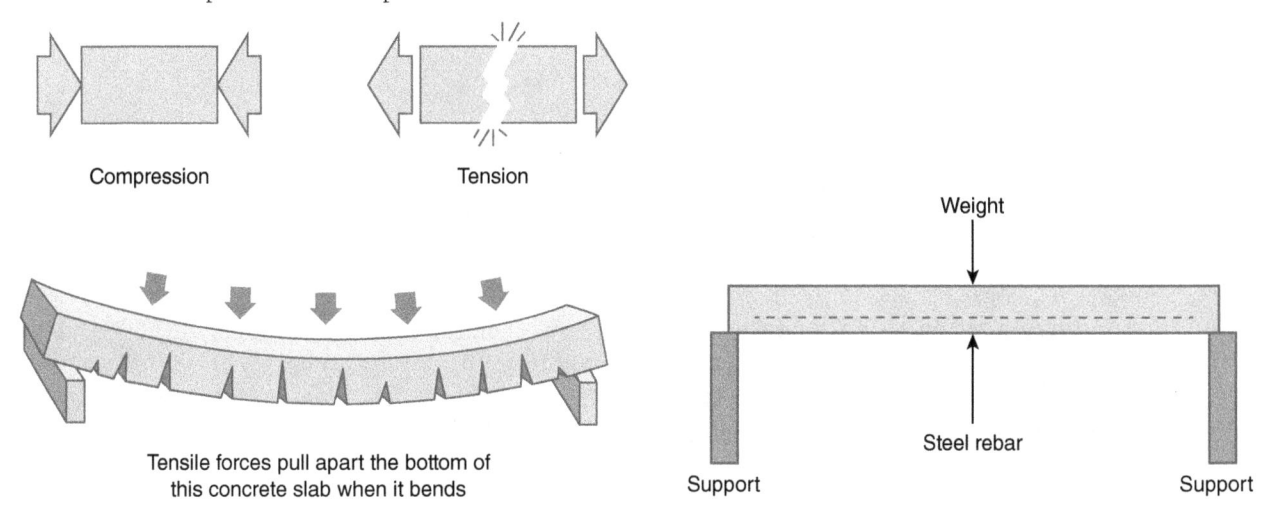

Figure 58 Strength in Tension and Compression

Figure 59 Reinforcing Beams

82. Answer: **D**. The single shackle connecting the load block hook to the rigging train is a single-point support. It will carry the weight of the entire load plus the weight of the rigging, which includes the strongback.

$$50{,}000 + 2400 = 52{,}400 \times 5 = 262{,}000 \text{ lbs}$$

The other shackles are in a parallel configuration and each carries one-half load plus rigging, or

$$50{,}000 + 2400 = 52{,}400 \div 2 = 26{,}200 \times 5 = 131{,}000.$$

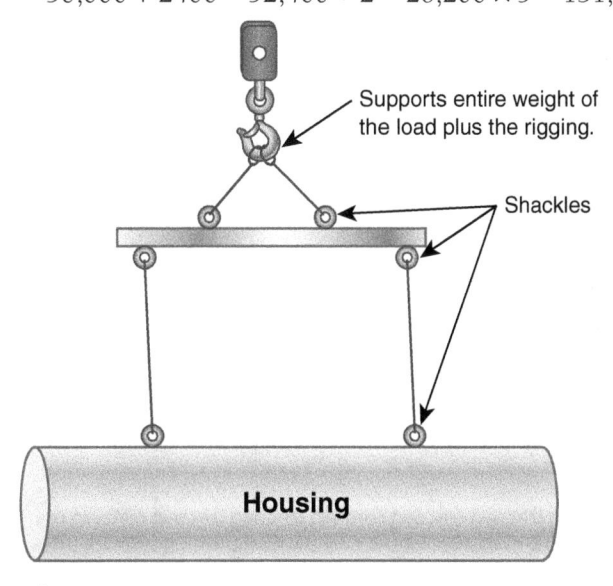

Figure 60 Supporting strength in rigging chain

83. Answer: **A**. The generally accepted factors used in determining the safety factor for the use of natural fiber rope such as manila, cotton, flax, asbestos, jute, silk, etc., are the size of rope, construction material (type of fiber), and the tensile or breaking strength (based on new, unused rope). For example, a new 3/8 inch diameter manila rope has a tensile strength of 1200 pounds and a recommended safety factor of 10, which makes the working load 120 pounds. A new 1 inch diameter manila rope has a tensile strength of 8000 pounds and a recommended safety factor of 7, which makes the working load 1150 pounds. Generally, manila rope from 3/16 inch to 3/8 inch requires a safety factor of 10; above 3/8 inch but less than 9/16 inch requires a 9 safety factor; above 9/16 inch but less than 3/4 inch has a safety factor of 8, and so on. These factors are guides, and judgment based on professional risk analysis must be used in many cases.
84. Answer: **A**. The purpose of an inverter is to convert direct current to alternating current. Selection C (rectifier) is used to convert AC to DC. Selection B (electrolytic capacitor) is just a particular type of capacitor, and selection A (transformer) is used to step up or step down electrical voltage.
85. Answer: **D**. Apply the formula and solve.

$$O_{Max} = 0.25 + (0.125D)$$

$$O_{Max} = 0.25 + (0.125 \times 6)$$

$$O_{Max} = 0.25 + 0.75$$

$$O_{Max} = 1$$

86. Answer: **C**. Local exhaust ventilation captures contaminant emissions at or very near the source and exhausts them outside. Since canopies are above the worker, the contaminant must travel very close to, and most of the time through, the worker's breathing zone.
87. Answer: **B**. The first principle of good storage practice for chemicals is segregation, including separation from other materials in storage, from processing and handling operations, and from incompatible materials.
88. Answer: **B**. Photoelectric smoke detectors respond faster (typically 30 minutes or more) to fire in its early, smoldering stage (before it breaks into flame). Photoelectric smoke detectors are best used in locations where smoldering fires or fires involving low-temperature pyrolysis PVC wire insulation may be expected. Fuel-loading platforms are protected by ionization detectors. Ionization detectors are more sensitive to the flaming stage of fires, so these detectors must be able to have a clear line of sight to the fire and must not be blocked.
89. Answer: **D**. A means of egress is a continuous path of travel from any point in a building or structure to the open air outside at ground level and consists of three separate and distinct parts:
    1. The way of exit access
    2. The exit
    3. The means of discharge from the exit
90. Answer: **C**. Fire-protective signaling systems are classified according to the functions they perform. The types and NFPA Standards are:
    - Central Station Alarm NFPA 71
    - Local NFPA 72A
    - Auxiliary NFPA 72B
    - Remote NFPA 72C
    - Proprietary NFPA 72D
    - Household Fire Warning NFPA 74
91. Answer: **B**. Fire resistive has structural members that will resist fire without collapse. In recent years, the classification of building has changed from descriptive terms to numerical or letter types of identification of construction classification.
92. Answer: **A**. Bonding is the process of connecting two or more conductive objects together by means of a conductor. Grounding (earthing) is the process of connecting one or more conductive objects to the ground and is a specific form of bonding. Grounding minimizes potential differences between objects and the ground.

93. Answer: **D**. The installation of the most suitable detector for the job is a very complicated subject and no one formula is entirely satisfactory. See NFPA 72 for additional information.
94. Answer: **B**. The air temperature in an area protected by a fixed temperature system is usually higher than the rated temperature because it takes time for the air to raise the temperature of the operating element to its set point. This is called thermal lag.
95. Answer: **D**. To prevent current flow, it is necessary to have all conductive surfaces at the same potential. This is only possible if all objects are grounded to the same reference point and bonded together.

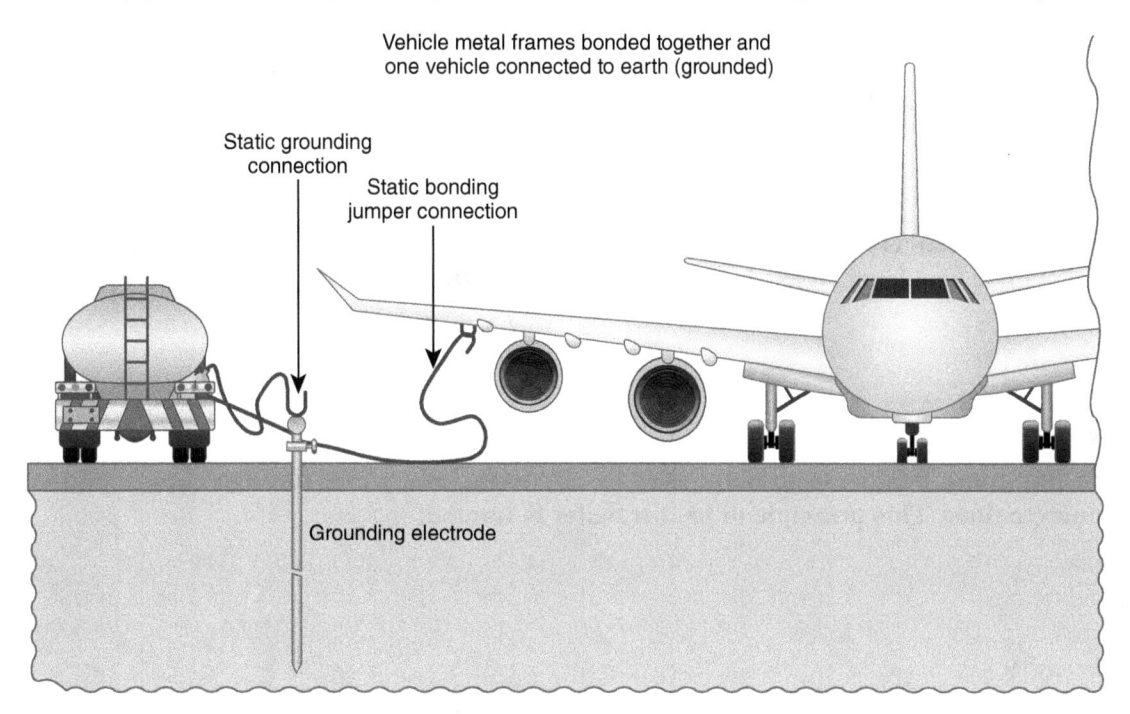

Figure 61 Bonding and Grounding

96. Answer: **A**. Fire-detection systems are commonly equipped with a monitoring system that warns of problems that may affect operation of the system. This is in effect a detection system watching a detection system.
97. Answer: **C**. Smoke-proof towers are the preferred method of providing a safe exit in high-rise occupancies. The addition of pressurized stair towers is an attractive feature and allows unrestricted entrance of firefighters to upper floors.
98. Answer: **B**. As a general rule, flammable and nonflammable gas bottles require a separation of 20 feet. A noncombustible barrier as high as the containers (usually 5 feet) having a fire-resistance rating of at least ½ hour is an acceptable substitute.
99. Answer: **D**.

$$D_1 \times f_1 = D_2 \times f_2$$

$$D_2 = \frac{D \times f_1}{f_2}$$

$$D_2 = \frac{700 \text{ ft} \times 4.40 \text{ psi}}{1.28 \text{ psi}}$$

$$D_2 = 2400 \text{ ft}$$

100. Answer: **D**. Fire sprinklers are designed to protect property by automatically delivering water to a fire. Generally, fire sprinklers are not considered life protection equipment. However, there are very few instances of multiple fatalities in buildings equipped with sprinklers. Additionally, the NFPA has developed a sprinkler standard for residential occupancies that has as its main goal "life safety." An automatic sprinkler system may be hazardous in an area used for storage of calcium chloride.

Self-Assessment Exam 6 Questions

1. A violent reaction that occurs when two materials come in contact with one another is termed:
   A. pyrophoric.
   B. hypergolic.
   C. pyrolysis.
   D. deflagration.

2. Which of the following *best* describes the purpose of hold harmless agreements?
   A. Prevent plaintiff from bringing suit
   B. Prevent hazardous materials from entering the market
   C. Prevent lawsuits
   D. Protect the court system

3. A facility has had an OSHA recordable accident experience of 673 mishaps a year and 42 are the result of vehicle accidents. What is the probability that the next incident will involve a vehicle?
   A. 0.03%
   B. 0.30%
   C. 6.2%
   D. 9%

4. In some buildings, heating is accomplished by circulating hot water through copper pipes contained in a concrete floor. This principle of heat transfer is termed:
   A. radiation.
   B. conduction.
   C. convection.
   D. differential.

5. In some system safety programs, computers use batch tasking to provide various reports throughout the life cycle of a project. Which of the following *best* describes the term *batch*, used in this context?
   A. Batch = β, which is the same as a Type I error.
   B. Batch is more than 10 programs executing at the same time.
   C. Batch is a basic unit of data along with bit and byte.
   D. Batch refers to the technique of executing a set of programs in series, one finishing before the next one starts.

6. An electrically actuated valve controlling hydraulic power to an aircraft control surface always goes to the open position should electrical power fail. This is an example of which of the following applications?
   A. Fail passive
   B. Fail active
   C. Fail neutral
   D. Fail redundant

7. Which of the following *best* describes the term *safety factor* when applied to a system/product safety effort?
   A. The extra margin of safety over intended use
   B. A scale from 1 to 10
   C. The product's cost factor
   D. Maximum strength over breaking strength

8. What is the failure rate of a device that has five components connected in parallel? Each component has a failure rate of 0.2.

   A. 0.4
   B. 2
   C. 0.00032
   D. 5×10^{-5}

9. A computer system controlling a chemical reactor in a plant has three components: the CPU, a storage disk, and the actuator. The failure probability on the CPU is 1×10^{-4}, the probability of failure on the storage disk is 1×10^{-1}, and the probability of failure on the actuator is 1×10^{-3}. What is the overall reliability of this control system?

   A. 98.01%
   B. 97.89%
   C. 89.9%
   D. 79.89%

10. Which of the following *cannot* require the recall of a manufactured product?

    A. State judge
    B. Federal judge
    C. NIOSH
    D. CPSC

11. A small business operation procures materials from three suppliers, assembles them, and then sells the machines under its own brand name. Supplier A delivers 13% of the components and has a defect rate of 3%; supplier B delivers 45% with a 5% defect rate; and supplier C provides 42% with a 3% defect rate. What is the probability that a recently returned product was configured with stock from supplier B?

    A. 200/390
    B. 100/390
    C. 90/390
    D. 225/390

12. Which of the following classes of materials *best* describes the compound $(CH_3)_2CHOH$?

    A. Ether
    B. Phenol
    C. Alcohol
    D. Organic acid

13. Which of the following organizations publishes the *most* standards within the United States?

    A. ANSI
    B. ASME
    C. FM
    D. NFPA

14. The probability that may be specified by the obvious nature of happenings is a/an _____ probability.

    A. a posteriori
    B. a priori
    C. obvious
    D. camouflaged

15. Which of the following is an ionizing radiation?
    A. Microwave RF
    B. UV
    C. IR
    D. X-rays

16. A supervisor orders a shutdown on a construction project for safety violations that do not exist. An employee's *best* course of action is to:
    A. shut down the project as ordered.
    B. resign the position immediately.
    C. advise the next level of management.
    D. write a letter of protest to the CEO.

17. During the assessment of a comprehensive computer system, which of the following would you expect to cause the *most* errors resulting in downtime?
    A. Computer hardware
    B. Power supply
    C. Inadequate grounding
    D. Computer software

18. The Mine Safety and Health Administration (MSHA) requires certain training for each new underground miner. Which of the following *best* describes the type of training?
    A. Performance-based training
    B. Specification-based training
    C. 180 hours of OTJ training
    D. 8 hours of classroom instruction

19. All of the following are duties that are part of a central safety committee's responsibilities *except*:
    A. it approves purchase requests for safety equipment.
    B. it reviews proposed new plant equipment.
    C. it is a liaison with management.
    D. it guides and directs the safety effort.

20. Which of the following *best* describes a supervisor's safety performance activity measure?
    A. Reporting incidents to management
    B. Identifying the financial impacts of losses associated with incidents
    C. Conducting incident investigation on reported incidents
    D. Performing safe work observations of employees and discussing the observations with them

21. A training supervisor has observed training delivered by a new staff trainer. In order to maximize the potential for improvement, the observation follow-up should be:
    A. discussed immediately with recommendations to develop the skills and confidence of the trainer.
    B. based upon a standardized instructor evaluation form.
    C. sent via e-mail for documentation.
    D. provided for the annual performance appraisal.

22. The *best* indicator of training effectiveness is:
    A. favorable student critiques.
    B. correct student responses to questions.
    C. an increase in job performance effectiveness.
    D. when testing meets expected norms.

23. **The *best* measurement of learning for job performance skills is:**
    A. documentation using written pre- and post-tests.
    B. documentation of observed job performance based on a criteria checklist.
    C. evaluation of each trainee through interviews.
    D. a perception survey.

24. **Formal observation, using criteria-referenced checklists, is a data collection method *best* used for:**
    A. measuring trainees' understanding of simple factual matter.
    B. complex performances such as operations or maintenance tasks.
    C. evaluations for which measurement costs are minimal.
    D. evaluating training results not defined as specific behaviors.

25. **When providing training for welders on fire characteristics of liquid hazardous chemicals, which of the following would *not* be discussed?**
    A. TLV
    B. Auto-ignition temperature
    C. Lower explosive limit
    D. Upper flammable limit

26. **One disadvantage of a lecture presentation is that:**
    A. the instructor has control of material presented.
    B. it presents large amounts of information in a short time.
    C. it offers limited audience participation.
    D. it is the most efficient way to teach knowledge-level objectives.

27. **When presenting statistical data for comparison at a presentation, which of the following would be the *best* choice of visual aid?**
    A. Table
    B. Organizational chart
    C. Bar graph
    D. Pie chart

28. **Calculate the incidence rate for a company if the recordable accidents are 60 and total man-hours are 1,750,000.**
    A. 6.9
    B. 8.8
    C. 9.2
    D. 9.5

29. **Which system identifies hazardous conditions, assesses their risk, and establishes effective risk control measures?**
    A. Risk control system
    B. Risk management system
    C. Loss-control system
    D. Loss management system

30. **One criterion that can be used to demonstrate commitment to continuous improvement is the use of:**
    A. proficiency assessments to determine appropriate pass/fail ratios.
    B. information from training evaluations when revising a course.
    C. summative evaluations for each learning objective.
    D. periodic third-party review, not less than annually.

31. **Which of the following encompasses the term *noncombustible*?**

    A. Fire proof
    B. Fire resistive
    C. Flame proof
    D. Fire retardant

32. **Current industrial fire pumps are of centrifugal design and pump water by centrifugal force from turbine vanes or a rotating wheel. The pumps may allowably be driven by which of the following?**

    A. Gasoline engines, steam engines, or electric motors
    B. Steam engines, diesel engines, or steam turbines
    C. Propane engines, diesel engines, or gasoline engines
    D. Electric motors, diesel engines, or steam turbines

33. **The National Institute for Occupational Safety and Health (NIOSH) is located within which federal agency?**

    A. Health and Human Services/CDC
    B. Department of Labor/OSHA
    C. Health and Human Services/PHS
    D. EPA

34. **According to NIOSH, to provide the most effective level of safety during confined space entry, which of the following correctly indicates the minimum amount of training necessary?**

    A. Recognition of hazardous materials, first-aid training, rescue training, and orientation on a self-contained breathing apparatus (SCBA)
    B. Confined space hazard recognition training, training for testing hazardous atmospheres, training on rescue procedures, training on PPE, and advanced first-aid training
    C. Confined space hazard recognition training, training for testing hazardous atmospheres, training on rescue procedures, training on PPE, and first-aid training
    D. Recognition of hazardous materials, advanced first-aid training, training on rescue procedures, and in-depth training on the use of self-contained breathing equipment

35. **If a commercial motor vehicle transporting hazardous materials (placarded) is equipped with dual tires on any axle, which of the following rules involving tire examination procedure is correct?**

    A. Tire examination must be done every hour or 50 miles.
    B. Tire examination must be done every 1½ hours or 75 miles.
    C. Tire examination must be done every 2 hours or 100 miles.
    D. Tire examination must be done every 2½ hours or 125 miles.

36. **A circuit protected at 20 amperes and loaded to 21 amperes is *best* protected by which of the following protection devices?**

    A. A thermal circuit breaker
    B. A magnetic circuit breaker
    C. A bolted fault fuse
    D. A GFCI

37. **A scaffold erected on a construction site will be loaded to 57 lb/ft². Which of the scaffolds listed below would be the proper choice for this loading?**

    A. Normal load scaffold
    B. Ordinary use scaffold
    C. Extra hazard scaffold
    D. Heavy-duty scaffold

38. All the following groups of hydrocarbons have a high chance of being flammable *except*:
    A. aliphatic hydrocarbons.
    B. aromatic hydrocarbons.
    C. halogenated hydrocarbons.
    D. ethers.

39. How many cubic feet of air does a normal worker, performing moderate work, breathe during an 8-hour-per-day, 40-hour workweek?
    A. 300 ft³
    B. 1500 ft³
    C. 1800 ft³
    D. 9000 ft³

40. The first stage of a spray finishing system applies a solvent coating to the surface of parts in a spray booth. The solvent has a VP of 176 mm Hg, a LEL of 2.3%, and produces 33 ft³ of vapor. Company standards require enough dilution air to reduce the vapor of flammable materials to 20% of the lower explosive limit. Given the above information, what volume of dilution air is required?
    A. 2800 ft³
    B. 8880 ft³
    C. 19,200 ft³
    D. 1500 ft³

    $$Q' = \frac{G}{C}$$

41. Which of the following would be the *most* appropriate sampling media for $CH_3(CH_2)_6OH$ and CHI_3?
    A. Midget Impinger – solution 0.6% HCl + 0.6% H_2SO_4
    B. Tared low-ash polyvinyl chloride filter (5 microns)
    C. Coated glass fiber filters (coating is H_2SO_4)
    D. Charcoal tube

42. What is the air velocity in a 10-inch circular duct with a flanged round opening if the hood has a 0.72 coefficient of entry and a static pressure of 2.25 in. w.g.?
    A. 4325 fpm
    B. 5400 fpm
    C. 6980 fpm
    D. 7500 fpm

    $$V = 4005C_e\sqrt{SP_h}$$

43. A small high-pressure cylinder used for breathing air is 0.250 ft³ in volume and weighs 15 pounds when empty. What is the weight of the cylinder when pressurized with dry air to 2200 psig?
    A. 15.8 lbs
    B. 17.5 lbs
    C. 19.5 lbs
    D. 20.8 lbs

    $$\frac{P_1V_1}{T_1} = \frac{P_2V_2}{T_2}$$

44. What is the volume of dilution ventilation required to reach the TLV of 200 parts per million, if a process is generating 0.5 cubic feet of material in a room 10 feet by 10 feet by 20 feet?
    A. 2950 ft³
    B. 2500 ft³
    C. 2750 ft³
    D. 2000 ft³

45. Fire-detection and alarm systems protect property and processes and are widely used in the United States. These fire-protection systems use three distinct types of fire alarm signals: supervisory, alarm, and _____.

    A. trouble
    B. activation
    C. warning
    D. sabotage

46. The term "dry chemical" fire-extinguishing agent is associated with flammable liquids. What material is the term "dry powder" associated with?

    A. Metaloids
    B. Metals
    C. Unusual chemicals
    D. Particulates

47. Which of the following *best* describes the coefficient of variation?

    A. Mean divided by square of standard deviation
    B. Standard deviation divided by mean
    C. Total of squares of all data points
    D. Square root of standard deviation

48. Which of the following equipment would be considered "intrinsically safe"?

    A. Battery-powered electrical equipment
    B. Low-voltage drop light
    C. Flashlight with pop-out bulb
    D. Windup wristwatch

49. **Most playground child injuries are caused by:**

    A. unsafe equipment and pinch points.
    B. children getting caught under or in-between equipment.
    C. falls to ground level.
    D. wear and tear resulting in equipment failure.

50. If a gas, with a molecular weight of approximately 90, evaporates from an enclosed process tank, where would it build up?

    A. Near the floor
    B. Near the ceiling
    C. Neither of the above; it will disperse uniformly.
    D. It is temperature dependent.

51. Diesel fuel has a specific gravity of 0.83 and one gallon produces 128,400 Btu during combustion. Given this information, how many Btus will one pound of diesel produce?

    A. 8300
    B. 100,300
    C. 116,300
    D. 18,600

52. It is mandatory to orally report serious accidents to an OSHA representative nearest to the site of the incident within 8 hours. The report must expressly include all of the following *except*:

    A. a phone number and contact person.
    B. the most probable cause of the incident.
    C. the number of fatalities and/or number of hospitalized employees.
    D. a description of the incident.

53. The discernment that a manufacturer is liable for injury, due to a defect in a product, without proof of negligence or even fault, is called:

    A. res ipsa loquitor.
    B. standard tort.
    C. strict liability.
    D. privity.

54. Standards that are specific or have application for a specific industry only are called:

    A. horizontal standards.
    B. performance standards.
    C. vertical standards.
    D. stipulation standards.

55. Under which of the following conditions would the Fault Tree Analysis be the *least* effective?

    A. Analysis before design
    B. Developing maintenance schedules
    C. Troubleshooting
    D. Developing emergency manuals

56. Which of the following is *not* a common design factor that is usually considered in system safety work?

    A. Risk analysis
    B. Redundant design
    C. Cost/benefit ratio
    D. Barrier design

57. Heat transfer occurs by three processes, which are:

    A. radiation, induction, and refraction.
    B. radiation, ionization, and convection.
    C. convection, conduction, and induction.
    D. convection, conduction, and radiation.

58. The system safety concept calls for risk management strategies based on identification, analysis of hazards, and application of remedial controls using a systems-based approach. This is different from traditional safety strategies that rely on which of the following?

    A. Control of conditions based upon past analysis
    B. Control of causes based upon epidemiological analysis
    C. Investigation of past accidents
    D. All responses listed

59. Which of the following Boolean algebraic expressions correctly shows a commutative law?

    A. $(A + \overline{A}) \bullet (A + B) = A + B$
    B. $A + B = B + A$
    C. $A(A + C) = (A \bullet B) + (A \bullet C)$
    D. $A + (B \bullet C) = (A + B) + (A + C)$

60. Given equal thickness of the following materials, which would be an effective shield for gamma but *not* neutron emanation?

    A. Water
    B. Lead
    C. Synthetics
    D. Concrete

61. _____ is the science that studies the patterns, causes, and effects of health and disease conditions in defined populations.
    A. Entomology
    B. Etymology
    C. Epidemiology
    D. Etiology

62. Small discussion groups are a useful adult training method and *best* described by which of the following statements?
    A. They make it easy for the instructor to control the quantity and type of information presented.
    B. They are likely to encourage participation and stimulate interest.
    C. There is very little risk of a dominant speaker controlling the discussion.
    D. They are inappropriate for teaching creative problem-solving skills.

63. The statement that is true when describing the discipline of Boolean algebra is:
    A. Boolean algebra follows well-known algebraic principles.
    B. Boolean algebra is uniquely suited to conditions that vary inversely with the amplitude of the logic applied.
    C. Boolean algebra is used in the study of symbolic logic.
    D. Boolean algebra is a logic science that uses algebraic zymology to depict "set theory."

64. Which of the following graphs correctly illustrates the strength vs. flexion curve for the human elbow?

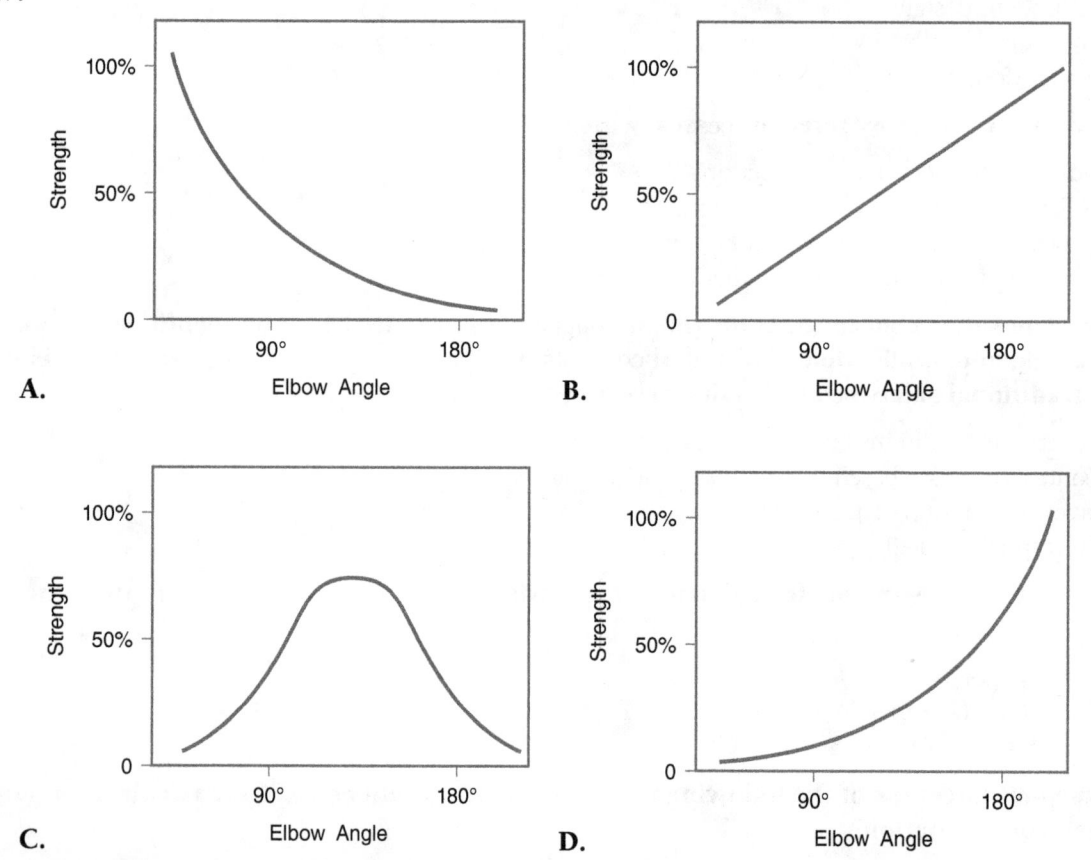

Figure 62 Strength vs. Flexion

65. **In a comparison of the capabilities of a computer and humans, which of the following is false?**
    A. Computers are better at voluminous searches of data.
    B. Humans are better at abstract judgment situations, such as emergency management.
    C. Computers are better at following random and variable strategy.
    D. Humans are better at exercising inductive reasoning, making judgments based on experience and reasoning.

66. **The *best* statement for establishing adult learner accountability in the classroom training situation is:**
    A. Objectives must be defined in operational terms.
    B. The trainer's style is most responsible for effective learning.
    C. The trainer must provide all facts and conclusions.
    D. Participants must know, accept, and take ownership for achieving the training objectives.

67. **The Process Safety standard, 29 CFR 1910.119, requires employers to establish a compliance audit capability. The standard requires employers to certify that they have evaluated compliance with process safety requirements at least every _____ years.**
    A. 3
    B. 2
    C. 5
    D. 4

68. **Which of the following is the *most often* recommended fundamental safety training for employees in an industrial setting?**
    A. First aid, supervisor's safety, and welding
    B. Welding, fork truck training, and back care
    C. Contingency, first aid, and vehicle operations
    D. Fire extinguisher training, first aid, and contingency

69. **Which of the following is *not* a principle for training adults?**
    A. Explain the purpose of the training session.
    B. Do not allow questions.
    C. Acknowledge the learners' experience and expertise.
    D. Do not talk down to learners.

70. **Calculate the WBGT index from the following information: outdoor globe temperature of 102°F, wet bulb temperature of 119°F, dry bulb temperature of 115°F.**
    A. 119.2°F
    B. 115.2°F
    C. 92°F
    D. 47°C

71. **Which group of employees is *most* likely to have the greatest probability of being involved in an on-the-job accident?**
    A. Line new hires with 1–3 years total experience
    B. Employees with 10 or more years of experience
    C. Office employees
    D. Functional and access needs employees

72. Under the HAZWOPER standard, 29 CFR 1910.120, owners of a hazardous waste site cleanup project are required to provide training for all the following *except*:
   A. training to general site workers.
   B. training on PPE and specialized equipment.
   C. training for contracted specialists responding to the scene.
   D. training on the safety, health, and other hazards present.

73. Environmental management is defined as:
   A. the organizing and controlling of affairs related to an organization's impact on the natural world, our surroundings, people, animals, and plants.
   B. the discipline of dealing with and avoiding risks, and supporting and rebuilding society.
   C. the identification, assessment, and prioritization of environmental risk (whether positive or negative), followed by coordinated and economical application of resources to minimize, monitor, and control the probability and/or impact of unfortunate events.
   D. ensuring proper climate control.

74. A process enclosure design retrofit is being evaluated at plants over which the health and safety manager has responsibility. The following formula has been devised to determine the cost effectiveness of several options. Using the formula below, determine which reduction offers the greatest cost/benefit ratio per dB.

   $C_X = 1,000,000 + 75,000X + 1500X^2$

   $A_X = \dfrac{C_X}{X}$

   Where: C_X = Total cost of retrofit
   A_X = Cost per dB
   A. 5-dB reduction
   B. 15-dB reduction
   C. 25-dB reduction
   D. 35-dB reduction

75. Your supervisor has asked you to calculate statistics on the accidents at one of your plants. The safety technician at the plant indicates that the total average number of accidents that occur during a given month is five. What is the probability that there will be exactly four accidents in the upcoming month?
   A. 0.0067
   B. 0.0033
   C. 0.0842
   D. 0.1755

   $P_{(r)} = \dfrac{(\lambda 1)^r e^{-\lambda t}}{r!}$

76. Which of the following is *not* a characteristic of integrated performance assurance, safety and health, and quality assurance programs?
   A. Require common intangible asset control
   B. Serve common underlying objectives
   C. Share common success and failure measures
   D. Use a common approach to achieve objectives

77. **Which of the following would be considered the primary talent of a safety professional?**
    A. Outsources as many responsibilities as possible
    B. Is recognized as the boss's "right-hand man"
    C. Displays continuous and flexible learning
    D. Strictly adheres to company policy guidelines

78. **Potential disadvantages of matrix management include all of the following *except*:**
    A. power struggles.
    B. increased costs.
    C. "groupitis."
    D. meeting attendance.

79. **The basic approach, according to many management systems, includes four sequential steps:**
    A. Plan, organize, develop, evaluate
    B. Plan, organize, implement, control
    C. Analyze, design, develop, implement
    D. Analyze, design, implement, evaluate

80. **What is the primary function of a loss-control system?**
    A. Assess risk, establish effective risk control measures, and eliminate risk.
    B. Establish effective risk control measures for hazardous conditions, establish effective control measures, eliminate risk.
    C. Identify hazardous conditions, assess their risks, and establish effective risk-control measures.
    D. Assure compliance with applicable regulatory requirements and eliminate residual risk.

81. **If a potential toxic hazard release is identified during a Preliminary Hazard Analysis (PHA) of a new process, what is the best procedure to determine how to protect against the hazard in case of a release or to determine if the hazard is present in a work area?**
    A. Conduct a site analysis and take air samples.
    B. Determine the effects of local meteorological conditions.
    C. Review the design with the engineering department.
    D. Use a computerized process flow sheet for initial evaluation of hazard releases.

82. **Based on the OHSAS 18001 guidelines that all management systems should be suitable, adequate, and effective, which of the following situations indicates that a management evaluation should be performed?**
    A. Profits are down from the preceding year.
    B. The ES&H Director position has been held by three individuals during the previous 18 months.
    C. The company's environmental performance has been questioned by a local "green" group.
    D. The company's safety performance is 40% lower than in the previous year.

83. **A manufacturer must keep records relating to product safety for what period of time?**
    A. As long as possible
    B. Life of the product guarantee
    C. Well beyond the life of the product
    D. Term of employment plus 30 years

84. The diagram shown below illustrates a parallel component arrangement where the failure of one, two, or three components would not result in output failure (all four components must fail to produce output failure). Assuming the failure rate is the same for all components, which of the following formulas should be used for computing the probability of failure for this system?

   A. $C^2 - F^4$
   B. $C_1 + C_2 + C_3 + C_4$
   C. $F(e^{-t/m})$
   D. $F_1 \times F_2 \times F_3 \times F_4$

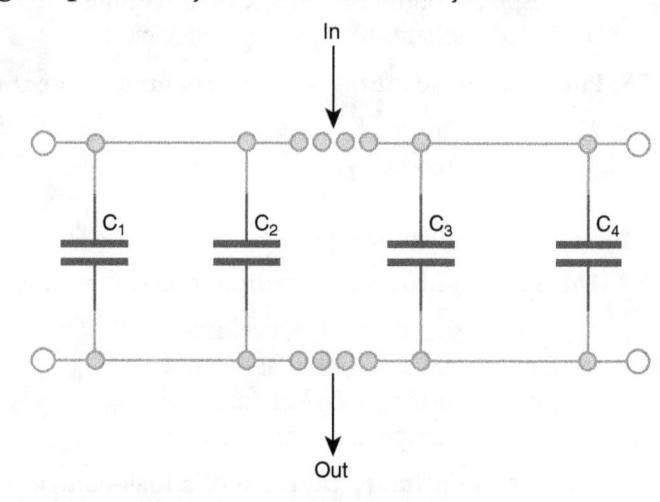

   Figure 63 Parallel Components

85. A company's Chief Executive Officer and General Manager ask the Safety Director where in the organizational structure is the best place for the safety function. The preferred placement of the safety function is in which department?

   A. Personnel
   B. Support
   C. Operations
   D. General Manager staff

86. Using the Management Grid® by Robert Blake and Jane Mouton, illustrating management styles by drawing a grid with a y-axis Concern for People and an x-axis Concern for Production, a 9,1 supervisor could be called a:

   A. country club manager.
   B. dictator.
   C. workaholic.
   D. company man.

87. The closed-loop system known as the behavior-based safety process includes identifying critical behaviors, problem solving to develop an action plan, measuring performance, and evaluating for acceptable progress. Identify the final step required to finish the loop.

   A. Nothing more is required; the loop is complete.
   B. Management must become involved in the process.
   C. Employee committees are formed to define penalties for no improvement.
   D. Accident and injury data is collected for inclusion in performance reports.

88. To discharge a capacitor safely, which tool should be utilized?

   A. A screwdriver to short-circuit the terminals
   B. An approved leakage meter
   C. A properly rated bleeder resistor or capacitor discharge tool
   D. A properly rated test light or lightbulb

89. **Which of the following is the best statement related to audit documentation?**
    A. Checklists must always be used.
    B. Forms to record supporting evidence must be documented.
    C. Audit sampling plans are generally not documented.
    D. Chain of custody is not a legal form of documentation.

90. **During a semi-annual inspection, what is the best chain inspection method?**
    A. Check links with a caliper and compare at least 10 links.
    B. Check for cracks in the end links.
    C. Compare twist on the end sections.
    D. Perform a detailed link-by-link inspection of the entire chain.

91. **What hand tool is most often misused?**
    A. Wrench
    B. Pliers
    C. Screwdriver
    D. Hammer

92. **Candlepower, the English standard for luminous intensity, is measured by the International System of units as:**
    A. candelas.
    B. luminescence.
    C. luminance.
    D. lumens.

93. **The *best* example of a proactive approach is which of the following?**
    A. Analysis of past injury/illness to identify trends
    B. Use of a medical history questionnaire to identify workers with preexisting conditions
    C. Implementation of a strength-testing protocol to select workers based on the physical demands of the job
    D. Observations and use of employee symptom surveys to identify problem jobs and tasks

94. **Single-celled organisms that can cause occupational illnesses are called:**
    A. viruses.
    B. RNA.
    C. protozoa.
    D. bacteria.

95. **In some people, the hepatitis B virus may develop into serious or fatal problems such as cirrhosis, liver cancer, or chronic liver disease. Which is the acronym for the hepatitis B virus?**
    A. HIV
    B. HCV
    C. HBV
    D. HAV

96. **A manufacturing area employee is working where presumed asbestos-containing material (PACM) or asbestos-containing material (ACM) is being used. If he/she requests information on PACM, the employee is entitled to:**
    A. the materials Safety Data Sheet (SDS).
    B. information as provided only for employees using ACM/PACM.
    C. training, as provided for all exposed employees and housekeeping staff who work in the area.
    D. training, as provided for all exposed employees who work in the area.

97. In some combustible gas meters, an electrical circuit consisting of a series of resistors is used to measure the mixture of combustible gas to air. The circuit is called the:

   A. combustible resistor circuit (CRC).
   B. Wheatstone bridge.
   C. combustible balancing circuit.
   D. hot wire detector (HWD).

98. To understand noise exposure experienced by all employees in a workplace with highly variable noise levels, which instrument should be used?

   A. Personal noise dosimeter
   B. Pressure-level meter
   C. Sound-level meter
   D. Integrating meter

99. A common and devastating result of some volcanic eruptions resulting in fast-moving currents of hot gases and rock at speeds greater than 50 mph/80 kmh, gas temperatures of 1000°C/1800°F, that hug the ground and travel downhill defines:

   A. a cyclonic event.
   B. pyroclastic flow.
   C. magma.
   D. lava.

100. A flood destroys your company's operations facility. After the emergency management issues are addressed, your company implements several plans to recover critical files and information that had been stored off-site; establish a temporary facility from which operations can be conducted; and inform customers of the situation and how they will be served. These plans are among examples of a comprehensive loss-control activity called:

   A. Emergency management/emergency response
   B. Situational awareness
   C. Disaster recovery/business continuity planning
   D. Business impact analysis

Self-Assessment Exam 6 Answers

1. Answer: **B**. Hypergolic describes a violent reaction, which occurs when two materials come in contact with each other. Pyrophoric materials ignite spontaneously when in contact with air. Pyrolysis is the process of decomposition in the presence of heat. Deflagration is a rapidly burning fire, which produces flame speed that travels slower than the speed of sound.
2. Answer: **C**. Hold harmless clauses in contracts between employers and manufacturers are common but rarely enforceable. In the standard clause, the employer agrees to hold the manufacturer or producer harmless in the event of a third-party lawsuit. In practice, the court rarely upholds the clause unless both parties are knowledgeable and are posturing from an equal position of strength.
3. Answer: **C**.

$$P = \frac{\text{Number of vehicle accidents}}{\text{Number of accidents}}$$

$$P = \frac{42}{673} = 0.062$$

$$P = 6.2\%$$

4. Answer: **B**. Convection is the transfer of heat by the circulation or movement of the heated parts of a liquid. The actual heat transfer principle here is that of *conduction*. When heated material flows parallel to the piping wall, a very thin layer of fluid clings to the wall and does not move. Heat is transferred through this stagnate layer to the laminar layer and on to the turbulent inner layer by *conduction*. There are only two general kinds of heat transfer: *conduction* and *radiation*. *Conduction* is the transmission of heat by molecular vibrations from one part of a body to another part of the same body or from one body to another body in physical contact with it. *Radiation* is the transmission of heat in the form of electromagnetic waves. Be careful not to confuse these principles on the test!
5. Answer: **D**. Batch processing refers to sequencing of various programs in order, one finishing before the other. One such application might involve sorting of an accident database on age in the following order:
   - First identifying location and injury
   - Requiring information formatting for a report
   - Printing of report so that it is available for review every week, month, etc.
6. Answer: **B**. This is an example of a fail-active device. It always fails open so that hydraulic power is available to control the vehicle.
7. Answer: **A**. The safety factor is that extra margin of safety designed into the product over and above its intended use.
8. Answer: **C**. For components in parallel, the total failure rate is the product of the individual components' failure rates: $0.2 \times 0.2 \times 0.2 \times 0.2 = 0.00032$ or 3.2×10^{-4}
9. Answer: **C**.
   $(1 \times 10^{-4}) + (1 \times 10^{-1}) + (1 \times 10^{-3}) = 1.01 \times 10^{-1} = 1 - 0.11 = 89.9\%$
10. Answer: **C**. NIOSH is the only agency listed that does not have some power in issuing a recall of consumer products in the United States.
11. Answer: **D**.

$$A = 13 \times 3 = 39$$
$$B = 45 \times 5 = 225$$
$$C = 42 \times 3 = \underline{126}$$
$$390$$

$$B = \frac{225}{390}$$

12. Answer: **C**. Alcohols are organic compounds in which a hydrogen atom has been replaced with the hydroxy (OH) group. In the case cited in this question, the compound is ethyl alcohol or according to the International Union of Pure and Applied Chemistry (IUPAC) is designated ethanol. Closely related are phenols (selection B) that are aromatic alcohols that are hydroxy derivatives of benzene. Selection A includes the ethers, which are also organic compounds that have an oxygen atom bridged between two alkyl or aryl groups. For example, methyl ethyl ether (methoxyethane) would have the chemical formula CH_2—O—C_2H_5. Selection D is an organic acid, which is a compound containing the carboxyl group (–COOH) and is often called carboxylic acid (i.e., formic acid has as a chemical formula HCOOH, acetic acid is CH_3COOH, etc.).
13. Answer: **A**. The American National Standards Institute, 1430 Broadway, New York, NY 10018, is by far the largest publisher of safety standards in the United States.
14. Answer: **B**. A priori probabilities are those that can be specified by the obvious and evident nature of the events from which they emerge. An example would be calculating the chance of getting a seven from a single roll of the dice. A posteriori probability is developed by conducting an experiment and observing the outcome. For example, it would be a posteriori probability to calculate the failure of an electronic component over time.
15. Answer: **D**. X-rays and gamma rays overlap and share a common region in the electromagnetic spectrum. This is the only possible ionizing radiation source among those listed.

16. Answer: **C**. Historically, several of these ethics questions have been included on the examination. The selection of an answer is very difficult because this workbook's authors differ in process approaches to these problems. However, the preferred answer in this case is to elevate the problem up the management chain until an executive is found who supports an individual inspector's decision. Supervisors must be alerted to specific concerns and plans to notify higher management.
17. Answer: **D**. Computer software causes many times more errors than any other single item listed. Some estimates run as high as 100 to 1. Although recent development techniques have reduced the amount of computer software errors, the ratio still remains high. This does not mean the overall error rate is high, simply that the ratio of software to hardware is high. Most computer downtime is actually for preventive maintenance, updating equipment or software, and housekeeping functions.
18. Answer: **B**. Throughout the history of the Mine Safety and Health Administration (MSHA), the organization has stressed the importance of training for miners. The training is expressly prescribed, "Every new underground miner shall receive no less than 40 hours of prescribed training." MSHA then lists the prescribed training complete with format. This is in contrast to the performance-based training required by recent legislation, such as the OSHA Hazard Communication Standard.
19. Answer: **A**. Safety committees to be effective should not be concerned with the day-to-day activities of the safety program within the company; that is, they should not purchase safety equipment, or investigate minor hazards or accidents. They should be responsible for direction of the overall safety effort and provide guidance for various program elements.
20. Answer: **D**. Author Dan Peterson explains that activity measures are leading (proactive) measures a line supervisor should do as part of his or her normal responsibilities in being accountable for the safety of employees. See *Techniques of Safety Management: A Systems Approach,* 4th edition.
21. Answer: **A**. Effective trainer feedback is done sooner versus later, is certain to happen, specific versus generic, positive versus negative, and perhaps most important, *useful*; it provides *actionable* information. Thus, "Good job!"; "You did that wrong"; and B+ are not feedback at all. We can easily imagine the new trainer asking him- or herself in response to these comments, "What *specifically* should I do more or less of next time, based on this information?" The new trainer would have no idea, and wouldn't know what was "good" or "wrong" about what he/she did.
22. Answer: **C**. Job performance is the most effective and final measure of any training program.
23. Answer: **B**. The best method to evaluate performance is on the job. A good method is the use of a criteria-referenced performance evaluation or proficiency assessment checklist.
24. Answer: **B**. Another means of providing employees with information about their skill development is to require business unit managers to conduct an assessment of each employee's level of knowledge, skills, and abilities relative to the level required for successful performance in the position. The Skill Gap Analysis can be administered using a survey instrument such as an observation checklist. A skill gap occurs when an employee is rated with a lower level of skill than the position requires. This assessment should be used for informational purposes only and should not be linked to the employee evaluation process. Employees can use the results of this assessment to track their skill development over time from their manager's perspective.
25. Answer: **A**. The Threshold Limit Value (TLV) as defined by the American Conference of Governmental Industrial Hygienists (ACGIH) refers to "airborne concentrations of substances and represents conditions under which it is believed that nearly all workers may be repeatedly exposed day after day without adverse health effects." Certainly information about TLVs should be included in welder training; however, this question referred to fire characteristics of hazardous chemicals. TLVs mainly concern health effects and are not indicators of flammability. Selection B, auto-ignition temperature, is defined by the National Fire Protection Association (NFPA) as "the lowest temperature at which a flammable gas or vapor-air mixture will ignite from its own heat source or a contacted heat source without the necessity of spark or flame." Selection C, the Lower Explosive Limit, is defined as "the minimum concentration of combustible gas or vapor in air below which propagation of flame does not occur on contact with a source of ignition." Selection D, Upper Explosive Limit, is defined as "the maximum concentration of vapor or gas in air above which propagation of flame does not occur."

26. Answer: **C**. One of the major disadvantages of lecture is that there is limited audience participation. The major advantage is that it is the most efficient way to teach knowledge-level objectives or when training a large group in one setting.
27. Answer: **C**. Bar charts are one of the simplest and most effective ways to display data to an audience.
28. Answer: **A**. The formula to calculate incident rate is recordable accidents times 200,000 divided by the total man-hours worked. This formula yields the rate of injuries per hundred full-time workers.

$$\frac{60 \times 200,000}{1,750,000} = 6.857$$

29. Answer: **C**. This is the definition of a loss-control system. Risk is defined as the combination of the severity of a defined exposure with its frequency of occurrence.

    The technique that effectively decreases a project's schedule risk without increasing the overall risk incorporates slack time into the project's critical path schedule early in project planning.
30. Answer: **B**. ANSI Z490.1-2009 Continuous Improvement.
    4.7.1 Training course revisions shall be made on a periodic basis in accordance with the written training plan.
    4.7.2 Training providers shall use information from training evaluations when revising a course.
31. Answer: **B**. The first term provided in the answers, "fire proof," is a contradiction. There is no such thing as fire proof. All known materials will suffer from effects of a fire if exposed to sufficient intensity and duration.

    The second term, "fire resistive," is generally considered to include noncombustible. Noncombustible is defined as "not capable of burning or supporting combustion." Fire resistive implies a resistance to an expected fire (i.e., within design limits). The term is usually used to indicate the ability of a structure or device to withstand effects of a severe fire for an extended period. Fire resistance is usually indicated in hourly periods determined by standardized fire tests using a time-temperature curve (e.g., one-hour fire wall). Fire resistive is at least one step above noncombustible. Thus, fire-resistive materials are always noncombustible but noncombustible materials may not always be fire resistive.

    The third choice, "flame proof," is a very ill-defined term, use of which is highly discouraged.

    Fire retardant is a useful term indicating a lesser degree of protection than "fire resistive." It is generally used to indicate treated interior and exterior building materials (e.g., fire-retardant plywood). Another term, "flame retardant," is also commonly encountered and is used to indicate the treatment of furnishings or decorations. Christmas trees are often treated to be flame retardant.
32. Answer: **D**. Current industrial fire pumps must be powered either by electrical motors, diesel engines, or steam turbines.
33. Answer: **A**. NIOSH is located within the Dept. of Health and Human Services, Centers for Disease Control.
34. Answer: **B**. The National Institute for Occupational Safety and Health (NIOSH) document, Criteria for a Recommended Standard Working in Confined Spaces, provides several recommendations for safely working in confined spaces. The major recommendations include:
    - Recognition: Training in what constitutes a confined space and what hazards may be present is essential to the establishment of a good accident prevention system.
    - Testing, Evaluation, and Monitoring: All confined spaces should be tested by a qualified person before entry. Tests should be made for oxygen, flammability, and toxic substances. Evaluation should consider methods of isolation, ventilation, PPE, communication, lock-out, etc. Monitoring should be continuously employed to determine if the atmosphere has changed while the work is being performed or during breaks in the work routine.
    - Rescue: Rescue procedures and training must be well thought out, developed, and implemented prior to entry. The rescue procedures should be practiced frequently enough to provide a level of proficiency that eliminates life-threatening rescue attempts and ensure a calm response to any emergency. Advance first-aid training is strongly recommended for all participants in the rescue phase of the operation.

The following example from the NIOSH research file demonstrates the need for an organized confined space entry control program.

Case Study: Four Fatalities, 40 Hospitalized

A 20-year-old construction worker died while attempting to refuel a gasoline engine–powered pump used to remove wastewater from a 66-inch-diameter sewer line that was under construction. The pump was approximately 3000 feet from where the worker had entered the line. The worker was overcome by carbon monoxide. Two co-workers who had also entered from another point along the sewer line were also overcome; however, one was able to escape. A 28-year-old state inspector entered from another point along the sewer line and died in a rescue attempt. The inspector's apprentice, 21 years of age, was also overcome and died attempting to rescue the inspector. All fatalities were due to carbon monoxide intoxication. In addition to the fatalities, 40 additional rescue, medical, and other construction personnel were transported to hospital facilities and treated for carbon monoxide poisoning that occurred while trying to rescue workers and inspectors.

In this example, there were serious mistakes made in every phase of operations. In the Recognition phase, it is obvious that no one on this job site considered the sewer line a dangerous confined space or was aware of the effects of carbon monoxide. Certainly the Testing, Evaluation, and Monitoring phase was deficient. No one, including the responding rescue team, was aware of the CO concentrations within the sewer line. The Rescue phase of this mishap produced 40 hospital cases, certainly evidence that the rescuers were not prepared for this type of incident. A rapid rescue and proper first aid might have spared all of the fatalities in this tragic incident.

35. Answer: **C**. If a motor vehicle that contains hazardous materials is equipped with dual tires on any axle, its driver must stop the vehicle in a safe location at least once during each two hours or 100 miles of travel, whichever is less, and must examine its tires. The inspection should spot any overheating, improper inflation, or general appearance discrepancies. Reference 49 CFR 397.17.

36. Answer: **B**. The magnetic circuit breaker operates on the amount of current passing through the circuit and is the best choice. The thermal circuit breaker operates on the principle of temperature rise or rate of temperature rise and is better suited for circuits with variable loading.

37. Answer: **D**. OSHA requires that a light-duty scaffold not be loaded in excess of 25 pounds per square foot; a medium-duty scaffold not be loaded in excess of 50 pounds per square foot, and a heavy-duty scaffold not be loaded in excess of 75 pounds per square foot. Therefore, a heavy-duty scaffold would be required for this loading.

38. Answer: **C**. Hydrocarbons are compounds that contain atoms of carbon and hydrogen only. They are broadly classified into two types: aliphatic and aromatic.
Aliphatic hydrocarbons are subdivided into saturated and unsaturated compounds and include the alkanes: methane, ethane, propane, and butane.
Aromatic hydrocarbons are derivatives of the parent compound benzene.
Ethers are members of a class of organic compound in which an oxygen atom has bridged between two hydrocarbon groups. Aliphatic ethers are highly volatile and extremely flammable.
Halogenated hydrocarbons are hydrocarbons derived from the basic methane structure in which one or more hydrogen atoms have been replaced with a halogen. Hydrocarbons that have been partially halogenated burn, but generally with much less ease than their nonhalogenated analogs. The fully halogenated derivatives such as carbon tetrachloride are noncombustible.

39. Answer: **B**. A normal worker during a moderate workday will breathe about 8.5 cubic meters, or 300 cubic feet of air. So for a 40-hour workweek, about 1500 cubic feet of air would be used.

40. Answer: **B**.
Step 1 Calculate 20% of the LEL.

Adjusted LEL = LEL × 20%

Adjusted LEL = 2.3 × 20%

Adjusted LEL = 0.46%

Step 2   Apply the formula and solve.
$$Q = G / LEL \times 100$$
$$Q = 33 / 0.46 \times 100$$
$$Q = 7174 \text{ ft}^3$$

The formula used for this problem is a modification of the general dilution formula. The process and rationale are shown below.

Step 1   The original formula solves for TLV, which is expressed in ppm, hence the multiplication by 10^6.
$$Q = \frac{G}{TLV} \times 10^6$$

Step 2   Substitute LEL for TLV, which is expressed in percentage, so multiply by 100.
$$Q = \frac{G}{LEL} \times 100$$

41. Answer: **D**. A charcoal tube is the only selection that would provide adequate sampling for $CH_3CH_2OCH_2CH_3$ (ethyl ether) or $CHCl_3$ (chloroform).

42. Answer: **A**.
$$V = 4005C_e\sqrt{SP_h}$$
$$V = 4005 \times 0.72 \times \sqrt{2.25}$$
$$V = 4325 \text{ fpm}$$

43. Answer: **B**.
Step 1   Determine the volume of air in the cylinder under pressure of 2000 psig.
$$P_1V_1 = P_2V_2$$
$$14.7 \times V_1 = 2014.7 \times 0.250$$
$$V_1 = \frac{2014.7 \times 0.250}{14.7}$$
$$V_1 = 34.26 \text{ ft}^3 \text{ of air}$$

Step 2   Compute the weight of 34.26 cubic feet of air.
$$34.26 \text{ ft}^3 \times 0.075 \text{ lbs/ft}^3 = 2.6 \text{ lbs}$$

Note: If unable to recall that the formula sheet indicates air weighs 0.075 lb/ft^3, one alternate conversion solution is to make a mole conversion and convert from grams to pounds. The molecular weight of air = 29 or 30 grams.

$$\frac{34.26 \text{ ft}^3}{1} \times \frac{1 \text{ liter}}{0.03531 \text{ ft}^3} \times \frac{1 \text{ mol}}{24.45 \text{ liter}} \times \frac{29 \text{ g}}{1 \text{ mol}} \times \frac{1 \text{ lb}}{454 \text{ g}} = 2.6 \text{ lbs}$$

Or, use the lb-mole conversion.
$$\frac{29 \text{ lbs}}{392 \text{ ft}^3} = \frac{X \text{ lbs}}{34.26 \text{ ft}^3}$$
$$X = \frac{29 \times 34.26}{392} = 2.5 \text{ lbs}$$

Step 3: Add 2.5 lbs to the empty weight of 15 lbs for a total weight of 17.5 lbs.

44. Answer: **B**.
    Apply the formula and solve. Note that the room size is not used in the equation.
    Note: Since there is no time indicated in the question, the answer is in ft³. If the contaminant had been generated at an hourly rate, the answer would have been in ft³/hr, etc.

    $$Q = \frac{G}{TLV} \times 10^6$$

    $$Q = \frac{0.5}{200} \times 10^6$$

    $$Q = 0.0025 \times 10^6$$

    $$Q = 2500 \text{ ft}^3$$

45. Answer: **A**. Protective signaling systems provide three categories of signals:
    - Alarm signals: Used to indicate water flow, manual station actuation, fire detector activation, discharge of a system, or other indication of a fire
    - Supervisory signals: Used to indicate time-critical input, such as guard check-in, or loss of water or agent pressure, valves in the wrong position, exit light not functioning, etc.
    - Trouble signals: Used to indicate a fault in the system, shorted wiring, loss of signal, ground fault, etc.

    Note: The preferred reference for additional study is NFPA 72, *Protective Signaling Systems*.

46. Answer: **B**. The designation "dry powder" has been especially chosen to indicate an agent's suitability for use on Class D (combustible metal) fires. The term "dry chemical" has been reserved for agents effective on A:B:C or B:C fires.

47. Answer: **B**. The coefficient of variation is a measure of the variation around the mean and is computed by dividing the standard deviation by the mean. An example of use would be when UCL of an exposure exceeds the PEL but the measured exposure does not. In this case, calculate the UCL and LCL using the coefficient of variation.

48. Answer: **D**. Intrinsically Safe equipment is defined as: "Equipment and wiring incapable of releasing sufficient electrical energy under normal or abnormal conditions to cause ignition of a specific hazardous atmospheric mixture." NFPA 70E, *Intrinsically Safe Apparatus for Use in Division 1 Hazardous Locations* has more information.

49. Answer: **C**. Unfortunately, it is estimated that 140,000 children nationwide will be injured on playground equipment this year. In fact, of all serious playground injuries, 9 out of 10 are the result of falls—causing head and/or internal injuries, fractures, and, in some cases, even death. A Consumer Product Safety Commission study of playground equipment–related injuries treated in U.S. hospital emergency rooms indicated that the majority resulted from falls from equipment. These were primarily falls to the ground surface below the equipment rather than from one part of the equipment to another part. Since the primary cause of injuries is falls to the surface, the surface properties will impact the extent of the injuries.

50. Answer: **A**. Determining where gases will accumulate is a complicated subject because of the tendency of gas to be dispersed by air movement. However, the best answer to this question is that the gas will sink to the floor, given the molecular weight (MW) of 90 (very heavy). Air has a MW of about 30. The National Fire Protection Association *Fire Protection Handbook* has additional information.

51. Answer: **D**. There are many types of diesel fuel. There's Low Sulfur #2, Ultra Low Sulfur #2, Low Sulfur #1, Ultra Low Sulfur #1, High Sulfur #1 & #2, Biodiesel #1 and #2, Premier Diesel Fuel, Low Sulfur Diesel Supreme, Low Sulfur Diesel #2 winterized blend, and many other blends and blend ratios of each. Usually they're about 6.5 lbs to 7.5 lbs per gallon. Seven pounds is commonly used because of the variation.

    Step 1   Determine the weight of one gallon of diesel.

    $$\frac{8.34 \text{ lbs}}{1 \text{ gallon}} \times 0.83 = 6.9 \text{ lb/gal}$$

Step 2   Determine Btu/lb.

$$\frac{128{,}400 \text{ Btu}}{1 \text{ gallon}} \times \frac{1 \text{ gallon}}{6.9 \text{ lbs}} = 18{,}608 \text{ Btu/lb}$$

52. Answer: **B**. The requirement to establish a "most probable cause" on a 8-hour report is neither realistic nor desirable, as it encourages speculation. OSHA 1904.8, Reporting of Fatality or Multiple Hospitalization Incidents, is quoted here for specific regulatory information.
    a) Within 8 hours after the death of any employee from a work-related incident or the in-patient hospitalization of three or more employees as a result of a work-related incident, the employer of any employees so affected shall orally report the fatality/multiple hospitalization by telephone or in person to the Area Office of the Occupational Safety and Health Administration (OSHA), U.S. Department of Labor, that is nearest to the site of the incident, or by using the OSHA toll-free central telephone number.
    b) This requirement applies to each such fatality or hospitalization of three or more employees that occurs within thirty (30) days of an incident.
    c) Exception: If the employer does not learn of a reportable incident at the time it occurs and the incident would otherwise be reportable under paragraphs (a) and (b) of this section, the employer shall make the report within 8 hours of the time the incident is reported to any agent or employee of the employer.
    d) Each report required by this section shall relate the following information: Establishment name, location of incident, time of the incident, number of fatalities or hospitalized employees, contact person, phone number, and a brief description of the incident."
53. Answer: **C**. Strict liability is the concept whereby the plaintiff need not show negligence or fault to prove liability.
54. Answer: **C**. A vertical standard applies to a single industry. A specification standard demands precise compliance with exacting codes, frequently detailing exact specifications for materials, sizes, etc. A performance standard reveals rules that must be complied with and leaves specific details up to the industry.
55. Answer: **A**. The technique of Fault Tree Analysis requires that the design be complete.
56. Answer: **C**. Cost/benefit analysis is generally not considered a system safety tenet.
57. Answer: **D**. Convection, conduction, and radiation are the three types of heat transfer.
58. Answer: **D**. The system safety concept calls for a risk management strategy based on identification, analysis of hazards, and application of remedial controls using a systems-based approach. System safety is always conducted before mishaps actually occur. This factor plus the fact that the system safety practitioner may use information from all other safety areas makes this discipline unique.
59. Answer: **B**. The only Boolean Commutative Law is selection B. Selection A is an example of a derivation of the distributive law. Selections C and D are also distributive laws. The laws are shown below for clarification, and the laws are also provided in the Formulae, Constants, and Conversions provided by the BCSP for use during examination. The easy solution to this problem is to simply look up the information and see which law applied.

Table 26 Boolean Postulates

	Commutative Laws
A + B = B + A	The total of the components having the characteristic A or B will be the same irrespective of the order.
A • B = B • A	

	Associative Laws
A(B • C) = (A • B)C	The elements having all the characteristics of A, B, and C will retain them irrespective of the order.

(Continues)

Table 26 Boolean Postulates (*Continued*)

A + (B + C) = (A + B) + C	The total of all the components in any subsets will be the same irrespective of the order.
Distributive Laws	
A(B + C) = (A • B) + (A • C)	The union of one subset with two others can also be defined as the union of their intersections.
A + (B • C) = (A + B) • (A + C)	The union of one subset with the intersection of two others can also be expressed by the intersection of the unions of the common subset with the other two.

60. Answer: **B**. Lead is the best shield listed for protection against gamma radiation.
61. Answer: **C**. Epidemiology is the branch of medicine that investigates the causes and control of epidemics. It is defined as all of the elements contributing to the occurrence or nonoccurrence of a disease in a population.
62. Answer: **B**. A discussion is usually effective in engaging learners and encouraging participation. Peer learning is one of the most direct benefits resulting from the discussion method. Discussions can involve small groups (2–8 participants) or be structured for larger groups. Typically, discussions center around problems, questions, ideas, or issues presented to the group for consideration and verbal exploration.
63. Answer: **C**. Boolean algebra was originally developed for the study of symbolic logic by an English mathematician, George Boole. In Boolean algebra, conditions are expressed with two values (e.g., on or off, true or false, hot or cold, up or down, right or wrong, etc.). This approach uses its own symbolism and is used extensively in safety and health accident investigation, Fault Tree Analysis, Venn diagrams, etc. A casual analysis of the Boolean postulates provided in the BCSP examination information booklet shows that the + symbol in Boolean is read "OR" and the • symbol is read "AND." This means that 1 + 1 does not equal 2 in Boolean logic, but 1 or 1 = 1, just as 1 and 1 would equal 1, and 1 and 0 must equal 0.
64. Answer: **C**. The chart shown in option A best illustrates the force vs. flexion curve for the human elbow. The chart shown in option C confirms that strength is rather low near the extreme position of the body segment and larger in intermediate positions.
65. Answer: **C**. Computers must follow programmed instructions. They have no inductive capability and cannot perform complex tasks that require subjective decision-making. They are very good at routine, repetitive tasking and mathematical calculations.
66. Answer: **D**. For adult learners to be held accountable, they must know, accept, and take ownership for achieving the training objectives.
67. Answer: **A**. OSHA requires employers to certify that they have evaluated compliance with process safety requirements at least every three years. Prompt response to audit findings and documentation that deficiencies are corrected is required. Employers must retain the two most recent audit reports. Additionally, 1910.119 requires each employer to have written operating procedures, to perform a process hazard analysis, and to conduct training.
    Process control sampling involves testing attributes and testing variables. An example would be inspecting a component for missing parts.
68. Answer: **D**. The three most often recommended fundamental training courses for general industrial workers are first aid, fire extinguisher, and contingency, meaning emergency procedures.
69. Answer: **B**. The following are the guidelines for teaching adults:
    a) Explain the purpose of the training session.
    b) Share the session organization.
    c) Demonstrate a fundamental respect for all learners.
    d) Acknowledge the learners' experience and expertise.
    e) Allow choices when possible.

    f) Avoid body language that is degrading.
    g) Do not talk down to learners.
    h) Maintain a high degree of decorum and mutual respect.
    i) Admit mistakes.
    j) Ensure that everyone can see and hear and has comfortable seating.

70. Answer: **B**. Apply the outdoor formula and solve.

$$WBGT = 0.7\,WB + 0.2\,GT + 0.1\,DB$$
$$WBGT = (0.7 \times 119) + (0.2 \times 102) + (0.1 \times 115)$$
$$WBGT = 83.3 + 20.4 + 11.5$$
$$WBGT = 115.2°F$$

71. Answer: **A**. According to the NSC, although statistical data differ, it is generally agreed that new employees are significantly more prone to work-related accidents.

72. Answer: **C**. OSHA 1910.120 requires an extensive safety and health plan that includes a safety and health training plan. Extensive requirements are outlined in the HAZWOPER standard on the various levels and complexity of training. Training for responding specialists, such as Hazmat teams, is required, but generally the responsibility for this training would fall upon their employer rather than the owner of the cleanup contract.

73. Answer: **A**. As defined by the Alliance of Hazardous Materials Professionals (AHMP) *Hazardous Materials Management Desk Reference 2005*, environmental management is the organizing and controlling of affairs related to an organization's impact on the natural world, our surroundings, people, animals, and plants. Environmental management requires strong administrative skills and an understanding of environmental regulations, the fate and transport of chemicals, and the interaction of people and processes. Environmental management also requires other business skill attributes such as an understanding of the costs and benefits of handling environmental issues. To understand environmental management, one must understand its unifying principles and the way the elements of environmental management contribute to the overall objective—achievement of environmental goals and improvement in environmental performance.

74. Answer: **C**. The formula given includes a constant design start-up cost of $1,000,000 and a cost per dB reduction of $75,000 combined with a cost per dB^2 of $1500.

    Step 1

$$C_X = 1,000,000 + 75,000\,X + 1500\,X^2$$

$$A_X = \frac{C_X}{X}$$

    For 5-dB reduction

$$C_5 = 1,000,000 + (75,000 \times 5) + (1500 \times 5^2)$$

$$C_5 = 1,412,500$$

$$A_5 = \frac{1,412,500}{5} = \$282,500 \text{ per dB}$$

    Step 2 For 15-dB reduction

$$C_{15} = 1,000,000 + (75,000 \times 15) + (1500 \times 15^2)$$

$$C_{15} = 2,462,500$$

$$A_{15} = \frac{2,462,500}{15} = \$164,167 \text{ per dB}$$

Step 3 For 25-dB reduction

$$C_{25} = 1{,}000{,}000 + (75{,}000 \times 25) + (1500 \times 25^2)$$

$$C_{25} = 3{,}812{,}500$$

$$A_{25} = \frac{3{,}812{,}500}{25}$$

$$A_{25} = \$152{,}500 \text{ per dB}$$

Step 4 For 35-dB reduction

$$C_{35} = 1{,}000{,}000 + (75{,}000 \times 35) + (1500 \times 35^2)$$

$$C_{35} = 5{,}462{,}500$$

$$A_{35} = \frac{5{,}462{,}500}{35} = \$156{,}071 \text{ per dB}$$

25-dB reduction offers the lowest price per dB.

75. Answer: **D**. Apply the Poisson distribution formula.

$$P(r) = \frac{e^{-\lambda t}(\lambda t)^r}{r!}$$

$$P_4 = \frac{e^{-5} 5^4}{4!}$$

$$P_4 = \frac{(0.00674) \times (625)}{4 \times 3 \times 2 \times 1}$$

$$P_4 = \frac{4.2125}{24} = 0.1755$$

76. Answer: **A**. Although industry generally separates the compliance, SH&E, and quality programs, these functions have many similarities, including:
    - Serving common underlying objectives, such as performance assurance or risk management
    - Using a common approach to achieve objectives, such as activity-specific evaluation or planning and oversight
    - Sharing common success and failure measures, such as cost, schedule, violations, or liabilities
    - The first step in establishing a good corporate quality plan is to determine customer requirements.
77. Answer: **C**. Managers who deliver under the high performance expectations of the current dynamic times must be well educated and continue that education during their career. They must be unrelenting in their efforts to develop, refine, and maintain their skills and competencies, which may not agree with their previous training.
78. Answer: **D**. Matrix management has the potential to include **power struggles**, which may result from the two-boss system. Team members may become too focused on themselves and develop "**groupitis**," losing sight of important program goals. The matrix often creates **increased cost** as overhead rises.
79. Answer: **B**. Many management experts use such terms as "planning, organizing, leading, and controlling the use of resources" or "planning, organizing, activating, and controlling."
80. Answer: **C**. As described in *Assurance Technologies*, a loss-control system must be able to identify the hazardous conditions as well as understand the real risks associated with those hazardous conditions. A loss-control system is incomplete if it solely identifies hazardous conditions and does not take action to understand the risks. Therefore, the actions taken are relative to the risks associated with the hazardous conditions.
81. Answer: **D**. According to the NSC's *Fundamentals of Industrial Hygiene*, a simple process flow sheet should be drawn to show how and where each toxic material is introduced and how it can be introduced into the work area. This could include evaluating the meteorological conditions and reviewing the process with

the engineering staff. After the process is online, safety managers should sample the area to identify any actual releases.

82. Answer: **D**. The purpose of adopting the OHSAS 18001 Health and Safety Management System is to maintain continuous improvement. If the management system finds a significant reduction in company safety performance, it should indicate that a comprehensive management review of the items is warranted.

83. Answer: **A**. Due to product liability claims, a manufacturer should keep product safety records as long as possible. Some states may have limits on the time period, while other states do not—and that is where lawsuits often originate.

84. Answer: **D**. Since the components are in parallel, the configuration indicates an "AND" gate situation—that is, C_1 and C_2 and C_3 and C_4 must fail before the output fails. The symbol for an "AND" gate is "*" which indicates multiplication; this leads to the correct answer. Multiply the failure rates of each component. $F_1 \times F_2 \times F_3 \times F_4$, or since the failure rates are all the same, F^4.

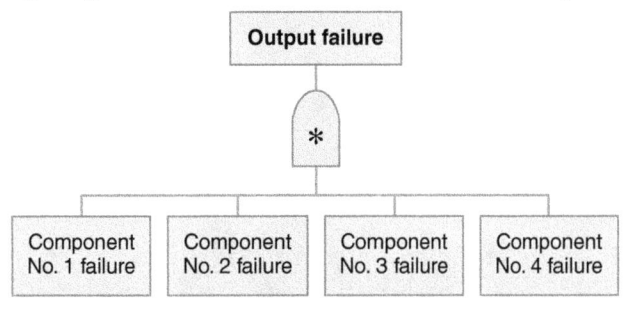

Figure 64 Output Failure "AND" Gate Example 2

Note: When dealing in probability of failure, the general rules are:
- Parallel construction indicates "AND" = multiplication
- Series construction indicates "OR" = addition

85. Answer: **D**. Several different answers could be acceptable. According to the NSC, the safety professional advises and guides management, supervisors, the foreman, employees, and such departments as purchasing, engineering, and personnel on **all** matters pertaining to safety. Formulating, administering, monitoring, evaluating, and improving the incident prevention program are additional responsibilities. The general safety and health professional belief is that the safety and health effort should report to a function with power and ability to control and correct problems, specifically, the General Manager. Root causes of mishaps can exist in any of the elements of a company, as can the interrelated causes of accidents. The best place for safety expertise, however, is in a staff function reporting to the senior executive.

86. Answer: **B**. The 1, 1 supervisor is indifferent. The 9,1 supervisor is the one who is interested more in production than in the interests of the employees and thus would be labeled a dictator or authority-obedience manager. A 9,9 would be considered a team manager; a 1,9 would be a country club manager; and a 5,5 would be considered a middle-of-the-road manager.

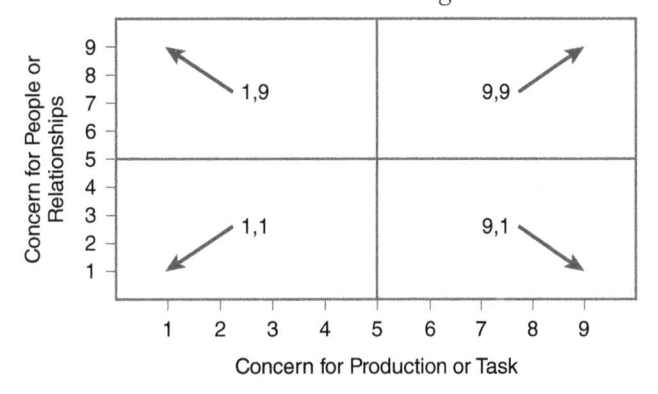

Figure 65 Management Grid

87. Answer: **A**. According to *The Behavior-Based Safety Process* by Krause, Hidley, and Hodson, the process is as shown below. If improvement progresses at an acceptable rate, then the process is working. If the improvement rate is unacceptable, the existing action plan must be modified.

    The behavioral approach uses operational definitions, measurements, and feedback on safety-related issues, along with goal setting as key components to improve safety.

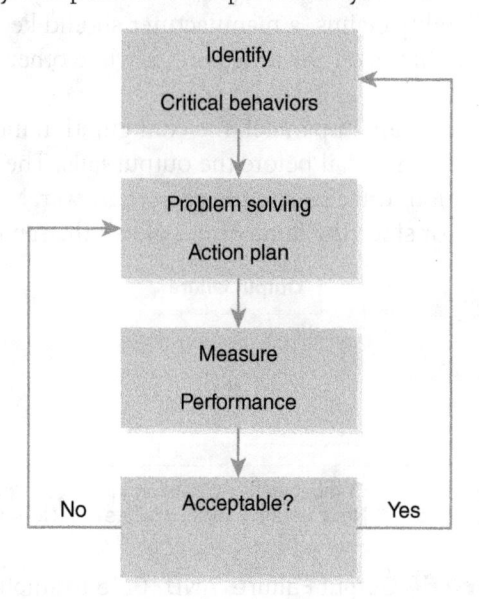

Figure 66 The Continuous Improvement Safety Process

88. Answer: **C**. It is essential that large or high-voltage capacitors be fully discharged before measurements are made, soldering is attempted, or the circuitry is touched in any way. Some of the large filter capacitors commonly found in line-operated equipment store a potentially lethal charge. Capacitors (like the high voltage of the CRT in a TV or video monitor) will retain a dangerous or at least painful charge for days or longer. The main filter capacitors in the low-voltage power supply should have bleeder resistors to drain their charge relatively quickly, but resistors can fail. There is no discharge path for the high voltage stored on the CRT capacitance, other than the CRT beam current and minimal reverse leakage through high-voltage rectifiers. In the case of old TV sets using vacuum tube HV rectifiers, the leakage was essentially zero. They hold their charge almost indefinitely.

    When a capacitor is safely discharged, some capacitors, due to their ability to leak, are "dead" after being safely discharged with a "bleeder resistor" of the right value for the job. Using a resistor that is underrated, wattage-wise, can result in the bleeder going open circuit during a discharge sequence, leaving some energy. High-voltage capacitors, or worse yet, high-energy/high-voltage capacitors, require correct wattage *and* correct resistance to be bled safely.

    Also, high microfarad low-voltage capacitors can vaporize a screwdriver and spray metal into a person's eyes. (An adequate voltage margin is also essential for resistors used in high-voltage circuits. Low-inductance capacitors that are used in energy pulse circuitry are often of the oil-filled high-energy/high-voltage type. This type can give a shock after it has been completely drained by a safe bleeding technique. **Never attempt to discharge a capacitor without protective goggles shielding eyes and gloves that are NFPA 70E compliant.** Using the right tools and materials for discharging the capacitor is very crucial. Discharging a capacitor simply means giving the stored electrical currents a path out of the apparatus.

    To discharge a small capacitor, touching the two lead terminals with the tip of screwdrivers with insulated handles should discharge; however, this is not recommended. Attach a properly rated resistor or capacitor discharge tool onto the capacitor's terminals to safely dissipate the stored electrical currents. To verify that the capacitor is completely discharged, use a voltmeter or test light.

89. Answer: **B**. The audit team members should collect and review the information relevant to their audit assignments and prepare work documents, as necessary, for reference and for recording audit evidence. Such work documents may include the following:
    - Checklists
    - Audit sampling plans
    - Forms for recording information, such as supporting evidence, audit findings, and records of meetings

    The use of checklists and forms should not restrict the extent of audit activities, which can change as a result of information collected during the audit.

    Note: Guidance on preparing work documents is given in Clause B.4.

    Work documents, including records resulting from their use, should be retained at least until audit completion, or as specified in the audit plan. Retention of documents after audit completion is described in 6.6 of ISO 19011. Those documents involving confidential or proprietary information should be suitably safeguarded at all times by the audit team members.

90. Answer: **D**. Chain inspections should be done visually in an attempt to detect any elongation or other defect. This is best accomplished with a link-by-link inspection. Overall measurements or caliper readings of a section are often misleading because not all links will be affected or damaged.

91. Answer: **C**. The two most common hazards associated with the use of hand tools are misuse and improper maintenance. Misuse occurs when a hand tool is used for something other than its intended purpose. Improper maintenance allows hand tools to deteriorate into an unsafe condition. According to the National Safety Council (NSC), the **screwdriver** is perhaps the most misused and abused tool in the workplace. Misuse can compromise the integrity of the tool by breaking the handle, bending the shaft or dulling the tip, making workers susceptible to hand injury when the tool is used correctly. To prevent injury and keep screwdrivers in shape, the NSC recommends:
    - Do not use a screwdriver as a punch, wedge, pinch bar, or pry.
    - Keep the tip clean and sharp to permit a solid grip on the tip of the screw.
    - Keep the handle of the screwdriver clean and intact to allow for a solid grip.
    - Never hold the piece you are working on in your hand. Always lay it on a workbench or place it in a vice.
    - Carry screwdrivers in toolboxes or work belts—never in your pocket. In wood and sheet metal, make a pilot hole for the screw.
    - Never use a screwdriver during electrical work unless it is properly insulated.

    A **hammer** is an impact tool used to drive items into material by way of manual or powered force and is a common source of injury, according to the NSC. All hammers should have a securely fitted handle suited to the type of head being used, the council notes. The handle, regardless of what it is made of, should be oil-free, shaped to fit the hand, and the correct size and length for the task. When using a hammer, protective eyewear should always be used to guard against flying chips, nails, or scales.

    Pliers are often misused as general-purpose tools. Their use should be limited to operations for which they were designed: gripping and cutting (never for loosening or tightening nuts). Always use wrenches on nuts and bolt heads, never use pliers. There are many types of pliers. The most commonly used are the 6-inch combination slip-joint pliers. The slip-joint permits the jaws to be opened wider at the hinge pin for gripping large-diameter objects. Some combination pliers are made with a side-cutter arrangement for cutting wire.

    Choose a **wrench** that properly fits the fastener that is to be turned. Using the correct size reduces the chances of wrench slippage. Always try to pull on a wrench (instead of pushing) in case the fastener suddenly loosens.

92. Answer: **A**. The International System of Units uses seven units as the basis for all other SI units:
    - Meter for length
    - Kilogram for mass
    - Second for time
    - Ampere for electrical current

- Kelvin for temperature
- Candela for luminous intensity
- Mole for substance amount

93. Answer: **D**. Both reactive and proactive worksite analysis approaches are used when identifying existing or potential ergonomic hazards and conditions. Reactive worksite analysis by definition means analysis of past incidences, while proactive means identification of problem jobs and tasks before injury or illness has occurred. Reviewing past injury records is an example of a passive or reactive approach, as you are analyzing incidences that have already occurred. Observations and symptom surveys are used to identify workers who might be in pain but have not yet reported an injury. Ergonomic interventions can be implemented before an injury occurs. Medical histories and strength testing are often used to screen workers who might be at risk of injury, but there is little data to show these techniques are effective.

94. Answer: **D**. Bacteria are single celled. Viruses do not have all the components of a cell; RNA (ribonucleic acid) is composed of organic compounds, not composed of cells; and protozoa are multicellular organisms, many of which are parasitic.

95. Answer: **C**. Hepatitis B virus (HBV). The hepatitis B virus infects the liver. In some individuals, HBV develops into serious or fatal problems, such as cirrhosis, liver cancer, or chronic liver disease. Some people have no problems or symptoms, yet become carriers of the virus. HBV is more common and is a much hardier virus than HIV; it can exist on a surface outside the body for up to 30 days. For this reason, it poses a greater hazard to an exposed individual than human immunodeficiency virus (HIV), hepatitis A virus (HAV), or hepatitis C virus (HCV).

96. Answer: **D**. According to 29 CFR 1910.1001:
1910.1001(j)(7)(i): The employer shall institute a training program for all employees who are exposed to airborne concentrations of asbestos at or above the PEL and/or excursion limit and ensure their participation in the program.
1910.1001(j)(7)(ii): Training shall be provided prior to or at the time of initial assignment and at least annually thereafter.
1910.1001(j)(7)(iv): The employer shall also provide, at no cost to employees who perform housekeeping operations in an area which contains ACM or PACM, an asbestos awareness training course, which shall at a minimum contain the following elements: health effects of asbestos, locations of ACM and PACM in the building/facility, recognition of ACM and PACM damage and deterioration, requirements in this standard relating to housekeeping, and proper response to fiber release episodes, to all employees who perform housekeeping work in areas where ACM and/or PACM is present. Each such employee shall be so trained at least once a year.

97. Answer: **C**. A Wheatstone bridge electrical circuit means the resistors are balanced and one leg of the circuit, called a hot wire, causes exposure to the suspect atmosphere. If a combustible mixture is present, a catalytic combustion increases wire resistance and causes an imbalance.

98. Answer: **D**. The simplest measuring device is the handheld sound-level meter if noise levels are fairly constant throughout the day. Sound-level meters are acceptable for assessing a workshop where employees spend most of their time in a fixed location next to a changing noise source(s).
But for workers who are mobile, a personal noise dosimeter that can follow workers where they go is preferred. If the noise is too variable to follow with a sound-level meter, an integrating meter may be used. This meter can integrate, or average, the changing noise levels over a period of time to produce a time average noise level.
Time averaging is the way the instrument makes its eyeball average reading, except that it does so scientifically, using a set of rules defined in the standards so that it is repeatable under many different circumstances.

99. Answer: **B**. This defines a pyroclastic flow, which is a hazard that can engulf an entire town with little warning.

100. Answer: **C**. According to *Risk Analysis and the Security Survey*, 3rd edition, business continuity planning is a key part of a loss-control program. Such plans should include recovering corporate information, setting up operations, and financing temporary operations until a new facility can be commissioned. Depending upon the risk of a natural disaster, some companies purchase business interruption insurance to help finance operations.

Reference List

ANSI Z136.1. Safe Use of Lasers. American National Standards Institute. 2007.
Adams, P. S., Brauer, R. L., Karas, B., et al. "Professional Certification: Its Value to SH&E Practitioners and the Profession." *Professional Safety* 49 (2004): 26–31.
ANSI/ASSP Z590.2. *Criteria for Establishing the Scope and Functions of the Professional Safety Position*. Des Plaines, IL: American Society of Safety Engineers, 2003.
ANSI/ASSP Z10. *American National Standard for Occupational Health & Safety Management Systems*. Des Plaines, IL: American Society of Safety Engineers, 2012.
BCSP. *BCSP Certifications at a Glance*. Champaign, IL: Author, 2014. Retrieved November 24, 2014, from http://www.bcsp.org/Portals/0/Assets/PDF/BCSP_AtAGlance.pdf.
BCSP. *Complete Guide to the ASP®*. Champaign, IL: Author, 2014. Retrieved November 24, 2014, from http://www.bcsp.org/Portals/0/Assets/DocumentLibrary/ASP-Complete-Guide.pdf.
BCSP. *Associated Safety Professional Role Delineation Report*. Champaign, IL: Author, 2014. Retrieved November 24, 2014, from http://www.bcsp.org/Portals/0/Assets/DocumentLibrary/BCSP_ASP_RDS[1].pdf.
Brauer, R. L. *Evaluating a Safety Degree Curriculum Using Job Analysis for Professional Safety Practice*. Champaign, IL: BCSP, 2005.
Brauer, R. L. *Career Success: Lessons Learned from a New CSP Salary and Demographic Survey*. Champaign, IL: BCSP, 2008.
Brauer, R. L. *Safety and Health for Engineers* (2nd ed.). Hoboken, NJ: Wiley & Sons, Inc., 2006.
Brodbeck, J. E., ed. *Motor Fleet Safety Manual* (4th ed.). Itasca, IL: National Safety Council, 1996: 7–50.
Centers for Disease Control and Prevention. *Crisis and Emergency Risk Communication*. Alanta, GA: Author, 2014: 2.
Code of Federal Regulations of the United States of America, U.S. Government Printing Office, 1998.
Das, J. C. *Arc Flash Hazard Analysis and Mitigation*. Hoboken, NJ: Wiley & Sons, Inc., 2012.
Environmental Protection Agency. Office of Policy, Planning, and Evaluation, United States. Inventory of U.S. greenhouse gas emissions and sinks, 1990-1994, U.S. Environmental Protection Agency, 1995.
ESD fundamentals, PART 3:Basic ESD Control Procedures and Materials" EOS/ESD Association, Inc. Retrieved from https://www.esda.org/esd-overview/esd-fundamentals/part-3-basic-esd-control-procedures-and-materials/
Finucane, E. W. *Definitions, Conversions, and Calculations for Occupational Safety and Health Professionals*. Boca Raton, FL: CRC Press, 2006.
Hagan, P. E. *Accident Prevention Manual: Administration & Programs* (13th ed.). Printed in the United States of America: National Safety Council Press, 2009.
Hagan, P. E. *Accident Prevention Manual: Engineering & Technology* (13th ed.). Printed in the United States of America: National Safety Council Press, 2009.
Hagan, P. E., Montgomery, J. F., et al. *Accident Prevention Manual for Business & Industry: Administration & Programs* (14th ed.). Itasca, IL: National Safety Council, 2015.
Haight, J. M. *The Safety Professionals Handbook: Management Applications* (2nd ed.). Des Plaines, IL: American Society of Safety Engineers, 2012.
Haight, J. M. *The Safety Professionals Handbook: Technical Applications* (2nd ed.). Des Plaines, IL: American Society of Safety Engineers, 2012.
Hazard Communication Safety Data Sheets, U.S. Department of Labor. Retrieved from https://www.osha.gov/Publications/HazComm_QuickCard_SafetyData.html.
HHS, USPHS, et al. *Biosafety in Microbiological and Biomedical Laboratories* (5th ed.). Washington, DC: US Department of Health and Human Services, 2009.
Hill, D. C. *Construction Safety Management and Engineering* (2nd ed.). Des Plains, IL: American Society of Safety Engineers, 2014.
ISO 9000/9001. Quality management, ISO. Retrieved from https://www.vanharen.net/blog/iso-9000-in-3-minutes/.
ISO 19011:2011. Conformity assessment techniques – Auditing. Retrieved from https://www.iso.org/sites/cascoregulators/documents/Annex%204%20-%20Conformity%20 assessment%20techniques%20-%20Auditing.pdf.
John, R. Monteith, Rogue Betrayer, Volume 2 of Rogue Submarine Series.
Jones, R. A., Mastrullo, K. G., et al. *NFPA 70E. Handbook for Electrical Safety in the Workplace* (2018 ed.). Quincy, MA: National Fire Protection Association, 2017.
Joseph A. S. *Developing Safety Training Programs: Preventing Accidents and Improving Worker Performance through Quality Training* (1st ed.). Hoboken, NJ: Wiley & Sons, Inc., 1994.
Krieger, G. R. *Accident Prevention Manual for Business & Industry: Environmental Management*. National Safety Council, 2000.
Manuele, F. *On the Practice of Safety* (3rd ed.). Hoboken, NJ: John Wiley and Sons, Inc., 2003.
Moser, P. "Rewards of Creating a Fleet Safety Culture." *Professional Safety* (2001): 39–41.
NFPA 70. Contents. May 2001. Retrieved from https://www.nfpa.org/Assets/files/AboutTheCodes/70/70-A2001-ROPDraft.pdf.
NFPA 101. Life Safety Code, National Fire Protection Association. 2009 edition.

NFPA 101. Life Safety Code, National Fire Protection Association. Retrieved from https://nationalfireinc.com/inspection-testing/emergency-exit-light.html.

NIOSH. *Assessing Occupational Safety and Health Training A Literature Review.* DHHS (NIOSH) Publication No. 99-145. Cincinnati, OH: Author, 1998.

Occupational safety and health for the Federal employee. U.S. Department of Labor, Occupational Safety and Health Administration, Office of Federal Agency Safety Programs, 1974.

OSHA 29 CFR 1904.7(b)(5)(ii)(F). U.S. Department of Labor. Retrieved from https://www.osha.gov/recordkeeping/tutorial/first-aid-list.pdf

OSHA 29 CFR 1904.8. Reporting of fatality or multiple hospitalization incidents. Retrieved from https://www.osha.gov/laws-regs/federalregister/1994-04-01-1.

OSHA 29 CFR 1910.23(e)(4). Retrieved from https://www.osha.gov/laws-regs/regulations/standardnumber/1910/1910.23

OSHA 29 CFR 1910.94(c)(6)(ii). U.S Department of Labor. Retrieved from https://www.osha.gov/laws-regs/regulations/standardnumber/1926/1926.57.

OSHA 29 CFR 1910.120 - Hazardous waste operations and emergency response.

OSHA 29 CFR 1910.178(l)(4).Training Assistance, U.S. Department of Labor. Retrieved from https://www.osha.gov/SLTC/etools/pit/assistance/

OSHA 29 CFR 1910.1001: 1910.1001(j)(7)(ii). U.S. Department of Labor. Retrieved from https://www.osha.gov/laws-regs/regulations/standardnumber/1910/1910.1001.

OSHA 29 CFR 1910.1200(d)(1). Retrieved from https://www.osha.gov/dsg/hazcom/HCSFinalRegTxt.html

OSHA 29 CFR 1910.1200. Retrieved from https://www.osha.gov/laws-regs/regulations/standardnumber/1910/1910.1200

OSHA 29 CFR 1910.1028. Retrieved from https://www.osha.gov/laws-regs/regulations/standardnumber/1910/1910.1028

OSHA Publication 3125. Ergonomics: The Study of Work. 2000. Retrieved January 29, 2015, from https://www.osha.gov/Publications/osha3125.pdf.

OSHA Publication 3182. Guidelines for Nursing Homes Ergonomics for the Prevention of Muscular Skeletal Disorders.

Petersen, D. *Techniques of Safety Management: A Systems Approach* (4th ed.). Des Plaines, IL: American Society of Safety Engineers, 2003.

Plog, B. A. *Fundamentals of Industrial Hygiene* (6th ed.). Printed in the United States of America: National Safety Council Press, 2012.

Prevention through Design, Centers for Disease Control and Prevention. Retrieved from https://www.cdc.gov/niosh/topics/ptd/default.html

Snyder, D. J. *Pocket Guide to Safety Essentials* (2nd ed.). Printed in the United States of America: National Safety Council Press, 2014.

Snyder, D. J., et al. *The Hazardous Materials Management Desk Reference* (3rd ed.). Bethesda, MD: Alliance of Hazardous Materials Professionals, 2014.

Stewart, J. H., et al. *Occupational Safety Calculations: A Professional Reference* (2nd ed.). Printed in the United States of America: Millennium Associates, 2007.

Threshold Limit Values for Chemical Substances and Physical Agents & Biological Exposure IndicesAmerican Conference of Governmental Industrial Hygienists. Itasca, IL: American Conference of Governmental Industrial Hygiene, 2015.

Threshold Limit Values for Chemical Substances Introduction, American Conference of Governmental Industrial Hygienists (ACGIH). Retrieved from https://www.acgih.org/tlv-bei-guidelines/tlv-chemical-substances-introduction.

Training Requirements in OSHA Standards and Training Guidelines, U.S. Department of Labor, Occupational Safety and Health Administration. 29 CFR 1910.120(e)(5), U.S. Department of Labor, 1992. Retrieved from https://www.osha.gov/laws-regs/standardinterpretations/2010-02-16-01910.120(q)(6).

Yates, D. W. *Safety Professional's Reference and Study Guide.* Boca Raton, FL: CRC Press, 2011.

Index

A

abduction, 109, 109f
absorption coefficient, 319
acceleration due to gravity, 53
Acceptable Quality Level (AQL), 203, 218
acceptable risk, 71, 74, 79
accident costs, 279, 291
    expected value of, 54, 60
accidents, 88, 183, 279, 291, 330, 334
    data collection system, 302
    financial method for reducing costs of, 91
    hidden costs of, 81
    investigations, 3, 124, 128, 316
    leading cause of, 237
    multicausal aspects of, 180
    powered industrial truck (PIT), 53
    precursor, 67
    prevention, 302
    proneness, 271
    release measures, 214
    reporting, 285
acclimatization to heat, 317
accountability, 130
    for environmental, safety, and health losses, 68
    for safety performance, 89
accredited certification vs. certificate program, 7
accurate data, 93
acetaminophen, 154
acetone, 160
    evaporation rate of, 42
acetylene
    cylinders, 287, 296
    oxidation of, 30
acidic industrial waste, 282
activated carbon, 198, 212
active learning, 184
activity-based trenching, 191
activity sampling technique, 96
addiction, 154
ADDIE, instructional design model, 174f, 176
additive effect, 150, 154
adduction, 109, 109f
adjacent building heating, 259
administrative and work practice controls, 105
administrative controls, 97, 101
adult learners, 14, 346
    accountability, 333
adult learning, 172, 177
adults learners, 228
adult training method, 332

advanced sciences and math, 19
    area and volume formulas, 22
    concentrations of vapors and gases formulas, 19
    electrical formulas, 21
    engineering control calculations, 22–25
    radiation formulas, 21
    structural and mechanical calculations, 22
    trigonometry functions, 22
advising management, 3
aerospace industry, 243
affected employee, 94
affliction of frostbite, 205
aging, 140
airborne
    concentration, 274
    hazards, 146
    substance, 155
aircraft control surface, 324
aircraft fueling operations, 310
Air Discharge Volume, 23, 48
air resistance, 53
air respirator, 153
airstream, 160
air temperature, 323
airtight enclosures, 219
air velocity, 329
aisles, 233
alarm
    condition, 111
    systems, 330
alcohol-resistant aqueous film-forming foams (AR-AFFF), 122
alcohols, 143, 339
    ingestion, 141
aliphatic hydrocarbons, 120, 342
Alliance of Hazardous Materials Professionals (AHMP), 353
allowable limits in table, 42
alloy steel, 221
Alternative Release Scenario, 135
aluminum metal dust, 154
alveoli, 158
alveolus, 158
American Conference of Governmental Industrial Hygienists (ACGIH), 149, 270, 340
American Industrial Hygiene Association (AIHA), 263
American National Standard for Occupational Health and Safety Management Systems, 72
American National Standards Institute (ANSI), 52, 72, 206, 285
American Society of Mechanical Engineers (ASME), 257, 294
ammonia, 148

analysis system, 226
analysis technique, 226
analytical skills, 180
analytic epidemiology, 241
"AND" gate, 355, 355f
andragogy, 177
anhydrous, 275, 288
animal products, 305
annual audiograms, 292
annual injuries, average cost of, 57
annual radiation, 238
antagonism, 154
antagonistic effect, 151
anthology, 242
anthracosis, 142
anthrax, 317
anthropometry, 107
antibodies, 141
applied study, 12–14
approaches to estimating, 65
a priori probabilities, 339
AQL. See Acceptable Quality Level (AQL)
aqueous film-forming foam (AFFF), 122
arc flash boundaries, 96, 96f
Arctic Fire, 122
aromatic hydrocarbons, 120, 198, 342
asbestos, 144
asbestos-containing material (ACM), 160, 337
as low as reasonably practical (ALARP), 71
ASME Code, 231
ASP. See Associate Safety Professional® (ASP)
aspect ratio, 282
ASP/GSP/CSP qualifications, 8–10
asphyxiants, 266
assessment methods, 151
Assigned Protection Factor (APF), 158
Associate Safety Professional® (ASP), 6, 7, 190
    certification process, 8, 8f
    exam study, 14
    select study references for, 17–18
    workbooks and workshops, 1
ASSP/ANSI Z10-2012, 75
assumption of risk, 193
atmosphere, 31, 197
atmospheric gases, 170
atomic mass, 297
attractive nuisance doctrine, 193
audiogram, 306
audio signal, 252
auditory ossicles, 219
audits/auditing, 77, 247
    comprehensive, 165
    conclusions, 69
    conduct of, 84
    criteria, 83
    documentation, 337
    document request for, 78t
    evidence, 84

objectives, 80, 83, 84
purpose of, 165
team, 80, 357
authorized employee, 94
authorized representatives of Board, 193
auto-ignition temperature, 246
automatic guillotine paper cutter, 308
automatic sprinkler systems, 267
    classifications of, 254
auxiliary system, 114

B

back belts (braces), 100
bacteria, 358
bacterial pneumonia, 157
baghouse, 221
balanced formula, 291
bar charts, 243, 341
bar, gravity of, 210
batch processing, 339
BCSP. See Board of Certified Safety Professionals (BCSP)
behavior-based approach, 75
behavior-based safety experts, 91
behavior change, 94
behavior sampling, 94, 96
benefits, 97
benzene, OSHA standard on, 298
benzopyrene, 154
Biological Exposure Indices Booklet, 292
biological oxygen demand (BOD), 165
biomechanical calculation, 106
biomechanics analysis, 100
biosafety levels (BSLs), 153, 157
black globe thermometer, 150
BLEVE. See Boiling Liquid Expanding Vapor Explosion (BLEVE)
blood vessels, 102
    compression of, 100
Board of Certified Safety Professionals (BCSP), 2, 6, 9, 192, 195
    ASP examination blueprint, 1–2
    certifications, 7
    Code of Ethics, 5–6t, 194, 195
    goal of, 10
BOD. See biological oxygen demand (BOD)
body of water, 161
body postures, 103
body segment, movement of, 102
body's internal heat, 259
boilers, 284
    inspection of, 270
Boiling Liquid Expanding Vapor Explosion (BLEVE), 122
boiling point, 281
bonding, 117, 297, 322, 323f
Boolean algebra, 332, 346
Boolean algebraic expressions, 331
Boolean Commutative Law, 345
Boolean expression, 53

Boolean logic and applications, 59
Boolean postulates, 345–346t
brachial plexus, 103
brainstorming, 184, 184t, 243
branch circuit loads, 244
Brauer, Roger, 75
British Thermal Unit (Btu), 265
bronchioles, 158
bronchioli, 158
brown lung disease, 139, 141
brucellosis, 317
BSCP, 6, 7
Btus, 330
budgeting, 65–66
Bureau of Labor Statistics (BLS), 108
butyl gloves, 147
byssinosis, 141

C

cadmium exposure, 298
calcium carbide, 115, 313
   use and handling of, 300
calibrations, 212
calorie, 278, 291
capacitor, 336
capture velocity, 23
carbon dioxide, 157
   agents, 120
carbon disulfide, 216
   characteristics of, 201
carbon monoxide (CO), 150, 157, 307
carbon tetrachloride, 140, 198, 304, 317
carcinogen, 257
carcinogenesis, 141–142
carpal tunnel syndrome (CTS), 101, 104, 306, 319
case study, 180, 180t
cataracts, 249
CBT. See computer-based training (CBT)
ceiling limit, 157
central safety committee, 326
centrifugal fans, 198, 212
certificate program, accredited certification vs., 7
certification, 2
   ASP, 9
   benefits of, 7–8
   primary advantage of, 7
   process of, 7–8, 162
Certified Safety Professional® (CSP) designation, 2, 6
cesium-137, 33
CESQG. See Conditionally Exempt Small Quantity Generator (CESQG)
CGIs. See combustible gas indicators (CGIs)
chain inspection method, 337, 357
chain of command, 130
chain slings, standard material for, 207
characteristic waste, 168
Charles's Law, 288

chemicals/substances, 144, 309
   asphyxiants, 253
   explosion, 119
   protective clothing, 155
   resistant gloves, 144, 147
   treatment, 251
Chemical Transportation Emergency Center, 271
child injuries, 330
chlorine, 148
chloroform, 140, 152, 154
chromium, 283
chronic wasting disease (CWD), 108
circuit breakers, 223
circular ducts, 266, 276
citation, 291
Class 3B laser, 147–148
Clean Air Act (CAA), 127
CLI. See Composite Lifting Index (CLI)
client/server database management, 264
closed-loop recycling, 163
closed-loop system, 336
cloud-to-cloud lightning discharges, 163
cloud-to-ground lightning, 163
coal mining, 110
coal workers' pneumoconiosis (CWP), 110
Cobalt-60, 32
codes of conduct, 4–5, 5
coefficient of correlation, 60, 60f, 236
coefficient of friction, 210, 276
coefficient of variation, 330
coefficients of correlation, 55
cognitive knowledge, testing methods for, 229
cohesiveness, 178
cold temperatures, 108
coliform bacteria, 165
collective bargaining, effectiveness in, 194
color blindness, 238
colorimetric tube, 147
colors, separation of, 290
combined audit, 78
combined exposure to several risk factors, 108
combustible dusts, 245–246
   workplace evaluation for, 110
combustible gas analyzers, 267
combustible gas indicators (CGIs), 202
combustible gas meters, 338
combustible liquid, 112
combustible material spill, 125
combustible mixture, 202
combustible sign, 130
combustible solvent, 207
Command Staff (CS), 125, 129
commercial motor vehicle, 221, 328
Commercial Motor Vehicle Safety Act of 1986, 207, 221
commitment, 80
common cause failure, 254
common killers, 267
common terminology, use of, 129

communication, 172, 173, 180, 239, 251
    barriers in, 181, 184, 229, 242–243
    defined, 264
    technique, 173
    type of, 178
company, incidence rate for, 263
compartmentalization of facility, 198
compensation losses, 55, 60
competency, 188
compliance, 78
    audit capability, 333
component failure, common causes of, 267
Composite Lifting Index (CLI), 100, 103
comprehensive audits, 165
comprehensive computer system, 326
comprehensive loss control, 127
comprehensive resource management, 130
comprehensive survey, 88
compressed air foam system (CAFS) extinguishers, 122
compression, 320–321, 321f
computer-based exam, 10–12
computer-based training (CBT), 187
computer, capabilities of, 262, 333
computer exam, 12
computer-generated statistical analysis, 301
computer software, 241, 340
computer system, 228, 325
computer test, procedures and policies for, 10–12
computer vision syndrome (CVS), 103
computers, 273
concrete-encased electrodes, 222
concrete structures, 308
Conditionally Exempt Small Quantity Generator (CESQG), 166
conduction, 150, 271, 339
conductive objects, 310
conduct measurement, 83
conference method, 179
confidentiality, 79
confined space, 127
conformance, 78
conjunctivitis, 248
construction hard hats, 255
containments, 157
contaminants, 265
content hazard, 243
continuous improvement, 247, 327, 356, 356f
continuous loads, 244–245
continuous noise, 149
contract tenosynovitis, 256
contributory negligence, 193
control
    radiant heat, 294
    type of, 104
convection, 150, 339
convection heat transfer, 271
copper-based dry powder, 121
cornea, 155
corporate environmental stewardship, 164

corporate experience, 98
corrosive placard, 125, 131f, 212
corrosives, 233
corrosive sign, 130
cost/benefit analysis, 75
cotton bail, mass of, 58
cotton bract disease, 139
course of action, 192, 195, 200, 307
    for crane operator, 125
covered process, 135
cradle-to-grave concept, 166
crash bar, 123
criteria-referenced checklists, 327
critical behaviors, identify, 83
critical incident technique, 94, 239
critical pressure, 252
Crosby clamps, 307
Crosby clips, 84, 84f
cross-sectional area, 22, 23
cross-sectional or prevalence studies, 314
cross-sectional studies, 271
CRT, 356
CS. See Command Staff (CS)
curie, 279, 291
curriculum, 2
customers, 87
    needs, 87
cutting drum bit maintenance, 114
cutting wheels, 203
CVS. See computer vision syndrome (CVS)
CWD. See chronic wasting disease (CWD)

D

damaging effects of corrosion, 206
Danger tag, 200
DART rate, 64–66
data logger, 146
Days Away Restricted or Transferred (DART) rate, 202
decay constant, 32
decibels, 47
decontamination, 144
deductive analysis technique, 84, 90
definite volume, 298
deflagration, 114, 233, 234
demonstration/practice strategy, 185t
Department of Transportation (DOT)
    hazard, 131
    oxidizer placard, 125, 130f
    regulations, 225, 302, 308
    reporting guidelines, 258, 270
deployment, 130
dermatitis, 145, 268
descriptive epidemiology, 241
Designated Geographic Area (DGA), 217
design principle, 107, 269
design retrofit, 334
destructive testing, 257

diesel fuel, 330, 344
diluted solution, preparation of, 308
dilution ventilation, 42, 151, 203, 217, 253, 329
    use of, 146
direct contact of solvents, 141
direct costs, 59, 91t
direct incident costs, 59
directional water spray systems, 114
disaster plans, 242
discounted cash flow technique, 71
disintegration constant, 32
dispatch, 130
disposal perspectives, 163, 164–165
distance, 23
    learning, 183, 187, 239, 251
distillation, 160
distribution system, integrity of, 161
diverters, 105
double-handled pinching, 101
double insulation, 221, 320
driver error, cause of, 88
drug testing, 211
drug use, 152
drum-mounted water sprays, 114
dry air, 298
dry bulb thermometer, 150
dry chemical, 121
    fire-extinguishing agent, 118, 330
dry friction, 311
dry lightning, 163
dry powder, 120, 330, 344
    designation, 120
dual pump arrangement, 54
ductility, 268
duct velocity, 22
due professional care, 79
dust, 245
    particles in respiratory system, 293f
dust explosion, 233
    destructiveness of, 246
    prevention of, 110

E

ear, 293
earthquake, 256
economic definitions, 164
effective management system, elements of, 73
effective risk
    communication, 128
    control, 67, 327
effective trainer feedback, 340
egress, means of, 322
electrical appliances, 232
electrical branch circuit, 232
electrical circuit breakers, 209
electrical conduit, 118
electrical current, 199

electrical distribution transformer, 206
electrical installation, 208
electrical systems, 222
electrical truck usage, 307
electrode systems, 222
electron flow detection systems, 220
electronically store data, 144
electrostatic air cleaner, 163
electrostatic discharge (ESD), 256
electrostatic precipitator (ESP), 163
elements
    of contract, 228
    vertical grouping of, 276
embryo, development of, 307
emergency, 125
Emergency Action Plan, 261
emergency management, 127, 338
    agencies, 137
    phase of, 125
emergency response/action plan, 3, 261
Emergency Response Guidelines (ERGs®), 263
emergency response information, 259
emergency response management (ERM), 124
emergency response sequence, 127
emissivity, 319
emphysema, 293
    medical condition of, 283
employees, 89, 304, 305, 333
    coaching, attributes of, 68
    controlling dermatitis of, 233
    exposure record, 141
    motivation, 68
    testing, 138
    unions, 191
employment opportunities, 7
EMR for workers' compensation insurance, 193
EMS. *See* Environmental Management Systems (EMS)
enclosed process tank, 330
endemic disease, 256, 268
end-of-service-life indicator (ESLI), 159
energy
    isolation program, 261
    traditional unit of, 252
engineering, 215
    controls, 97, 104
environmental audit, 161
Environmental Audit Protocol, 165
environmental ethics, 164
environmental management, 81, 334
    guidelines, 162, 169
Environmental Management Systems (EMS), 164
    system, 66, 77
environmental protection, 3
environmental protocol, 161
environmental regulations, 168
environmental risks, 136
EPA modifications, 53
EPA/OSHA levels of protection, 155t

epicondylitis, 283, 294
epidemiological studies, 227, 241
    morbidity and mortality data for, 203
epidemiology, 346
equalization, 163
equal volume of water, 50
equipment, 81
equipment-grounding conductor, 207
ergonomic problems, 151
ergonomic risk factors, 101
ergonomics, 3, 107, 222, 242
    definition of, 208, 229
    description of, 208
ERGs®. *See* Emergency Response Guidelines (ERGs®)
ERM. *See* emergency response management (ERM)
ERPs, 288
errors
    classification of, 242
    types of, 229
ERV. *See* expiratory reserve volume (ERV)
ESD. *See* electrostatic discharge (ESD)
ESLI. *See* end-of-service-life indicator (ESLI)
ESP. *See* electrostatic precipitator (ESP)
ethanol (ethyl alcohol), 154
ethers, 120
ethics, 4–5, 5, 194
    employer codes of, 195
evaluating, 3
event tree analysis, 226
evidence-based approach, 79
exam graphic user interface, 16
examination, 13
    blueprint, 12–13
exam review screen example, 17
excessive leaning, 101
exclusive remedy, 193
excursions, 157
exhaust ventilation, 151, 322
exit device, 123
exothermic redox reaction, 234
expiratory reserve volume (ERV), 266
explosion proof, 256, 269, 284
explosive atmosphere, 203
exposure, 71
    assessment, 79
    incident, 150
    risk, 205
    time, 42
express warranty, 236
extension, 109, 109f
external audits, 77–78
external distractions, elimination of, 13
external radiation exposure, 145, 148, 148t
eye, 155, 282
    damage to, 265
    injury, 144
    protection area, 191
    strain, 101

eyeballs, involuntary movement of, 249
eyelids, 248

F

fabric filtration, 207
face-to-face communications, 178
face ventilation, 114
facilitators, 188
Factory Mutual Engineering Corporation, 262
fail-safe designs, 85
Failure Mode and Effects Analysis (FMEA), 85, 95, 316
Failure Mode Effects and Criticality Analysis (FMECA), 81
Failure Modes and Effects Analysis (FMEA), 226, 303
fair presentation, 79
fatality, 202, 231
fault tree analysis (FTA), 60f, 84, 95–96, 236, 236f, 331, 345
"fault tree" symbols, 82, 82f
federal dust standard, 114
Federal Hazard Communication Standard, 268
Federal Motor Vehicle Safety Standards, 281
fellow servant rule, 193
"fellow servant" rule, 190
female, 268
    workers, 255
FEV1, 219
fibers, 293
fibrosis, 146
film-forming fluoroprotein (FFFP), 122
filtration devices, 160
financial principles formulas, 25
fire, 112
    detection system, 310, 323, 330
    extinguishers, 284
    hazards, 111, 115
    hydrant, 293
    prevention and protection, 110
    protection, 2
    resistive, 341
    structural damage from, 254
    theory of, 126
firefighting, 259, 269
    agents, 257
    booster pumps, 203
    measures, 212
    standpipe systems, 203
The Fire Protection Handbook, 207, 232
fire-protection systems, 311
fire sprinkler systems, 111, 115, 198, 230, 311, 323
fire-suppression agent, 287
fire tetrahedron, 119, 123
firewalls, 117, 117f
fire water tank, 287
first-aid measures, 212
first-aid treatment, 274
first responder awareness, 185–186
fish kills, 283
fixed-temperature, 132

flame proof, 341
flame retardant, 341
flame symbol, 132
flammable and combustible liquids, 218, 218t
flammable atmosphere, 203
flammable inside storage locations, 111
flammable liquids, 113, 203, 205, 288
flammable storage cabinet, 256
flash hazard analysis, 90
flash point, 234, 246
   defined, 118
   of liquid, 120
flash protection boundary, 96
flat metal shape, 209, 209f
flat plate materials, 306
fleet formulas, 64
flexion, 109, 109f
floor loading, 88
flow testing, 118
fluid friction, 311
fluid pressure, 249
foams, 122
foot controls, 102
Forced Vital Capacity (FVC), 219
foreseeability, 193, 248
forklift operators, 245, 285
fork truck accidents, 60
Frequency-Independent Lifting Index (FILI), 103
Frequency-Independent Recommended Weight Limit (FIRWL), 103
fresh water, weight density of, 49
friction, 201, 297, 311
   loss, 210
frostbite, 142, 220
   affliction of, 140, 205
frozen tissue, 212
fuel, 112, 113
   storage tanks, 40
   tank, 209
fume, 122
functional test, 116
fusible lead, 212

G

gamma globulin proteins, 139
gamma radiation, 282
gas, 122, 288
   cylinder, 31, 258
   gravity of, 312
gasoline, 305
General Industry Standards, 262
GFCI, 119. *See* ground fault circuit interrupter (GFCI)
GHS. *See* Globally Harmonized System (GHS)
glaucoma, 248–249
Globally Harmonized System (GHS), 89
   pictograms and hazard classes, 94f
   symbols, 93

   Working Group, 93
globe thermometer, 145
glove materials, 214
"go-ahead" evaluation, 248
Graduate Safety Professional (GSP), 1
graphite-based powder, 121
gravity, 224
   acceleration due to, 53
   of water, 275
greenhouse effect, 163
greenhouse gas, 170
grinders, 203
grinding operations, 219
grinding wheel, 284
gross hazards, 259
ground fault circuit interrupter (GFCI), 14–15, 15f, 123
   significant knowledge about, 15
ground fuel tank requirements, 208–209t
grounding, 117, 297, 322, 323f
   programs, 257
group, 263
   cohesiveness, 172
   discussion, 98
   training, expected outcome of, 264
guided (facilitated) discussion strategy, 178t

H

half-mask respirator, 154
half-value layers, 294
halogen, 276
halogenated derivatives, 120
halogenated hydrocarbons, 160, 342
halon-replacement clean agents, 120
halons, 120
hammer, 357
hand coupling, 239
hand tool, 337
Hawthorne studies, 259, 271
hazard, 69–70, 70, 76, 78, 85, 89, 99
   analysis, 90
   assessment, 73
   classification, 267
   control, sequence for, 200
   definition of, 91
   degree of severity, 88
   diamond, 207
   identification, 73, 78, 212, 254
   identifying, 260
   recognition, 2
   symbols, 93
Hazard and Operability (HAZOP) analysis methodology, 95
Hazard Communication Guidance for Combustible Dusts, 113–114
Hazard Communication Standard (HCS), 213
hazardous chemical, 304
hazardous conditions, 67
hazardous energy, 89, 94

hazardous material incident, 155
Hazardous Material Label, 126, 126f
hazardous materials, 160, 161, 162, 199, 234, 283
 emergency responders, 135
 incidents, 127
 management, 3
 placards for shipping, 162
 specialist, 186–187
 technician, 186
hazardous substances, 128
Hazardous Waste Operations and Emergency Response (HAZWOPER), 185
hazardous wastes, 161, 166, 168, 182
 disposing of, 162
 profiles, 160
 regulations, 162, 167–168t, 168
 transportation, 161
 treatment of, 251
Hazen-Williams empirical formula, 210
HAZWOPER standard, 200, 334
health and safety information, 182
health and safety training, 181, 260
health hazard, 2, 206, 305
health physicist, 158
hearing
 ability, 140
 conservation program, 204
 loss, 138
 protection, effectiveness of, 42
 receptor for, 293
 threshold of, 199
heat
 detectors, 132
 gain, source of, 271
 lightning, 163
 of material, 287
 related illness, 204
 stress measurement, 258
 treatment, 300
heating, 276
heatstroke, 253, 255, 266, 268
 symptoms of, 219
heat transfer, 145, 331
 principle of, 324
 types of, 150
Heinrich's domino theory of accidents, 226
helmet, types of, 249
hematoxins, 143
hepatitis B virus (HBV), 337, 358
hepatotoxins, 143
Herzberg, Frederick, 86
hidden costs, 86
hierarchy of controls, 68, 73–74, 95, 163
highballing, 65
higher-order needs, 178
high-pressure utility systems, 208
hold harmless (indemnity) agreement, 193
Holter monitor, 147
hoods on grinding and cutting operations, 218

horizontal line of sight (HLOS), 102, 257
hot-mill or aluminized gloves, 147
human
 behavior, 179
 body, 144
 capabilities of, 262, 333
 characteristics, 173
 error, 226
 kinesiology, 107
hurdle rate, 72
HVAC system, 146
hydraulics formulas, 26
hydraulic systems, 277
hydrocarbons, 42, 118, 120, 329, 342
hydrogen ions, 251
hydrostatics, 26
hydrostatic testing, 288
hygiene factor, 82
hypergolic, 246, 338
hypothermia, likeliness of, 141

I

ibuprofen, 154
identification techniques, 98
identify critical behaviors, 83
ignitable dust
 probability of, 233
igniting, 286
ignition source, 246
ignition sources, 117
illness, 140, 145
ILO-OSH 2001, 73
Immediately Dangerous to Life or Health (IDLHs), 30, 33, 157
impact-type noise, 149
implied warranty, 240
incidence rate, 64, 272, 327
incident, 79, 99
incident action planning, 130
Incident Commander (IC), 129, 133
Incident Command System (ICS), 125, 129
 Organizational Chart, 129f, 134f
incident energy calculations, 96
incident rate, 274
 recordable, 64
incidents, 279
independence, 79
independent effect, 150
indicators, 74
indirect costs, 55, 57, 59, 86, 88, 92t
 of incident, 53
individual audit, 83
individual preference, 215
indoor air quality, primary sources of, 151
industrial cleaning solvent, ideal flash point for, 288
industrial contaminants, 155
industrial effluents, 201
industrial facility, 263
industrial fire hydrant, 118

industrial fire pumps, 218, 328
industrial hygienist, 41, 158
industrial inspection, 201
industrial motor vehicle, 41
industrial safety, 260
    inspection, 118
    work, 260
industrial settings, 258
    ventilation in, 281
industrial toxicologist, 157
infection, 153
    in humans, 140
inflammation, 138
information, 130
    collecting and verifying, 80
    technology equipment, 113
ingredient, composition/information on, 212
injuries
    accident analysis, 279
    and illnesses, 243
    reduction of, 280
inspections/audits, 2
inspector test pipe outlet, 112
inspiratory reserve volume (IRV), 266
instructional content, 171
instruction, pitfalls of, 188
instructors, 177, 251
    behaviors, 239
insurance, 97
    company in business, 228
    protection, 190
    rates, 189, 291
integrated communications, 130
integrated performance assurance, 211, 334
integrity, 79
intelligence management, 130
interaction, 273
interactive computer-assisted training, 183, 239, 251
interactive learning, 180
interactive training method, 181
intermittent noise, 149
internal audits, 77–78
internal corrosion, 220
internal friction, 311
International Air Transport Association (IATA), 166
International Association for Impact Assessment (IAIA), 166
International Electrotechnical Commission (IEC), 147
International Labor Organization Guidelines on Occupational Safety and Health Management Systems, 73
International Maritime Organization (IMO), 165–166
International System of Units, 337, 357
intrinsic beliefs, 93
intrinsic safety, 218, 330
    equipment, 344
inverse square law, 39, 252, 253
ionizing radiation, 148–149t, 245, 249, 326
ionizing radiation shield, 284
irritants, 147
ISO 9000 ("quality management"), 85

ISO 14000 ("environmental management"), 85
isopropyl alcohol, 152

J

job elements, systematic analysis of, 289
job performance, 273, 340
    learning for, 327
job safety analysis, 271, 289, 315
jockey pump, 126, 133
joint audit, 78

K

key persons, 279
kidneys, 139
kinesiology, 107
kinetic energy, 298
kinetic friction, 216
knobs, 102
knowledge, 274

L

lacrimators, 144
ladder, 40
    slipping against building schematic, 44f
lagging indicators, 75
landfill gas (LFG) recovery, 170
Large Quantity Generator (LQG), 167
laser, 147
    hazard, 147
Latex gloves, 147
Law of Disuse, 184
Law of Effect, 183
Law of Frequency, 183
Law of Intensity, 184
Law of Learning, 181
Law of Primacy, 184
Law of Readiness, 183
Law of Recency, 183
Laws of Learning, 183
lead-acid batteries, 285
leadership, 80
Leadership in Energy and Environmental Design (LEED) certification process, 169
leading indicators, 74, 84
learner reaction, 171
learning
    objectives, 262
    process of, 14
    strategies, 173, 188
    styles and techniques, 188
    technique, 15
lecture, 273
    disadvantages of, 341
    method, 263
    presentation, 327
    strategy, 177, 177t

legal contract, 193
   mandatory elements for, 190
Legionnaires' disease, 153, 157
lens, 155
lesson plans, formats for, 184–185
leukemia, 227, 241
liability, 190
Liaison Officer, 129
license renewal, 208
Life Cycle Assessment (LCA), 162, 168–169
life safety, 246
Life Safety Code, 202, 217, 309
lifestyle change for better, 154
Lifting Index (LI), 100, 103
ligaments, 102
light, 33
   curtain reaction time, 43
   hazard, 212
   intensity, 265
   quality of, 256
Light Hazard Occupancy, 198
lightning, 160
   bolt, 163
limited approach boundary, 96
limit switches, 102
liquid hazardous chemicals, 327
listed hazardous waste, 168
listening, 187
liver-damaging substances, 140
load, 40
   boom indicator, 308
local exhaust ventilation, 253, 266, 266f, 292
local fire alarm system, 114
local fire department, 126
loss, 90
   of consciousness, 205
   exposures, 97
   prevention, 99
   reduction, 96
loss control system, 69, 97, 335, 341
   primary function of, 91
Lot Tolerance Percent Defective (LTPD), 204
Lot Total Percent Defective, 219
lowballing, 66
Lower Explosive Limit (LEL), 30, 33
lower flammable limit, 33
lower-order needs, 178
LPG hoses, 205
lubricated friction, 311
lungs, 153, 283
   parenchyma, 158

M

machine guards, 206, 220, 294
machine reaction time, 43
magnetic circuit breaker, 342
magnitude of force, cotton, 52
manageable span of control, 130

management, 87, 192
   authority, 82
   function of, 259
   grid, 355, 355f
   leadership, 73
   and safety systems, 68
   system, 68, 69, 77, 335, 355
management by objectives (MBO), 86, 129, 271
manual lifting, 101
   acceptable weights for, 103
manufactured product, 325
manufacturer to consumer, 228
margin of safety, 208
Maslow's hierarchy of human needs, 172, 179f, 304, 316
Material Safety Data Sheets (MSDSs), 212
matrix management, 354
   potential disadvantages of, 335
Maximal Voluntary Ventilation (MVV), 219
maximum use concentration (MUC), 154, 159
McGregor's theory, 280, 292
means of egress, 112
measurement, units of, 249
measures of system, 68
mechanical or physical treatment, 251
media, 176
median value, 54, 58
medical attention, 261
melanomas, 205
Ménière's disease, 141
mercury, 143
   exposure, 140
mesothelioma, 139, 141
metabolic heat load, 278f
metal fume fever (MFF), 139, 141, 306, 319
metallic mercury, 143
metals, 296
   flammable, 286
   safety, 113
methane, 30
methanol, 143
methylene chloride, 309
MET-L-KYL/PYROKYL, 121
mid-level supervisors, 291
milk, 305
mill fever, 139
Mine Safety and Health Administration (MSHA), 234, 246, 326, 340
minimum attractive rate of return (MARR), 71, 72
   definition of, 67
mishap, 71
mists, 122
   rapid vaporization of, 221
mitigation, 71, 129
mixtures, 168
modification rates, 193
modular organization, 129
Monday fever, 141
monoammonium phosphate, 121
morality, 5

most probable cause, 345
motivation, 75
motivational factor, 82
movable-barrier devices, 275
movement, defining, 109, 109f
mucous membrane, 146, 248
multiple-choice answers, 242
multiplexing, 230, 243
muscles, 102
musculoskeletal disorders (MSDs), 107–108
    examples of, 106t
mutagens, 148

N

naphtha, 31
naphthalene, 143, 212, 212f
narcosis, 156
National Electric Code (NEC), 119, 208, 222, 287
national experience rate for SIC-100, 56
National Fire Protection Association (NFPA), 112, 202, 215, 221, 340
    smoke management by, 124
    standards, 207, 284
National Highway Traffic Safety Administration (NHTSA), 292
National Incident Management System (NIMS), 127, 133, 134
National Institute for Occupational Safety and Health (NIOSH), 49, 140, 142, 151, 238, 284, 294, 328
    employees, 280, 292
    lifting equation, 28, 28f, 250
National Institutes of Health (NIH), 153
National Pollution Discharge and Elimination System (NPDES), 216
National Research Council (NRC), 136
National Safety Council (NSC), 124, 187
    Environmental Management Accident Prevention Manual, 165
natural disasters, 132
natural fiber, 286, 322
    safety factor for, 309
natural rubber, 147
NEC Class II hazard classification, 123, 123t
needs assessment, 230, 243
negligence, 193
neon, 289
neoprene, 147
    gloves, permeability of, 145
    latex, 147
nephrotoxins, 141, 143
nerves, 102
    compression of, 100
net present worth (NPW), 71
neutralization, 293
neutrons, 311
    emanation, 331
    radiation, 139, 142
    shielding, 257, 270
NFPA 704 System Hazard Diamond, 221

NIOSH. *See* National Institute for Occupational Safety and Health (NIOSH)
nitrile/natural rubber, 147
noise, 265
    attenuation, 306
    control barriers, effective design for, 204
    exposure, 149, 282, 338
    formulas, 23–24
    hazard, 145, 149
    issue, component parts of, 200
    problem, 214
noise reduction rating (NRR), 49
noncombustible, 328
nongovernmental organizations (NGOs), 134
nonhazardous waste, 168
nonintact skin, 146
non-steady noise, 149
normal distribution, 231
    distribution in, 54
notes and modifications, 28–29
NSC. *See* National Safety Council (NSC)
NTSB, 190
Nuclear Regulatory Commission (NRC), 233, 237
numbness, 140
    of fingers, 205
nystagmus, 249

O

obvious peril, 194
occupancy, classifications for, 217, 217t
Occupational and Educational Eye and Face Protection, 268
occupational dermatitis, 141
occupational diseases, 101, 255
occupational eye disorder, 237
occupational health, 138, 181
    and safety, 4
Occupational Health and Safety Management Systems (OHSMS), 68, 73, 75, 99
Occupational Health Assessment, 79
occupational illness, 144, 337
occupational noise
    exposure, 255
    measurement, 281
Occupational Safety and Health Administration (OSHA), 51, 155, 206, 230, 232
    accordance with provisions of, 232
    citations, 237, 280, 301
    classification for incident, 263
    compliance officers, 228, 280
    DART, 272
    Hazard Communication Standard, 235, 246, 254
    hearing conservation program, 204
    inspection, 306
    issued citation, 227
    noise standard, 204
    occupational noise exposure standard, 268
    operational procedures, 228
    promulgation of, 279

Occupational Safety and Health Administration (OSHA) (*Continued*)
 publication training guidelines, 176
 Right of Entry, 241
 standards, 48
 State Plans, 201
 300 summary form, 261
 29 CFR1910.1200, 208
 violation, 227
 Voluntary Protection Program (VPP), 73, 202
Occupational Safety and Health Program, 227
octave-band analyzers, 243
"off-site consequence analysis" (OCA), 135
OHSAS 18001, 73, 77
oncogenesis, 139, 141–142
one-way communication, 172, 183
on-scene incident commander, 187
on-the-job injuries, 301
on-the-job training (OJT), 182
operational safety rules, 281
operational stereotype, 312
operator control, precision for, 100
OPIM, 290
optic nerve, 152, 155
oral communications, 273
ordinary construction, 268
organic, 265
 chemicals, classes of, 202
 materials, 252
 peroxides, 202
Organization Behavior Model (OBM) approach, 75
OSHA. *See* Occupational Safety and Health Administration (OSHA)
ossicles, 219
Otis-Lennon Mental Ability Test, 261, 273
overall failure probability, 82
overcurrent device, 111
overcurrent protection, 120
overexertion injuries, 103
overhead conveyor system, 52
overhead crane, 40
overlapping systems, 160
overloading, 120
oversimplified attributes, 82
oxidizers, 111, 115, 312
oxidizing agents, 115, 298
 concentration, 126
oxygen, 33
 concentration, 246
 content, 31
 cylinders, 113

P

paint spray booth, 201, 287
panic bar, 123
panic device, 123
panic hardware, 119

parallel and series design, 239
parallel components, 336, 336f
 arrangement, 238, 238f
parallel redundant, 241
parallel system, 87
parenteral contact, 146
Pareto charts, 69, 76–77, 77f
Pareto principle, 91
parking lots, 208, 222
particular audience, 174
Pascal's Law, 289
pathologists, 158
Pearson VUE centers, 10
perchloric acid, 296
performance feedback, 83
Performance Oriented Standard, 72
periodic monitoring, 155
periodic testing requirements, 112
peripheral nervous system, 150
Permissible Exposure Limits (PELs), 30, 157, 257, 270
personal equation, 179
personal experience, 98
personal protective equipment (PPE), 97, 105, 148, 153, 200, 245
personnel injury, 232
pH, 212, 297
 scale, 30, 34, 34f
phenobarbital, 154
photoelectric (optical) presence-sensing device, 51
photoelectric smoke detectors, 309, 322
physical change, 93
physical characteristics, 102
physical definition, 164
physical hazards, 151
physics formulas, 24–25
physiological calculation, 106
physiology, 107
pictogram, 197, 197f
pipe sprinkler system, 112
pitot tube measuring device, 282
placards, 160, 163, 197
plan-do-check-act process, 75, 75f
plant manager encounter, 145
pleural cavity, 158
pleurisy, 317
pliers, 357
pneumatic systems, 277
pneumoconiosis, 139, 283
point-of-operation hazards, 264
point-of-operation protection, 295, 309
poisonous gases, 297
Poisson distribution, 277, 354
pollution prevention, 160, 165
polychlorinated biphenyls (PCBs), 161, 165
polyvinyl alcohol (PVA), 147
polyvinyl chloride (PVC), 147
population standard deviation, 55
population stereotype, 312

portable fire extinguishers, 121f
portable lifting device, 105f
    engineering control of, 105
PortaCount®, 147
postconsumer recycled content, 164
post-indicator valve (PIV), 116
postural analysis system, 101
potassium bicarbonate, 121
potential disaster, preparing for, 125
potential hazard, 81
potentiating effect, 151
potentiation, 154
potter's rot, 282
powered industrial truck (PIT), 208, 285
    accident, 53
power supply system, 310
power transmission, safeguarding of, 286
pre-action systems, 267
preconsumer recycled content, 163
pre-emergency management planning, 127
Preliminary Hazard Analysis (PHA), 335
premiums, 97
preparedness, 128
presbycusis, 142
presence-sensing devices, 275
pressure, 212
    relief panels, 295
    testing, 206, 220, 269
    vessels, 284
presumed asbestos-containing material (PACM), 337
prevention action, 79
prevention through design (PtD), 95, 102–103
preventive maintenance, 316
primary behavior model, 68
prioritizing scoring method, 78t
private, 248
Private Fire Brigade, 207
privity, 236, 248
proactive approach, 337
proactive worksite analysis approaches, 358
probability, 70, 325
Process Safety Management (PSM), 127, 135
process variations, 90
product
    development, 237
    features, 87
    liability, 237
    safety, 3, 228, 335
production accident, 234
professionalism, 4–5
    defined, 5
professionals
    defined, 4
    ethics, 5, 192
    liability, 190
    responsibility, 194
    safety studies, 2
    training, 190

profit margin, 60
program audits, 301
program evaluation, 247
programmed or instructional learning, 242
progressive companies, 292
project budgeting method, 57
project management, 80, 280
proof of negligence, 331
proprietary, 114
prospective experience rating, 193
prospective studies or cohort or incident studies, 314
protection devices, 328
protective signaling systems, 111, 344
protons, 311
psychology, 68
psychophysical, 100
psychophysical calculation, 106
Public Company Accounting Oversight Board (PCAOB), 77
Public Information Officers (PIOs), 129, 137
public relations manager, 230
public resists change, 128
pullback devices, 275
pulmonary alveoli, 158
pulmonary function testing, 205
puncture wounds, 155
pupil, 155
push bar, 123
push buttons, 102
pushing force, 276
pushing tasks, 210
pyroclastic flow, 358
pyrophoric metals, 256
pyrophoric substance, 268
Pythagorean theorem, 22f

Q

qualified electrical workers, personal protective equipment for, 97t
Quality and Environmental Management Systems audits, 77
quality of illumination, 268
question-and-answer study method, 14
quick opening devices, 116

R

radiant heat transfer, 271
radiation, 33, 150, 339
    protection, 249
radioactive isotope, 32
radioactive materials, 317
radioactive powder, 304
radioactive sign, 130
radioactivity, 32
ramp
    slope of, 298
    suggested maximum angle for, 244f
random sample, 197

Rapid Entire Body Assessment (REBA), 103–104
Rapid Upper Limb Assessment (RULA), 104
rate compensation, 132
rate of reaction, 255
rate-of-rise, 133
　　detector, 126
Raynaud's phenomenon, 219
reaction, 174
　　time, 52
reactive worksite analysis approaches, 358
readability, 215
recognition, 86, 91
recommended weight limit (RWL), 103, 239
record, 79
　　keeping, 3
recordable incident rate, 64
recovery, 128–129
recreational drugs, 154
recycling activity, 165
reduction of job stress, 152
redundant design philosophy, 228
reeving methods, 44f
refresher training, 222
Registered Nurse (RN), 263
regulatory compliance, 2
relative density, 220
relative humidity (RH), 269
reliability, 178
　　of system, 226
remote alarm system, 114
renovation, 160
residual risk, 71
residue, 118
res ipsa loquitur, 194, 248
resist change, 136
Resource Conservation and Recovery Act (RCRA), 168
respirators, 253, 265
　　maintenance program, 305
respiratory bronchioles, 158
respiratory protection, 152
　　devices, 281
　　workplace level of, 158
responders, 118
response, 128
responsibility for safety, 301
restraints, 275
restricted approach boundary, 96
retention, 176
　　training methods for, 171
retina, 155
retrospective experience rating, 193
retrospective or case control studies, 314
retrospective rating, 189, 302
retrospective studies, 259, 271
revolution clutch, 233
reward and punishment system, 82
Reynolds number, 265

rigging chain, 321, 321f
risk, 69, 70, 73, 74, 79, 99, 341
　　analysis, 70, 97
　　avoidance, 98
　　communicators, 137
　　defined, 76
　　level of, 70
　　management, 71, 97, 133
　　perception, 137
　　prioritization, 75
　　reduction, 99
　　remaining after preventive measures, 67
　　retention, 98
　　transfer, 97, 98
risk assessment, 70, 70f, 75, 79
　　matrix, 78t
　　methods, 90
　　studies, 239
risk communication (RC), 71, 136
Risk Management Program (RMP), 135
Rodger's Muscle Fatigue Assessment, 104
Roentgen equivalent man (REM), 258, 271
role-playing technique, 173
role-play strategy, 180, 180t
root cause analysis (RCA), 71
Root Cause Analysis report, 280
rotating vane anemometer, 215–216
rotational speed, 23, 41
rotator cuff, 294
round ducts, 253
routes of entry, 281
Ruthenium (Ru), 32

S

sacrificial anode, 296
safe distance, 51
safeguarding devices, 264
safeguards, varieties of, 284
safety, 71
　　behavior, 89
　　committees, 54, 226, 259, 340
　　conference planning committee, 191
　　considerations, 302
　　consultants, 5, 194
　　culture, 86, 91, 194, 250
　　factors, 51, 215
　　function, 336
　　hazard, 234
　　and health training, 229, 262
　　inspection, 191
　　lanyards and lifelines, 231
　　levels of, 220
　　management of, 82, 87
　　manager, 192
　　motivation in, 93
　　occupational health and, 4

officer, 129
philosophy of, 4, 4t
posters, 229, 242
precaution, 205
principles of, 3–4t, 260, 272
priority, 88
processes, 235
profession, primary focus of, 2
specifications, 285
state, 67
through design, 95
trainers, 173, 194
Safety Data Sheets (SDSs), 31, 199, 212
safety professionals, 2–3, 3, 3t, 4t, 5, 113, 182, 190, 192, 227, 303, 355
assignment of, 240
ethics for, 5
primary talent of, 335
roles and responsibilities, 2
safety programs, 86, 302
audits, 235
management, 82, 240
managing, 3
safety-related workplace behaviors, 80
safety relief devices, 288
safety sampling/searching, 95, 247, 260, 272
practice of, 235
safety training, 182, 235
for employees, 333
instructor, 173
primary benefit of, 181
program, 171, 181, 261
session, 182, 264
technique, 173
safety violations, 200
construction project for, 326
sample standard deviation, 303
sampling inspection, 218
Sarbanes-Oxley Act of 2002, 77
scaffolding platform, 285
scaffolds, 328
screwdriver, 357
security, 3
self-contained breathing apparatus (SCBA), 255, 307
sensitizers, 148
sensorineural hearing loss, 142, 297, 318, 319f
series redundancy, 241
severity, 70, 95
SH&E
professionals, 113, 210
training and information, 302
shipments, 279
short-term exposure limit (STEL), 156
siderosis, 142
sign, 87
signaling systems, 309
signal words, 93

silica dust, 144, 212
silica particle, 277
silicosiderosis, 142
silicosis, 142, 292
silver shield, 147
simple parallel circuit, 32, 32f
simple series circuit, 31, 31f
single-celled organisms, 337
single point failure, 226, 240, 240f
Single-Task Lifting Index (STLI), 103
Single-Task Recommended Weight Limit (STRWL), 103
6-dB Noise Rule, 47
size, decreasing order of, 42
skid-resistant material, 204
skin, 152, 205
absorption, 155
contact, 212
exposure, recommended treatment for, 199
friction, 311
layers of, 277, 289
notation, 156
slot hoods, 216
Small Quantity Generator (SQG), 166
SMART model, 72
smoke, 122
management, 128
proof towers, 323
SMR (Standardized Mortality Ratio), 219
social definition, 164
social responsibility programs, 164
sociocusis, 142
sodium bicarbonate, 121
sodium carbonate-based powder, 121
sodium chloride, 121
solar heat load, 41
solid airborne contaminants, 199
solid surfaces, 297
sound, 33
intensity levels, 47–48
occurrence of, 219
power levels, 47–48
pressure levels, 47–48
sound level, 48
meters, 199, 292, 358
source reduction, 165
space entry operations, 235
SPAN CertBoK™ Exam Learning Management System (LMS), 1
SPAN Ham Radio Station, 211, 211f, 225f
span of control, 67, 74
specific gravity, 313
in modern scientific usage, 205
speech-level interference, 231
split core ammeter, 212
sponsoring organizations, 6
sprays
finishing system, 329
rapid vaporization of, 221

sprinkler system, 97, 111, 112, 116, 133, 212, 254
square ducts, 253
staff safety professional, 94
stainless steel welding, 220
stairwell design, 310
standard deviation, 54, 58, 58f, 231, 247, 300
    of mean, 55, 58
    population, 55
standards, 331
    hydrostatic test, 231, 264
standby systems, 241
statement of warranty, 227
static electricity, 119, 122, 206, 220
static friction, 216, 311
static pressure, 248
statistical analysis, 235
statistics calculations, 26
steady noise, 149
stereotype, principle of, 299
Stoddard solvent, 31
stoichiometry, 227, 241
stonemason's disease, 282
storage, 115
storage tanks, 162
strength vs. flexion curve, 332, 332f
stress management, 151
stress of sling, 40
strict liability, 193, 248, 345
structural damage from fire, 310
structural performance, 257
Structured Query Language (SQL), 274
student-instructor interaction, 172
student reaction to instruction, 239
subsonic explosion, 110
substances, 265
    properties of, 153
substantial property losses, 202
sulfur dioxide, 299
sulfuric acid, 301
supervisor controls, 273
supervisor's safety performance, 326
sustainability, 160
    definitions of, 164
sustainable development, 164
    concepts of, 164
    definitions of, 164
synergism, 154
synergistic effect, 151, 154
systematic samples, 212
system life cycle, 163, 170
system/product safety effort, 324
system safety, 170, 267, 331
    analysis, 260
    concept, 331, 345
    programs, 324
    techniques, 81, 230
systems-based approach, 331

T

tannic acid, 140
target audience, 174
target organs, 150
task responsibility, 191
tasks, 276
    assessment of, 303
t-distribution, 231, 243
teaching adults, guidelines for, 241–242, 346
Technique for Human Error Rate Prediction (THERP), 239
temperature changes, 275
temporary depression, 214
tendons, 102
tenosynovitis, 268
tensile strength, 278, 291
tension, 320–321, 321f
teratogens, 148, 320
terminal bronchioles, 158
testing techniques, 12–14
tetrachloroethane, 143
thallium, 143
thermal anemometer, 215
third-party audits, 78
thoracic outlet syndrome, 103
Threshold Limit Value (TLV), 36, 43, 153, 154, 156,
    201, 204, 214–215, 219, 257, 270, 281,
    292, 304, 340
threshold quantities, 135–136
tidal volume (TV), 219, 253, 266
"time -distance-shielding," 276
time-distance-shielding principle, 258
time-weighted average (TWA), 49
    concentration, 30, 33
    exposure, 42
tinnitus, 138
toggle switches, 102
tolerable risk, 74
toluene, 31
tort, 193, 248
Total Case Incidence Rate (TCIR), 217
total lung capacity (TLC), 266
total pressure, 276, 289
toxic gases, 297
toxic materials, 152, 155, 292
toxic substance, 146, 154
TQM manager functions, 86
trachea, 158
traditional disease classifications, 107
traffic formulas, 25
trainer criteria, 188
training, 3, 182, 185
    adults, 333
    approaches, 230
    effectiveness, 262, 326
    of employees, 292
    environment, 176
    and instructional systems design models, 175f

method, 181
needs analysis, 182
needs assessment, 254
objectives, 183, 184, 187, 262, 273
personnel, 234
presentation, 264
program, 172, 174f, 188
purposes, 178
session, 172
speed and quality of, 188
for welders, 200
transfer of command, 130
transmissible spongiform encephalopathy (TSE), 108
traumatic vasospastic disease, 219
triangle relationship, 44
triangular prism, 278
trichloroethylene, 140, 304
tuberculosis, 146
two-hand tripping devices, 275
two leg sling, 45f

U

U-bolt, 84f, 85
unacceptable risk, 71
underground storage tanks (USTs), 169
unfired pressure vessels, categories of, 257
Unified Command, 129
unimpaired hearing, 277
unit conversion prefixes, 50
unit conversions, 27
United Nations Environment Programme (UNEP), 166
unity of command, 130
universal precautions, 277, 290
unprotected eyes, 253
upper explosive or flammable limit, 33
U.S. Environmental Protection Agency, 136

V

validation, 79
value of money over time, 57
vapor pressure, 216, 252, 265
vector-borne infection, 142
vehicle accidents, 324
velocity, 23, 52
pressure, 43
tractor trailer to reach, 52
ventilation system, 40, 204, 237, 252, 309
characteristics in, 252
hood design, 201
source of, 40
work, 276
verbal communication, 263
verification, 79
vertical groupings, 289
vertigo, 138
vibration, 108

video display terminals (VDTs), 151
vinyl, 147
chloride, 270
violations, categories of, 248
violent reaction, 324
virus, 144
visible spectrum, 155
visual delivery, 231
viton, 147
voice inflection, 264
volatile liquid, 201
volumetric flow rate, 22, 23

W

warning labels, 236, 258
warning signs, 83, 199
waste
creation of, 161
destruction of, 163
management hierarchy, 169, 169f
minimization, 165, 168
reduction, 165
stream, 161, 165
volume and toxicity of, 170
waste to energy (WTE), 170
wastewater stream, 165
water, 111
pipes, 222
Specific Gravity (SG) of, 50
treatment, adequacy of, 161
water-supply valves, 212
water-type extinguishers, 122
wavelength, 152
Weapons of Mass Destruction (WMD), 119
weight density of fresh water, 49
weight of cylinder, 329
weight of specific volume, 50
well-constructed training objective, 182
wellness program, 152, 154
wet bulb globe temperature (WBGT), 46
heat load, 278
index, 41, 199, 333
wet chemical, 122
Wet Globe Temperature (WGT) index, 270
wet pipe system, 111
Wheatstone bridge circuit, 217, 267, 358
white fingers, 140
wildfires, natural cause of, 160
windpipe, 158
wire rope, 81, 206
wood, 245, 296
workday case incident rate, 56
worker behaviors, 90
worker participation, 73
workers compensation, 189, 280, 301
losses, 60
costs, 52

Workers' Compensation Act, 301
workload criteria, 102
workplaces, 238
    communication, 172
    conditions, 150
    electrical safety standards, 90
    hazard assessments of, 36
    injuries, 211
    safety, 82
    tripping hazards, 258

work safely, 88
Worst-Case Release Scenario, 135
wrench, 357

Z

zero-based budgeting, 66
zero energy state procedure (ZESP), 305
zero mechanical state (ZMS), 317

CPSIA information can be obtained
at www.ICGtesting.com
Printed in the USA
JSHW050759300622
27467JS00004B/16